One Planet, One Health

PUBLIC AND SOCIAL POLICY SERIES

Marian Baird and Gaby Ramia, Series Editors

The Public and Social Policy series publishes books that pose challenging questions about policy from national, comparative and international perspectives. The series explores policy design, implementation and evaluation; the politics of policy making; and analyses of particular areas of public and social policy.

Australian social attitudes IV: the age of insecurity
Ed. Shaun Wilson and Markus Hadler

Globalisation, the state and regional Australia
Amanda Walsh

Markets, rights and power in Australian social policy
Ed. Gabrielle Meagher and Susan Goodwin

One planet, one health
Ed. Merrilyn Walton

Risking together: how finance is dominating everyday life in Australia
Dick Bryan and Mike Rafferty

Wind turbine syndrome: a communicated disease
Simon Chapman and Fiona Crichton

One Planet, One Health

Edited by Merrilyn Walton

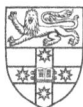

SYDNEY UNIVERSITY PRESS

First published by Sydney University Press

© Individual authors 2019

© Sydney University Press 2019

Reproduction and communication for other purposes

Except as permitted under the Act, no part of this edition may be reproduced, stored in a retrieval system, or communicated in any form or by any means without prior written permission. All requests for reproduction or communication should be made to Sydney University Press at the address below:

Sydney University Press
Fisher Library F03
University of Sydney NSW 2006
AUSTRALIA
sup.info@sydney.edu.au
sydney.edu.au/sup

A catalogue record for this book is available from the National Library of Australia.

ISBN 9781743325377 paperback
ISBN 9781743325360 epub
ISBN 9781743325391 mobi

Cover image by Conor Ashleigh. The treasurer of the cattle group in Karang Kendal hamlet, Java, Indonesia, washes one of his cows in a small creek.
Cover design by Miguel Yamin.

Contents

List of figures

List of figures

List of tables

Foreword

As human pressures on our planet increase, the sustainability of our way of life, our continuous push for development and so-called progress is under threat. Human contributions to declining ecosystems and the reality of climate change are no longer debatable. Already countries in different parts of the world are unable to support populations as a result of droughts, famine, conflict, epidemics and lack of infrastructure.

Nature is revealing to us the interdependence of environmental, animal and human health and emphasising that our resources are finite. This concept is embedded in the title of this unique book, *One Planet, One Health*. The following chapters bring together different academic and real life perspectives and examples, beginning with the post-industrial history and concepts of One Health and including a consideration of legal, gender and ethical issues and constraints, case studies, the importance of surveillance and interdisciplinary research and climate change.

The University of Sydney's Marie Bashir Institute for Emerging Infectious Diseases and Biosecurity has as its central vision reducing the health and socioeconomic impacts of emerging infectious diseases through the lens of One Planet, One Health. Our remit encompasses interdisciplinary research, capacity building and advocacy with governments, professions and communities. I am delighted that we have been able to bring together the perspectives of distinguished authors under the editorship of Professor Merrilyn Walton. I trust that you, the readers, will find the book informative and possibly contentious in parts, but always thought-provoking and stimulating.

Tania C Sorrell AM, FAHMS

Deputy Dean, Sydney Medical School and Head,
  Westmead Clinical School
Professor and Director, Marie Bashir Institute for Infectious Diseases &
  Biosecurity, University of Sydney
Director, Centre for Infectious Diseases and Microbiology,
  Westmead Institute for Medical Research
Service Director, Infectious Diseases and Sexual Health, Western Sydney
  Local Health District

Preface

By most measures, human health is better now than ever before in human history. Since 1950, global average life expectancy has risen 25 years to its current level of 72 years, and infant mortality rates have decreased substantially from around 210 per thousand live births to just over 30 per thousand now.

However, these gains in human health have been unequally distributed, and alongside them, and overall development gains made in the same period, we have witnessed environmental degradation on a massive scale. Pollution, deforestation, biodiversity loss, and climate change are among the striking examples of the damage caused by collective human endeavour.

The report of the Rockefeller Foundation–Lancet Commission on Planetary Health found that continuing environmental degradation threatens to reverse the health gains achieved during the last century. The consequences are far reaching, ranging from the emergence and spread of infectious diseases like SARS, Ebola, and Zika, to malnutrition, conflict, and displacement.

Those who are the least responsible for driving these changes – poor people in developing countries – are the most vulnerable to them. In short, we have been mortgaging the health and wellbeing of future generations to realise economic and development gains in the present.

But, the Commission report does conclude that solutions are within reach. They will require, however, a redefinition of prosperity to focus on quality of life and improved human health, together with respect for the integrity of the natural environment. The report identified three sets of challenges:

- First, conceptual challenges, which include the pressing need for genuine measures of progress which go beyond gross domestic product to measure human development and the state of environment.

- Second, governance challenges, such as how governments and other institutions recognise and respond to threats, especially when faced with uncertainty and the need to pool resources.

- Third, the report identified research challenges, such as ignoring the social and environmental context of human health, and the relative lack of cross-disciplinary research.

Planetary health is about safeguarding the health and wellbeing of current and future generations through good stewardship of Earth's natural systems, and by rethinking the way we feed, move, house, power, and care for the world. It requires us to challenge received wisdom, to acknowledge the interdependence of all species, and to think, and to act, in more integrative ways.

To respond effectively to the health challenges of the Anthropocene, we need to grapple with the global transitions that are currently shaping our lives – demographic, epidemiological, food, energy, urban, economic, cultural and ecological. Humanity can chart a safe, healthy and prosperous course ahead by addressing unacceptable inequities in health and wealth within the environmental limits of the Earth however, to do so, will require the generation of new knowledge, the implementation of wise policies, decisive action, and inspirational leadership.

As a member of the Rockefeller Foundation–Lancet Commission on Planetary Health, I am delighted see this timely book *One Planet, One Health* published by Sydney University Press. The book will be a valuable resource for policymakers, practitioners and students interested in learning more about planetary health, and concerned about the need for urgent action in the interest of planetary health.

Anthony Capon

Inaugural Professor of Planetary Health and Director, Planetary Health Platform, The University of Sydney

Works cited

Whitmee S, Haines A, Beyrer C, Boltz F, Capon AG, de Souza Dias BF, et al. (2015). Safeguarding human health in the Anthropocene epoch: report of The Rockefeller Foundation-Lancet Commission on planetary health. *Lancet* 386:1973–2028.

From the editor

Merrilyn Walton

The genesis for this book has been my involvement with an interdisciplinary team working with hard-to-reach rural communities in South-East Asia and the Pacific, and the challenges we faced in explaining our One Health approach to funding bodies. Government organisations and peer reviewers, unfamiliar with One Health methods, asked what did agriculture have to do with human health? While interdisciplinary research is now actively encouraged in some universities, research institutes, and policy and funding bodies yet to fully understand how One Health methods, while complex in nature, offer an alternative way to solve intractable problems that have thus far eluded solutions.

This book is a window into the interconnectedness of the sentient beings on the planet and the world they inhabit. It will provide readers and researchers with the fundamentals underpinning One Health. Governments concerned for the livelihoods of hard-to-reach rural communities in all countries know these communities suffer despite efforts to improve their situations. Millions of dollars of aid money directed to improving livelihoods in low-resource countries have yet to make a significant difference. Lack of will is not the problem. *The human development report: human development for everyone* (United Nations Development Programme 2017) reported uneven human development, with millions struggling with hunger, poverty, illiteracy, and malnutrition: one in three people is malnourished, more than one in ten lives in extreme poverty, and the same number cannot read or write. The 2017 Save the Children Report, *Short changed: the human and economic cost of child undernutrition in Papua New Guinea*, argues that reducing poverty and improving livelihoods of people, particularly emphasising the nutrition crisis, is a priority. These grave findings should not be surprising: the speed of population growth, reduced areas for food production, water scarcity, emerging infections, and other anthropogenic changes are making the planet unstable, with increasingly unequal access to safe environments and food security for many inhabitants in the poorest countries.

A 2016 study of Australian funding outcomes published in *Nature* showed that research involving multiple disciplines is less likely to be funded when compared to projects with a narrow, more specialised focus (Bromham, Dinnage and Hua 2016). Governments, statutory funding bodies and universities are structured according to specific disciplines – public health experts or agriculturalists or vets – and are less familiar (or comfortable) with a holistic approach. Peer review of interdisciplinary research requires a more expansive view, one that accepts and anticipates that the usual metrics may not always be appropriate or helpful. Academic track records across a range of disciplines will not fit one model, nor will the research methods be familiar to all. One Health projects also take more time and usually cost more than research funded under the Australian Competitive Grants Category 1 schemes such as the Australian Research Council and the National Health and Medical Research Council or Public-Sector Research Income grants under Category 2. The two- to three-year time frames typical of these research grants are too short for projects aiming to improve human–animal–environmental health.

Over the last decade, we have come to better understand unintended consequences of progress: climate change, habitat destruction, food insecurity, wealth inequality, species extinction, and zoonosis. Addressing these consequences and facing new challenges demand we respond but not by doing the same thing over and over. Yet there is evidence that we continue to repeat errors from the past. When the railroad network in India was built under British rule in the 19th century it paved the way for trade and mass travel, symbolising the ingenuity of the British in the post-industrial world. But railways also paved the way for infectious diseases, shocking labour conditions, and changed landscapes – unintended side effects that remain today. Raw sewage dropped from trains enabled the spread of disease by organisms (vectors) that transmit disease between humans or from animals (birds, insects, rodents) to humans; sewage also penetrated the underground water table. Trains also harbinger epidemic diseases such as cholera and influenza. The unintended consequences of human actions are found everywhere, not just in India and not just in the last century. Plastic bags in the Pacific Ocean, constituting around 80 per cent of marine debris, are being consumed by marine life as they fragment into smaller and smaller pieces, causing environmental devastation. The Green Revolution of the mid-20th century achieved spectacular success bringing agricultural technologies to poor countries where famine and starvation were frequent occurrences. However, the success in providing adequate carbohydrate nutrition was followed by a complacency regarding agricultural sustainability and food quality, resulting in environmental degradation and the double burden of malnutrition now afflicting all countries.

Tackling problems from just the perspective of a human, or of an animal, or of the land are unintended consequences of the 20th-century obsession with specialisation. This approach fails to recognise the interconnectedness of humans, animals, ecosystems and climate. Planetary Health, EcoHealth, and One Health are terms in this book that describe methods for solving these universal problems. The different terms express similar themes: multidisciplinary, transdisciplinary, interdisciplinary collaborations, a system approach, close engagement with communities, knowledge transfer, gender equity, and sustainability.

The Global Research Council meeting in New Delhi in 2016 identified interdisciplinarity as a key feature in future research and advocated increased support from governments and funding bodies, noting that their role in shaping interdisciplinary research is paramount (Lyall et al. 2013). Universities emphasise multidisciplinary research, but in reality One Health projects still occur opportunistically through networking rather than from an organised structured framework. Designing a One Health intervention involves more actors than traditional siloed research – the communities of interest must be engaged from the beginning – including identifying the problem they want to solve. This adds to the complexity and cost.

This book is for governments, health, agricultural and environmental administrators, bureaucrats, philanthropic organisations, and funding bodies as well as the general reading public, particularly in low- and middle-income countries. Written for non-specialist readers, it explains what One Health is and how it works. Its practical approach shows the benefits when people with different skills and knowledge work with communities to resolve problems.

To date, One Health funded initiatives have emphasised the human–animal interface, prompted by the urgency of containing the spread of disease from animals to humans (zoonosis). This book is not just about zoonoses because much has already been written about emerging and re-emerging infections; there is general acceptance that most emerging infections are caused by anthropogenic influences on the ecology (Lindahl and Grace 2015). How to contain the spread of infections remains a vexed issue. The 2018 Bangkok Statement acknowledged that despite advances in knowledge and practice, epidemics and pandemics remain a threat (Prince Mahidol Award Conference 2018). Attendees at that conference also called for the removal of 'the professional, bureaucratic and cultural barriers, as well as the obstacles inherent within social, economic and political processes, that silo human health, animal health and the environmental sectors from effective multi-sectoral partnership and actions'.

This book describes different pathways to a sustainable planet. Attention to natural systems and understanding how the parts of different systems interrelate is a core understanding for One Health research and a theme in all chapters. To understand one component of the system it is also necessary to understand how the other parts relate and interact. This interdependence is what specialisation neglects.

Why the urgency

In mid-2017 scientists from around the globe signed for the second time a 'Warning to humanity'. The first notice signed in 1992 by 1,500 scientists included most of the living Nobel laureates in the sciences.

Back then they drew attention to the destruction caused by ozone depletion, human population growth, climate change, biodiversity destruction, forest loss, and ocean dead zones, concluding that 'humans were on a collision course with the natural world' (Ripple et al. 2017). In 2017, the stratospheric ozone layer had stabilised but stalled progress prompted the second notice. This call for action sets out the steps to the sustainability of humanity, other species, and environs.

Readers will appreciate that One Health is not new, first appearing in the 19th century when industrialisation and overcrowded cities were hosts to cholera epidemics. The origins of that disease were uncovered by environmental and health workers who discovered that water, sewage and drainage all played a role in spreading the disease. Since these public health advances, the 20th and 21st centuries have seen the development of specialisation and a move away from the polymaths. Specialisation happens in many domains including biology but in humans it refers to the process of accumulating expert knowledge or skill in a particular area. There have been unquestionable benefits from specialising (antimicrobial medicines, vaccines, surgical advances, technology) but there have also been unintended consequences. Becoming an expert in an area has often been at the cost of working with multiple disciplines – work that necessarily understands the relevance of context and the interrelatedness of different components in any system. While the authors in this book are specialists in their domains of study and work in different professions, countries and environments, they share a common humanity in their wish to improve the health of the planet and the health of humans, animals and the environment.

Acknowledgements

I thank the authors of the chapters for their enthusiasm for One Health and for coming together in such a collaborative way to share their experience knowledge and vision for the health of the planet and its inhabitants. Professor Tania Sorrell, the Director of the Marie Bashir Institute for Infectious Diseases and Biosecurity, was supportive of this project from the beginning. I thank her for that support and showing leadership in multidisciplinary research. Sydney University Press, in particular Agata Mrva-Montoya, is thanked for their patience and confidence that the book would eventuate.

Finally, I especially thank Robert Pullan (Australia) and Chas Alexander (United Kingdom), two professional writers who knew little about One Health; they provided editorial assistance particularly in relation to the use of clear English.

Works cited

Lindahl, J., and D. Grace (2015). The consequences of human actions on risks for infectious diseases: a review. *Infection Ecology & Epidemiology* 5(1): 1–38.

Lyall, C., A. Bruce, W. Marsden, and L. Meagher (2013). The role of funding agencies in creating interdisciplinary knowledge. *Science & Public Policy* 40(1): 62–71.

Prince Mahidol Award Conference (2018). Bangkok statement: a call to action. Prince Mahidol Award Conference, Bangkok, 29 January–3 February.

Ripple, W., C. Wolf, M. Galetti, T. Newsome, and E.A.M. Alamgir (2017). World scientists' warning to humanity: a second notice. http://scientistswarning.forestry.oregonstate.edu/.

Save the Children (2017). *Short changed: the human and economic cost of child undernutrition in Papua New Guinea.* Carlton, VIC.: Save the Children Australia. http://bit.ly/2UUxjGj.

United Nations Development Programme (2017). *Human development for everyone.* New York: United Nations Development Programme.

1
One Health/Ecohealth/ Planetary Health and their evolution

Grant A. Hill-Cawthorne

Miasmic theory

Recent years have seen an increase in One Health publications, with 276 published in 2016 compared to only three in 1990. The term 'One Health' is relatively new but the concept is ancient. Hippocrates, a Greek physician (c. 460–c. 377 BC) theorised in his text 'On airs, waters and places' that disease was caused by environmental factors, putting forward the theory that bad air is equivalent to pestilence. Galen expanded the theory, postulating that individuals' susceptibility to illness is an interplay between the environment and the balance of four humours in the body.

Miasmic theory, a term derived from the Greek word for stain or defilement, has been around for over 2,000 years and was popularised in the 17th century with the publication of Nathaniel Hodges' treatise on the 1665 plague in London when he described how air has the potential to propagate the plague. Pestilence in the air was thought to be a major cause of the Black Death in 14th-century Europe (Garcia-Ballester 1994).

Giovanni Maria Lancisi, an Italian physician and epidemiologist, was struck by the co-localisation of malarial outbreaks and swampy marshes and noted in his essay 'On the noxious exhalations of marshes' that the humid air and presence of insects around marshy areas may be related to the increased incidence of disease (Mitchill and Miller 1810). While the 'mal aere' he described and modern-day malaria may not be the same disease, his linking humid, close air and febrile symptoms may represent an early connection with malaria in areas where the vector is potentially present. However, this may not be the earliest record of mosquitoes being blamed for disease: a plate in the *Hortus sanitatis* displays an unwell man lying under a tree with insects all around him (Figure 1.1 Meydenbach 1485). Putrid marshes have remained a concern in England since Lancisi's first observations. In 1774 Rev. Dr Priestly wrote to Sir John Pringle expressing unhappiness with Dr Alexander of Edinburgh's conclusion that 'there is nothing to be apprehended from the neighbourhood of putrid marshes', noting in his letter that, when left alone, water turns black with emanating bubbles. These were perhaps the first examples of links made between the environment and human health.

Hygiene theory

This link between polluted air (miasma) and disease underpinned reforms to sanitary conditions throughout Western Europe during the Victorian period. In the early 1800s, the industrial revolution in the United Kingdom led to an explosion in migration from rural to urban areas to fill the ever-increasing factories, particularly in northern England. This increase in urban population quickly overwhelmed the rudimentary drainage systems, setting up the perfect storm for the second cholera pandemic emerging from the Ganges River delta region of India. By 1830 cholera had reached Orenburg Oblast in Russia's south-west, close to Kazakhstan (Henze 2010). As miasma theory still dominated thinking about disease at the time, the UK-imposed quarantine orders for ships sailing from Russia. But in December that year, the water-borne disease (*Vibrio cholerae*) surfaced in Sunderland (UK) via a ship travelling from the Baltic and soon after in the other big port cities of Gateshead and Newcastle. By the end of 1831 over 6,500 people had died in London from the disease; the following summer around 20,000 people died.

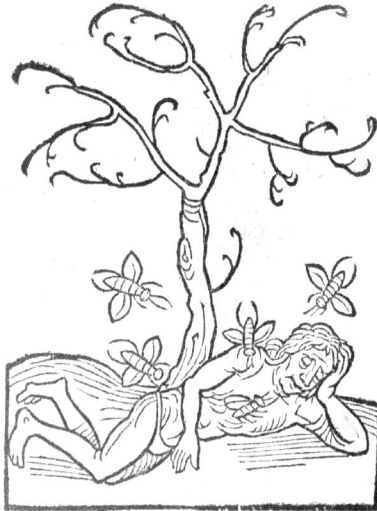

Figure 1.1 Unwell man surrounded by insects (Meydenbach, *Hortus sanitatis*, 1485). Made available by the Wellcome Trust Wellcome Images collection via Wikimedia Commons (https://bit.ly/2AQppoj).

The sudden appearance of cholera in Russia and the UK during 1831–32 in the context of poor communication (and understanding) by municipal authorities was of major public concern which was partly fuelled by the scandal of the murders by William Burke and William Hare, who killed 16 people to supply corpses for dissection by Dr Robert Knox in Edinburgh. In 1826, 23 corpses were discovered on the docks of Liverpool waiting to be shipped to Scotland for dissection. Crowds, particularly in Liverpool, were angry with the medical profession and saw cholera as yet another way for people to be removed to hospitals and killed for dissection.

Sir Edwin Chadwick, a lawyer and social reformer, focused attention on sanitation in an attempt to improve the poor laws. His report, *The sanitary condition of the labouring population,* published in 1842 with a commissioned supplement in 1843, led to the establishment of the Health of Towns Commission which he chaired. A year later branches of the

3

Health of Towns Association were established in Edinburgh, Liverpool and Manchester. Another major outbreak of cholera in England and Wales in 1848 killed 52,000 people, prompting the government to enact the *Public Health Act 1848* to bring the supply of water, sewerage and drainage, and environmental health regulations under the control of one local body, with local health boards overseen by the General Board of Health. Public health improved with the spread of activities across England and Wales. Local movements in public health spurred people to think about the health of their communities, as demonstrated by the petition for an inspection in Durham by the city council, cathedral, university and doctors. Local board powers were extensive, covering sewers, street cleaning, public toilets, water supply and burials. A decade later these powers also included fires and fire prevention, removing dangerous buildings and providing public bathing houses (*Local Government Act 1858*). These two 19th-century acts, in recognising the relationship between poverty and ill health, particularly in urban areas, are the foundations for the recently published Millennium Development and Sustainable Development Goals and the discipline of planetary health.

Cholera is also associated with the birth of microbiology and epidemiology. The third cholera pandemic in the Ganges delta in 1852 led to over a million deaths. Before Louis Pasteur's work on germ theory, a little-known Italian anatomist Filippo Pacini, who performed autopsies on cholera victims in Florence, noted when he examined the intestinal mucosa under a microscope the presence of small comma-shaped microorganisms which he called Vibrio. Even though the Paris Academy of Sciences published his *Microscopical observations and pathological deductions on cholera* in 1854, it was 82 years before he was credited with the discovery. This was despite his 'A treatise on the specific cause of cholera, its pathology and cure' being reviewed in 1866 in the *British and Foreign Medico-Chirurgical Review*. But acceptance of the role of *vibrio cholerae* in transmitting cholera did not happen until it was rediscovered by Robert Koch in 1884.

Miasma theory was ultimately disproved by John Snow when he proved the environmental connection to cholera. Prior to the Broad Street cholera outbreak in 1854, Snow published 'On the mode of communication of cholera' in 1849, in which he set out his theory that cholera is spread from person to person, making the connection that the disease 'is communicated by something that acts directly on the alimentary canal … excretions of the sick at once suggest themselves as containing some material … accidentally swallowed'. He placed the main route of transmission as direct faecal to oral and likened the transmission to recent studies in intestinal worm diseases. He also theorised that cholera could be disseminated by emptying sewers into drinking water, noting the presence of contaminated drinking water and significant cholera outbreaks in the two cities of Dumfries-Maxwelltown and Glasgow. He also gave circumstantial evidence to support his theory based on the epidemiology of cases in London, but it was his 1855 treatise based on the Broad Street cholera outbreak that proved his theory.

The 1854 Broad Street cholera outbreak killed 616 people; the disease resurfaced after significant outbreaks in London in 1832 and 1849 killing 14,137 people. Snow was sceptical of William Farr's theory that the outbreaks were caused by miasmata from the soil of the River Thames. Having pinpointed the source to a public water pump at Broad Street after talking to locals, he persuaded the local authorities to remove the pump handle. He then constructed one of the first Voronoi diagrams used in health by marking all affected houses with a dot. The well had been dug less than 1 metre from an old cesspit that had begun to leak, with the cholera bacterium supplied by the washing of an infected baby's nappies into the cesspit.

John Snow also performed one of the first double-blind trials on water supplies. He noted that houses adjacent to one another often received their water from different suppliers. He used statistics to demonstrate that fatalities were higher among customers of certain water suppliers. Snow proved that the Southwark and Vauxhall Waterworks Company was taking water from sewage-contaminated sections of the Thames and redistributing it as drinking water. However, as is frequently the case in public health, policy changes were not immediate. With the crisis passing and the urgency resolved, the authorities reinstated the handle on the Broad Street pump. But another 11 years passed before Snow's theory was accepted. A further 1886 outbreak in Bromley-by-Bow in East London enabled William Farr, previously a proponent of miasma theory, to apply his specialist skills in biostatistics to link the high mortality rates to the Old Ford Reservoir in East London. Local residents were immediately instructed to boil their drinking water. Farr also built on Snow's work on cholera, coining the term 'zymotic diseases' to describe acute infectious diseases. 'Zymotic disease' originated from the term 'microzymas', proposed by Antoine Béchamp as a potential cause of contagious diseases, and was used until bacteriology was better established in the early 20th century. Farr also identified urbanisation and population density as public health issues.

Beyond germ theory

John Snow's demonstration that cholera was a water-borne disease was followed by Louis Pasteur's experiments in 1860–64 to prove that the source of the microorganisms that grew in nutrient broths was environmental and not through spontaneous generation (Ligon 2002). Fourteen years later Pasteur discovered *Streptococcus* by demonstrating that blood from a woman dying of puerperal fever could be cultured and that it contained the same microorganism that he had previously observed in furuncles (skin abscesses) (Pasteur 1880).

This discovery heralded germ theory and the observation that infectious diseases were caused by an aetiologic agent. Robert Koch, in the late 19th century, made further progress when he created his famous postulates (conditions which must exist before a particular bacteria can be said to cause particular diseases) based on his work on anthrax. This work was critically important for the development of the specialties of microbiology and infectious diseases, and their spin-offs such as asepsis and antisepsis, but unintended was the narrowing of the concept of infections, their causes and prevention. As with most post-19th century science, specialists replaced polymaths. Early public health was resplendent with multidisciplinary ideas and One Health concepts, but these were lost to the greater struggles of diagnoses and treatments of specific conditions.

Rudolf Virchow, practising against the trend towards specialisation, was a polymath physician and pathologist living in Germany in the 19th century. His scientific contributions, in addition to establishing public health in Germany, built on his belief that medicine was both a scientific discipline and a social science. Revered as the father of cellular pathology, he was also widely known for his political views likening individual people to cells and the state to the organism. Curiously, Virchow refuted the idea that infections were caused by microorganisms, believing instead they were a result of cellular abnormalities and wider social situations. Curious because he also described the transmission cycle for *Trichinella spiralis*, which led to meat inspection. In all respects he was a proponent of microscopic examination and his work on cellular pathology, in particular comparing pathologies between humans and animals, was published as his great work *Cellular pathology* (Virchow 1859).

Virchow's focus on comparative pathology led him to establish connections between human and animal diseases, for which he is claimed to have labelled zoonoses, from the Greek for 'animal' and 'sickness'. In the mid-1850s he is believed to have said 'Between animal and human medicine there are no dividing lines – nor should there be … The object is different but the experience obtained constitutes the basis of all medicine'. The observation of comparative anatomy, physiology and pathology had been made by John Hunter, who co-founded the Royal Veterinary College in London, and Sir Jonathan Hutchinson, who contributed to the idea of animal models of disease.

One Medicine

If Virchow did coin the term zoonosis, he left unclear which diseases he thought were the origin of transmission; he may simply have been referring to his work on trichinellosis (a disease caused by eating raw or undercooked meat infected with the larvae of a worm). Nevertheless his writings influenced physicians such as Sir William Osler, who studied with Virchow for some time in Germany before returning to Canada. Osler's appointment in the Medical Faculty of McGill University was as a lecturer to medical and veterinary students from the Montreal Veterinary College, which later became affiliated with McGill. This vet college later amalgamated into Osler's Division of Comparative Medicine but Osler continued to teach medical and vet students in Philadelphia and Johns Hopkins University. Osler is famous for his contributions to the establishment of medical residency and his textbook *The principles and practice of medicine*. But he has also been credited with coining the term 'One Medicine' to describe his interest in comparative pathology. While there is no evidence in his writings for this, the concept was clearly established in his mind.

One Medicine first appeared when Calvin Schwabe, a veterinary epidemiologist at the University of California, Davis (UC Davis), introduced the term in his book *Veterinary medicine and human health*, 3rd edition (Schwabe 1984). In his earlier edition, he described veterinary medicine as 'the field of study concerned with the diseases and health of non-human animals. The practice of veterinary medicine is directly related to man's wellbeing in a number of ways' (Schwabe 1964).

Schwabe based his idea of One Medicine on his observations of the close relationship, for both good health and ill health, between humans, domestic animals and public health. His ideas were further developed when he established a Master of Preventive Veterinary Medicine at UC Davis, which taught the principles and strategies of mass disease control and prevention in animals. He noted that:

> Traditional veterinary medicine is concerned in varying degrees with problems in agriculture, biology and public health. These have been the three natural avenues of development for veterinary medicine. Until recent years, however, progress in extension of organised veterinary interests in public health has been frustrated by 'accepted beliefs' – long held in the Western world – on the presumed biological uniqueness of man. These erroneous notions have thwarted a general appreciation of veterinary contributions to the development of a science of general medicine.

James Harlan Steele continued to lead multidisciplinary approaches to health and medicine and today is widely regarded as the father of veterinary public health, earning his doctorate of veterinary medicine from Michigan State University and master of public health from Harvard. During World War II in Puerto Rico and the Virgin Islands he co-ordinated milk and food sanitation programs to reduce the risk from brucellosis and bovine tuberculosis. After the war, the US Centers for Disease Control and Prevention (CDC) discussed with him the role of vets in combating zoonotic infections as it was clear they constituted a significant health risk but little attention had been given to surveillance or research. Steele subsequently wrote the seminal report *Veterinary public health* in 1945, which examined zoonotic disease risks and how medicine may benefit from veterinarian knowledge and advice. This led to a new position of Veterinary Medical Officer in the Public Health Service. Steele, as chief veterinary officer in the CDC, established the veterinary public health program. He initially focused on rabies but later expanded to bovine tuberculosis, brucellosis, Q fever, psittacosis, salmonellosis and other food-borne diseases. He also integrated veterinary public health into the Pan American Health Organization (PAHO) and later the World Health Organization (WHO). In these ways, he brought One Health into the mainstream, embedding it within health policy and disease prevention and response.

EcoHealth

Ecosystem health, or EcoHealth, is a systems-based approach to promoting health and wellbeing with a focus on social and ecological interactions. Originating in North America, it claims to add to disciplinary knowledge by conducting pre-study meetings with affected communities to include social dimensions in the overall solution. The International Development Research Centre, established in 1970 as a Canadian federal Crown corporation, is a significant investor in international development. Jean Lebel, the current president, has written extensively on ecosystem approaches to health, focusing on the following three principles: transdisciplinary approach, participation and equity.

Strong support came from the EcoHealth Alliance, which began as the international arm of the Jersey Wildlife Preservation Trust in the Channel Island of Jersey; it is now named the Durrell Wildlife Conservation Trust. Wildlife Preservation Trust International, which started in 1971, became the Wildlife Trust in 1999 and in 2010 changed into the EcoHealth Alliance. During this time, it morphed from an organisation focused on captive breeding of endangered species to one with an environmental health and conservation remit. The main focus of the EcoHealth Alliance is on conservation medicine, defined as an

9

interdisciplinary field focused on the relationships between human and animal health, and the environment.

One of the best-known outputs of the then Wildlife Trust was an examination of the impact of human population growth, latitude, rainfall and wildlife richness on emerging infectious diseases (EIDs). While some of their findings were skewed by the distribution of EID laboratories, vector-borne pathogens tended to be in tropical and subtropical regions and zoonotic pathogens were much more likely to originate from wildlife than from non-wildlife reservoirs.

EcoHealth work is exemplified by the United States Agency for International Development (USAID) Emerging Pandemic Threats (EPT) program, which was facilitated by the emergence of severe acute respiratory syndrome (SARS) coronavirus and influenza A(H5N1). While USAID previously centred on A(H5N1), the Pandemic Influenza and Other Emerging Threats Unit launched the EPT 2009 program comprising four projects: Predict, Prevent, Identify, and Respond, operating in 20 countries. The EcoHealth Alliance is an implementing partner of the PREDICT project, and focuses on the detection and discovery of zoonotic diseases at the wildlife–human interface. The target countries are strengthening surveillance and laboratory capacity to monitor wildlife and people who have contact with wildlife so potential emerging pathogens can be identified early. The EcoHealth Alliance covers bio surveillance, deforestation, One Health, pandemic prevention and wildlife conservation.

One Health

With comparative medicine driving One Medicine in the veterinary world, the CDC, PAHO, and WHO lead a public health approach within a multidisciplinary framework called One Health. One Health involves collaborating disciplines working towards optimal health for the planet – its people, animals and the environment. This makes it distinct from One Medicine by taking a health rather than curative approach and stepping away from the narrow focus on animals and the environment for the benefit of humans. During the 1980s the concept of sustainable development – for people, animals and ecosystems – required health to be inclusive of these components. One Health describes people and agencies that link human, animal and environmental health through multi-sectoral and transdisciplinary approaches. Together, they tackle global health issues by prioritising the health of both humans and animals, and protecting these populations from infectious diseases and disease spread. Since 2000 One Health has had a pivotal role in health system strengthening, by integrating health services, particularly in hard-to-reach communities. One Health methods were seen as a better way to achieve the Millennium Development Goals following the WHO ministerial summit in Mexico City in 2004.

The 12 Manhattan Principles of One Health were also formulated in 2004 as a result of the Wildlife Conservation Society and the Rockefeller University bringing health experts together in a 'One World, One Health' event to discuss current and future emerging diseases, particularly Ebola virus, avian influenza virus and chronic wasting disease. This was followed by an article in *Foreign Affairs*, supporting the need for multidisciplinarity in approaches to infectious diseases, citing HIV and SARS as examples of emerging zoonotic infections.

Another leap by the One Health movement occurred in 2007, when Roger Mahr, then president of the American Veterinary Medical Association (AVMA), and Ronald Davis, then president of the American Medical Association, discussed how vets and medical doctors can work together. A One Health Initiative Task Force was set up and chaired by Lonnie King, then director of the National Center for Zoonotic, Vector-Borne and Enteric Diseases at the CDC; the US Assistant Surgeon General, William Stokes, was an invited member. This culminated in a report by the task force, which laid much of the groundwork for One Health (King et al. 2008). The recommendation to establish a National One Health Commission (OHC) as a non-profit organisation was implemented in 2008. Its mission was to "educate" and "create" networks to improve health outcomes and wellbeing of humans, animals and plants, and to promote environmental resilience through a collaborative, global One Health approach'. The OHC is training the next generation of One Health leaders.

The Roadmap to the OHC One Health Agenda 2030 says the only way to achieve the Sustainable Development Goals (SDGs) is through a multidisciplinary One Health approach. This work originated from a European Union funded initiative called the Network for Evaluation of One Health. Of particular note was the adaptation of a previous SDG figure placing the SDGs within a framework of wellbeing, infrastructure and natural environment (Waage et al. 2015) but highlighting some SDGs will naturally come into conflict with others, particularly goals 8, 9 and 12 on economic growth, industrialisation, and production and consumption, respectively (Figure 1.2). The importance of the political opportunity the SDGs represent for embedding a One Health approach – one that integrates the silos of EcoHealth, eco-public health, ecosystems and planetary health (see below) – has been highlighted by Queenan et al. (2017). This incorporates a whole-of-society approach to policy making and integrating One Health actions through health services, diagnostics, surveillance, and so on.

Core competency domains for One Health have been developed as a result of three independent initiatives: the Bellagio Working Group (Rockefeller Foundation and the University of Minnesota), the Stone Mountain Meeting Training Workgroup, and the USAID RESPOND initiative. They came together in 2012 in Rome to synthesise the competencies. While the sets of competencies remain separate, they all have overarching themes of management, communication and informatics, values and ethics, leadership, team and collaboration, roles and responsibilities, and systems thinking.

In addition to the OHC, in 2008 a One Health Initiative comprising a website developed by an autonomous team of people began highlighting information and research in One Health. This team originally founded by two physicians and a vet expanded to include public health expertise. This focus brings human and animal health together, although environmental health comes under its umbrella. Similar to the OHC, its main purpose is communication, information and education.

The One Health Platform has its own journal, *One Health*, which provides a forum for researchers, identifies research gaps and also raises awareness and disseminates information. It also organises the One Health Congress, the fifth of which was held in Saskatoon, Canada, in 2018. In an attempt to reduce the silos among these multidisciplinary initiatives, the 2016 Congress was a joint congress between the One Health Platform congress and the International Association for Ecology and Health.

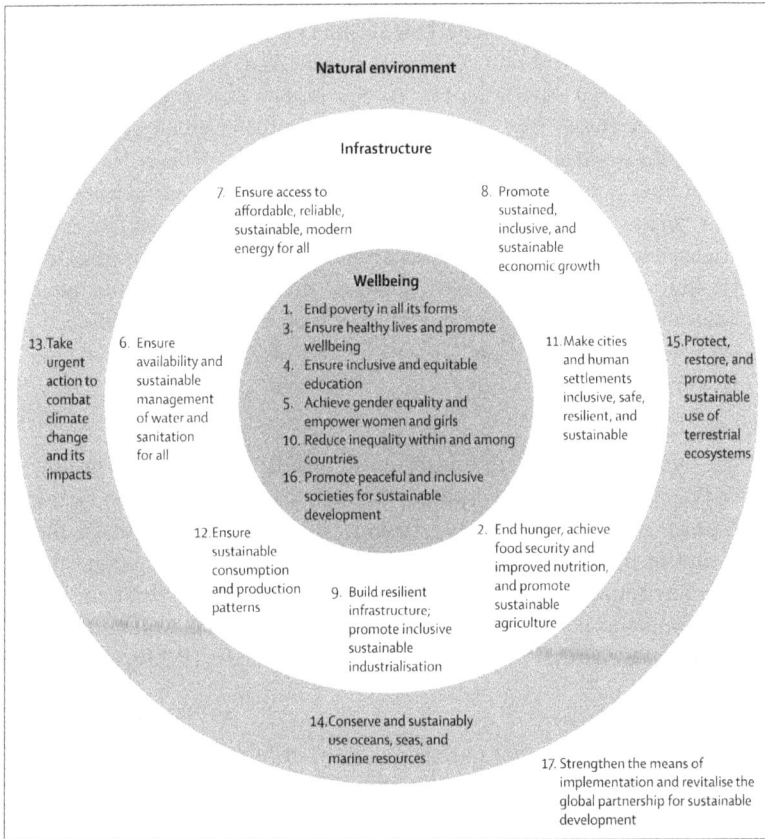

Figure 1.2 Governing the UN Sustainable Development Goals: interactions, infrastructures, and institutions (Waage et al.2015).

New kid on the block: planetary health

In 2015 the Rockefeller Foundation–Lancet Commission on Planetary Health published a series of papers, flagshipped by 'Safeguarding human health in the Anthropocene epoch' (Whitmee et al. 2015). The commission defined planetary health as

---

Box 1.1: Global One Health Day Initiative

The One Health Platform in collaboration with the OHC and the OHI has initiated a Global One Health Day, the first held on 3 November 2016. The goal of One Health Day is to focus the world on One Health interactions and for the world to 'see them in action'. With multiple self-started activities around the globe, it hopes to give One Health advocates opportunities to join forces in educational activities and events that bring together academicians and health professionals from different backgrounds. The One Health events offer educational programs in both academic and non-academic settings by inviting professionals from a variety of disciplines to discuss One Health topics and share their knowledge and experiences at One Health events.

---

the achievement of the highest attainable standard of health, wellbeing, and equity worldwide through judicious attention to the human systems – political, economic, and social – that shape the future of humanity and the Earth's natural systems that define the safe environmental limits within which humanity can flourish. Put simply, planetary health is the health of human civilisation and the state of the natural systems on which it depends. (Whitmee et al. 2015)

This commission first met in Bellagio, Italy, in July 2014 and was chaired by Sir Andrew Haines, former director of the London School of Hygiene and Tropical Medicine. It consisted of experts in environmental health, medicine, biodiversity and ecology. The three key challenges were a conceptual need to account for future harms to health and environment, a continuing lack of transdisciplinary research, particularly on the social and environmental drivers of ill health, and issues around global governance. While planetary health has multiple overlapping principles and ideas with both One Health and EcoHealth, it has been put forward by the *Lancet* as a new science. It is also being touted as the natural successor to public and global health. While global health built upon international health by focusing on the need to improve health through achieving equity, planetary health takes this further by incorporating the foundation upon which we live.

Richard Horton's manifesto on planetary health has been criticised for excluding One Health but this may be misguided as the way planetary health has been framed is as a co-movement with One Health and EcoHealth. Unlike much of One Health literature, the commission focused more on climate change, ocean acidification, freshwater usage, land use and soil erosion, pollutants and the loss of biodiversity; and less on zoonotic transmission between humans and animals (Whitmee et al. 2015). As well as human effects on the environment, the commission looked at human factors such as consumption, population growth, technology and urbanisation. Like other movements described above, planetary health sees itself as the implementer and integrator of the SDGs. The propositions put forward also go much further than previous movements, with increased focus on public and global policy and less on information and education.

In response to the commission, Harvard University and the Wildlife Conservation Society in 2015 founded the Planetary Health Alliance, which aims to support the development of a 'rigorous, policy-focused, transdisciplinary field of applied research aimed at understanding and addressing the human health implications of accelerating change in the structure and function of Earth's natural systems'. The alliance comprises a consortium of over 60 universities and NGOs with a similar purpose to the other multidisciplinary initiatives: to educate, inform, convene meetings, and build networks and best practices.

Where to next?

With lots of players, initiatives and ideas, there appears to be agreement for multi- or transdisciplinary approaches to earth's current challenges. If the SDGs are to be achieved we need to work differently and avoid the vertical siloed approach that the MDGs often elicited. The approach needs to be systems-based and policy-informing and move far beyond the simple recognition that many emerging infectious diseases are zoonotic to addressing the many challenges as set out by the Rockefeller Foundation–Lancet Commission (Whitmee et al. 2015). While it appears that planetary health encapsulates One Health and EcoHealth, these disparate groups need to join to be effective in the policy arena. Irrespective of the name, there needs to be recognition that modern public/global health needs a composite of human, animal and ecological health. This premise was uncontested in the early days of public health. The scientific basis for miasma theory may have been flawed, but the recognition that an ill environment causes illness in people and that root causes need addressing still pertains to modern-day Planetary Health. We have come full-circle from the polymaths of public health with an interest in methodologies and human/animal/environmental health, to the need to bring these disciplines back together and co-ordinate their work.

Works cited

Bailey, B. (2011). *Burke and Hare: the year of the ghouls*. London: Random House.

Bathurst, W.L. (1831). *London Gazette* (18807): 1026–1027.

Burrell, S., and G. Gill (2005). The Liverpool cholera epidemic of 1832 and anatomical dissection – medical mistrust and civil unrest. *Journal of the History of Medicine and Allied Sciences* 60(4): 478–98.

Byrne, J. (2004). *The Black Death*. London: Greenwood Publishing Group.

Calman, K. (1998). The 1848 *Public Health Act* and its relevance to improving public health in England now. *BMJ* 317(7158): 596–8.

Cardiff, R.D., J.M. Ward, and S.W. Barthold (2007). 'One medicine – one pathology': are veterinary and human pathology prepared? *Laboratory Investigation* 88(1): 18–26.

Chadwick, E. (1843). *Report on the sanitary conditions of the labouring population of Great Britain*. Beccles, UK: W. Clowes & Sons.

Cook, R.A., W.B. Karesh, and S.A. Osofsky (2004). One World, One Health. http://www.oneworldonehealth.org.

Elsevier (2017). One Health. http://bit.ly/2BWg5kw.

Frankson, R., et al. (2016). One Health core competency domains. *Frontiers in Public Health* 4(4): 239.

Garcia-Ballester, L. (1994). *Practical medicine from Salerno to the Black Death*. Cambridge, UK: Cambridge University Press.

Henze, C.E. (2010). *Disease, health care and government in late imperial Russia: life and death on the Volga, 1823–1914*. London: Taylor & Francis.

Hodges, N. (1720). *Loimologia, or, An historical account of the plague in London in 1665: with precautionary directions against the like contagion.* London: E. Bell & J. Osborn.

Horton, R. (2013). Planetary health – a new vision for the post-2015 era. *Lancet* 382(9897):1012.

Horton, R., et al. (2014). From public to planetary health: a manifesto. *Lancet* 383(9920): 847.

Jones, K.E., et al. (2008). Global trends in emerging infectious diseases. *Nature* 451(7181): 990–3.

Jordan, T.E. (1993). *The degeneracy crisis and Victorian youth.* New York: SUNY Press.

Kahn, L.H., et al. (2014). A manifesto for planetary health. *Lancet* 383(9927): 1459.

Karesh, W.B., and R.A. Cook (2005). The human–animal link. *Foreign Affairs* 84(4): 38–46.

Kennedy, E. (1869). *Hospitalism and zymotic diseases: as more especially illustrated by puerperal fever, or metria. Also, a reply to the criticisms of seventeen physicians upon this paper.* London: Longmans, Green.

King, L.J., et al. (2008). Executive summary of the AVMA One Health Initiative Task Force report. *Journal of the American Veterinary Medical Association* 233(2): 259–61.

Klauder, J.V. (1958). Interrelations of human and veterinary medicine. *New England Journal of Medicine* 258(4): 170–7.

Lebel, J. (2003). *Health: an ecosystem approach.* Ottowa, ON: International Development Research Centre.

Ligon, B.L. (2002). Louis Pasteur: a controversial figure in a debate on scientific ethics. *Seminars in Pediatric Infectious Diseases* 13(2): 134–41.

Mackenbach, J.P. (2009). Politics is nothing but medicine at a larger scale: reflections on public health's biggest idea. *Journal of Epidemiology & Community Health* 63(3): 181–4.

Mackenzie, J.S., M. McKinnon, and M. Jeggo (2014). One Health: from concept to practice. In *Confronting emerging zoonoses: the One Health paradigm,* A. Yamada, L.H. Khan, B. Kaplan, T.P. Monath, J. Woodall, and L. Conti, eds., 163–189. Berlin: Springer.

Meydenbach, J. (1485). *Hortus sanitatis.* Mainz, Germany: J. Meydenbach.

Mitchill, S.L., and E. Miller (1810). *The medical repository, comprehending original essays and intelligence relative to medicine, chemistry, natural history, agriculture, geography and the arts; more especially as they are cultivated in America; and a review of American publications on medicine and the auxiliary branches of science,* 3rd edn. New York: Collins & Perkins.

Nolan, R.S. (2013). LEGENDS: the accidental epidemiologist. http://bit.ly/2L1N0Hs.

One Health Commission (2017). Mission/Goals. http://bit.ly/2L0g0PG.

One Health Initiative (2017). One Health Initiative will unite human and veterinary medicine. http://bit.ly/2RAvOuN.

One Health Platform (2016). The 4th International One Health Congress & the 6th Biennal Conference of the International Association for Ecology and Health. http://oheh2016.org/.

Pacini, F. (1866). A treatise on the specific cause of cholera, its pathology and cure. *British & Foreign Medico-Chirurgical Review* 38: 167–8.

Pacini, F. (1854). *Osservazioni microscopiche e deduzioni patologiche sul cholera asiatico*. Florence: F. Bencini.

Pasteur, L. (1880). On the Extension of the Germ Theory to the Etiology of Certain Common Diseases. *Comptes rendus de l'Académie des Sciences*, xc: 1033–44.

Planetary Health Alliance (2017). Planetary Health Alliance. http://bit.ly/2RAuEzr.

Priestley, J. (1774). On the noxious quality of the effluvia of putrid marshes. A letter from the Rev. Dr Priestley to Sir John Pringle. *Philosophical Transactions* 64: 90–5.

Queenan, K., et al. (2017). Roadmap to a One Health agenda 2030. *CAB Reviews* 12(014): 1–17.

Schultz, M.G. (2008). Rudolf Virchow. *Emerging Infectious Diseases* 14(9): 1480–1.

Schultz, M.G. (2014). In Memoriam: James Harlan Steele (1913–2013). *Emerging Infectious Diseases* 20(3): 514–5.

Schwabe, C. (1964). *Veterinary medicine and human health*, 1st edn. Baltimore: Williams & Wilkins.

Schwabe, C. (1984). *Veterinary medicine and human health*, 3rd edn. Baltimore: Williams & Wilkins.

Singer, M. (2009). *Introduction to syndemics*. San Francisco: Jossey-Bass.

Snow, J. (1849). *On the mode of communication of cholera*. London: Wilson & Ogilvy.

United States Agency for International Development. Emerging pandemic threats. http://bit.ly/2RFS7PV.

Virchow, R. (1848). Der armenarzt. *Medicinische Reform* 18: 125–7.

Virchow, R. (1859). Die cellularpathologie in ihrer begründung auf physiologische und pathologische gewebelehre. Berlin: August Hirschwald.

Virchow, R. (1860). Uber Trichina spiralis. *Virchows Arch. Pathol. Anat.* 18(3–4): 330–46.

Waage, J., et al. (2015). Governing sustainable development goals: interactions, infrastructures, and institutions. In *Thinking beyond sectors for sustainable development*, J. Waage and C. Yap, eds., 79–88. London: Ubiquity Press.

Walker, L., H. LeVine, and M. Jucker (2006). Koch's postulates and infectious proteins. *Acta Neuropathologica* 112(1): 1–4.

Whitmee, S., et al. (2015). Safeguarding human health in the Anthropocene epoch: report of the Rockefeller Foundation–Lancet Commission on Planetary Health. *Lancet* 386(10007): 1973–2028.

Zinsstag, J., E. Schelling, K. Wyss, and M.B. Mahamat (2005). Potential of cooperation between human and animal health to strengthen health systems. *Lancet* 366(9503): 2142–5.

2
One Health and global security into the future

Martyn Jeggo, Kerry Arabena and John S. Mackenzie

Global health, broadly, is an organising framework through which the effects of identity, social position, policies, institutional practices and geography of multiple populations of people intersect with the health of animals and our changing environments. This framework, best reflected in the Manhattan Principles, was developed in 2004 at the Wildlife Conservation Society's meeting on 'One World, One Health: building interdisciplinary bridges to health in a globalized world' (Cook, Karesh and Osofsky 2004). The 12 principles (Box 2.1) recognise that human, animal, and environmental health are not mutually exclusive. Each is shaped by the relationships between them.

The principles recognise that decision-making processes are integral to maintaining the integrity of biodiversity, food supplies and economies and acknowledge the impact of decisions on relationships between ecosystem resilience and patterns of disease emergence and spread. The principles also embed global disease prevention, surveillance, monitoring, control and mitigation in biodiversity conservation work and call for holistic, integrative and ethical approaches to minimise social inequity. They acknowledge the overlapping agendas linking human, environmental and animal health, and call on the global community to unite on global security. Since 2004, EcoHealth and One Health scientists and advocates have been

Box 2.1: The Manhattan Principles

1. Recognizing the link between human, domestic animal, and wildlife health, and the threat disease poses to people, their food supplies and economies, and the biodiversity essential to maintaining the healthy environments and functioning ecosystems we all require.

2. Recognizing that decisions regarding land and water use have real implications for health. Alterations in the resilience of ecosystems and shifts in patterns of disease emergence and spread manifest themselves when we fail to recognize this relationship.

3. Including wildlife health science as an essential component of global disease prevention, surveillance, monitoring, control, and mitigation.

4. Recognizing that human health programs can greatly contribute to conservation efforts.

5. Devising adaptive, holistic, and forward-looking approaches to the prevention, surveillance, monitoring, control, and mitigation of emerging and resurging diseases that fully account for the complex interconnections among species.

6. Seeking opportunities to fully integrate biodiversity conservation perspectives and human needs (including those related to domestic animal health) when developing solutions to infectious disease threats.

7. Reducing demand for and better regulating the international live wildlife and bush meat trade, not only to protect wildlife populations but to lessen the risks of disease movement, cross-species transmission, and the development of novel pathogen–host relationships. The costs of this worldwide trade in terms of impacts on public health, agriculture, and conservation are enormous, and the global community must address this trade as the real threat it is to global socio-economic security.

8. Restricting the mass culling of free-ranging wildlife species for disease control to situations where there is a multidisciplinary, international scientific consensus that a wildlife population poses an urgent, significant threat to human health, food security, or wildlife health more broadly.

9. Increasing investment in the global human and animal health infrastructure commensurate with the serious nature of emerging and resurging disease threats to people, domestic animals and wildlife. Enhanced capacity for global human and animal health surveillance and for clear, timely information sharing (that takes language barriers into account) can only help improve coordination of responses among governmental and non-governmental agencies, public and animal health institutions, vaccine/pharmaceutical manufacturers, and other stakeholders.
10. Forming collaborative relationships among governments, local people, and the private and public (i.e. non-profit) sectors to meet the challenges of global health and biodiversity conservation.
11. Providing adequate resources and support for global wildlife health surveillance networks that exchange disease information with the public health and agricultural animal health communities as part of early warning systems for the emergence and resurgence of disease threats.
12. Investing in educating and raising awareness among the world's people and in influencing the policy process to increase recognition that we must better understand the relationships between health and ecosystem integrity to succeed in improving prospects for a healthier planet. (Cook, Karesh and Osofsky 2004b)

lobbying investors and collaborators to address emerging threats to human health, food security, animal populations and environments.

The challenges for this century are multi-factorial and traverse human, animal and environmental health imperatives, driven by rapid social, cultural and ecological change. We need to understand the impact of these factors as well as the need to enhance global human and animal health surveillance with clear, timely information sharing, taking language barriers into account. Improved co-ordination of responses among government and non-government agencies, public and private sectors, local and Indigenous people, animal health institutions, vaccine/pharmaceutical manufacturers, and other stakeholders are prerequisites. In addition to co-ordination, deep understanding of the principles of complexity and diversity is required if programs are to be effective. The development of early warning systems, appropriate engagement, and knowledge translation and dissemination strategies are all required core competencies.

Many groups and organisations (see Table 2.1) have embraced the continuity of human, animal and environmental health as a reality for 21st-century thinking and action, and employ practical and theoretical resources to tackle challenges to global security. The principal difference between these groups is the primacy given to either the environment, human beings, animals or the earth system that binds them together.

This chapter describes these different groups: their origins, distinctiveness and how their overlapping agendas intersect. Their distinction is as important as their convergence – each group has an explicit way of articulating thought, speech, aesthetic appreciation, judgements and approaches for addressing current threats and creating future opportunities for global security. Looking into the future, however, is as much about understanding our historical capacity for living in natural systems as it is about future megatrends, including digital immersion. In this chapter, we explore how these groups can collaborate as a rallying point for inter-sectoral reform and future collaborations for the next generation of researchers, policy makers, educators and practitioners.

The One Health world

At the start of the 21st century, One Health experienced a revival with the spread of zoonotic diseases, in particular the 2003 SARS pandemic and the spread of highly pathogenic avian influenza (HPAI) H5N1 outbreaks (Mackenzie, McKinnon and Jeggo 2014). The Manhattan Principles were devised around this time (Cook, Karesh and Osofsky 2004), leading to One Medicine and One World continuing under the banner One Health (Zinstagg et al. 2005). The movement grew internationally under a tripartite agreement between the World Health Organization (WHO), the Food and Agriculture Organization (FAO), and the World Organization for Animal Health (OIE) in 2010 (WHO

Acronym	Full title of organisation
ACCAHZ	ASEAN Coordinating Centre for Animal Health and Zoonoses
CDC	Centers for Disease Control and Prevention
EC	European Council
FAO	Food and Agriculture Organization
IAEH	International Association for Ecology and Health
IDRC	International Development Research Centre of Canada
IMCAPI	International Ministerial Conference on Avian Pandemic Influenza
OHC	One Health Commission
OHCEA	One Health Central and Eastern Africa
OHI	One Health Initiative
OHP	One Health Platform
OIE	Office International des Epizooties (World Organization for Animal Health)
PHA	Planetary Health Alliance
PMSEIC	Australian Prime Minister's Science, Engineering and Innovation Council
UNICEF	United Nations International Children's Emergency Fund
UNSIC	United Nations System Influenza Coordination
USAID	United States Agency of International Development
WB	World Bank
WHO	World Health Organization

Table 2.1 Organisations and their acronyms.

2010). Commitment to a One Health approach in managing zoonotic diseases is evident worldwide with the creation of specific One Health entities both nationally and regionally (Mackenzie et al. 2013; Mackenzie, McKinnon and Jeggo 2014). Many countries now recognise the importance of a One Health approach to combat the rise of antimicrobial resistance (AMR), and ensure food safety.

A number of seminal activities over the past decade have shaped One Health, none more so than the publication of the Manhattan Principles, which has enhanced the uptake of One Health and EcoHealth thinking internationally. Concern about the potential risks to human and animal health of emerging zoonotic diseases and especially the possibility of an influenza pandemic, has also been a critical factor. These concerns underpin the development of national and regional One Health centres now established in many countries. The strategies to translate One Health concepts into practice originate from two meetings in 2009 and early 2010 – the first, 'One World, One Health: from ideas to action' (Public Health Agency of Canada 2009), was organised by the Public Health Agency of Canada, and the second, 'Operationalizing "One Health": a policy perspective – taking stock and shaping an implementation roadmap' (CDC 2010), was organised by the Centers for Disease Control and Prevention (CDC). A number of One Health groups associated with promotion, governance and information activities provide the mechanisms for unifying the One Health community, including sharing concepts and activities and giving support through co-ordinating roles such as that provided by the One Health Commission (OHC) in the US, the One Health Initiative (OHI), and the One Health Platform (OHP). Finally, and most relevant for sustainability, the inclusion of One Health concepts into medical and veterinary education is essential for breaking down silos and ensuring that knowledge of One Health is explicit in the education of the next generation of veterinarians, clinicians, and relevant biological disciplines.

Emerging diseases as a driver of One Health

Among global health security issues, the emergence and spread of epidemic-prone infectious diseases (EIDs) is a major international concern and plays a pivotal role in the development of One Health – not least because of the significant economic impact of outbreaks (Forum on Microbial Threats 2015; Institute of Medicine (US) Committee on Emerging Microbial Threats to Health in the 21st Century 2003). The term 'EIDs' has become synonymous with previously unknown infectious diseases, such as the Nipah virus in Malaysia in 1999 (Field et al. 2001) and SARS, which appeared suddenly in South Asia in 2003 (Forum on Microbial Threats 2004), and with known infections that are either increasing in incidence and geographic spread as exemplified by dengue and West Nile viruses (Mackenzie, Gubler and Petersen 2004), or expanding their host range as demonstrated by H5N1 avian influenza (Beato and Capau 2011). Evidence indicates increased risks from EIDs to humans, to animals and to the environment. Such diseases require national and international approaches for effective management.

Factors contributing to disease emergence include travel and the movement of people (particularly by air), international trade in live animals and fresh animal products, changes in land use and agricultural production, developments in technology capable of detecting new diseases, and the spread of exotic vectors to colonise new habitats thereby making new areas receptive to the spread of infections. The greatest challenge for the 21st century may well be climate change, which will have as yet uncharacterised effects on disease patterns and emergence, through its impact on the ecology of hosts, vectors and pathogens (Lafferty and Mordecai 2016; McMichael 2015) as well as the need to provide food and safe water to an ever-increasing world population.

In an effort to define EID threats to Australia, an expert working group of the Australian Prime Minister's Science, Engineering and Innovation Council (PMSEIC) was formed in 2009 to advise about epidemics. Their 2009 report concluded that 'it is a matter of when, not if, a lethally catastrophic epidemic will happen' and recommended 'the Government establish cross-portfolio arrangements essential for effective implementation ... as a matter of immediate priority' (PMSEIC 2009).

The role of One Health in managing risks from infectious diseases is now widely accepted in the United States, the European Community, and by the World Bank and WHO (Direction Générale de la Mondialisation, du Développement et des Partenariats 2011; Institute of Medicine 2012; World Bank 2010; WHO 2014). All agree that effective global surveillance is an essential ingredient for detecting EIDs, and is best achieved by a global alliance of networks established by the WHO, FAO and the OIE – such networks provide early detection of, and enable early response to, EIDs (Vallat 2009; WHO 2010). Notwithstanding these collaborative efforts, major gaps still exist in the surveillance of wildlife diseases where surveillance, if it exists, is devoid of depth or detail, with most outbreaks recognised by occasional widespread deaths among particular species.

The One Health approach was accelerated by the global threat of an avian influenza pandemic caused by pathogenic influenza A virus H5N1 (HPAI H5N1) and the risks such a pandemic would pose to human health. The United Nations, in collaboration with the FAO, OIE, WHO, United Nations System Influenza Coordination (UNSIC), United Nations International Children's Emergency Fund (UNICEF), the World Bank and other international and national agencies, instigated a series of International Ministerial Conferences on Avian and Pandemic Influenza (IMCAPI) to discuss the spread, transmission and possible containment of HPAI H5N1. While these conferences were directed primarily at HPAI H5N1, by 2008 it was clear that the intention was to extend to the wider context of EIDs as evidenced by the IMCAPI held in Sharm el-Sheikh, Egypt, in October 2008, where the 'Strategic framework for reducing risks of infectious diseases at the animal– human–ecosystems interface' was developed (IMCAPI 2010). The framework documented the necessity of a holistic One Health approach in response to HPAI H5N1 and other zoonotic disease emergencies to manage risks and minimise the global impact of epidemics and pandemics. A spirit of collaboration developed in the international community, resulting in part from IMCAPI and the cross-sectoral leadership shown by the WHO, FAO and OIE when they published their tripartite concept note 'Sharing responsibilities and coordinating global activities to address health risks at the animal–human–ecosystems interfaces', which aligned strategies and streamlined resources (WHO 2010). The 2010 IMCAPI in Hanoi, shortly after the publication of the concept note, concluded with the Hanoi Declaration, which proposed a multi-sector array of national measures to detect new diseases that might cross from animals to humans. Agreement was also reached to promote international surveillance, diagnosis and rapid response – noting that country strategies should be aligned nationally and regionally (IMCAPI 2010).

One Health: food safety and antimicrobial resistance

The risks from food contaminated with pathogenic microorganisms are well established. Early One Health approaches managed risks after the product had left the farm (post-farm gate), applying detection processes for infectious agents and chemical contamination linked to food production processes. However, the increasing impact of food-borne pathogens such as *Escherichia coli*, *Salmonella* spp., and *Clostridium difficile*, along with the risks associated with bovine spongiform encephalopathy (mad cow disease), have led to a number of whole-of-food-production-chain approaches. Appreciating the risks of these food-borne pathogens to humans and the need to manage them in animals (or plants) has necessitated a One Health approach (Lammie and Hughes 2016; Silva, Calva and Maloy 2014).

Mitigating risks for humans, animals and environments has not been without controversy, particularly in the use of antibiotics and the subsequent increase in AMR. The One Health approach has polarised rather than unified debate between human and animal health experts as to the underlying cause(s) of the growing microbial resistance that has persisted over many years. Influenced by the significant value of antibiotics as growth promoters in intensive livestock production systems, it was some time before the underlying issues were recognised and addressed, establishing a clear nexus between AMR, food safety, and agriculture (Review on Antimicrobial Resistance 2015). Had the One Health framework been used earlier, the nexus might have been identified through systems of political and scientific decision-making underpinned by a collectivist approach to disease emergence.

National and international activities promoting the One Health paradigm

National and international organisations proactively support One Health approaches to pandemic and emerging zoonotic disease threats. A number of initiatives have been supported by the World Bank, particularly in the avian and human influenza arena through its report *People, pathogens, and our planet* (World Bank 2010). The European

Community supports One Health in the Asian area, through the European External Action Service's Asia and Pacific Department (European Union 2016). In addition, regional groups operate across Africa and Asia, such as the Southern African Centre for Infectious Disease Surveillance's One Health Virtual Centre Model (Rweyemamu et al. 2013), the One Health Central and East Africa network (OHCEA 2016), the One Health Network South Asia, and the recently announced ASEAN Coordinating Centre for Animal Health and Zoonoses (ACCAHZ) (Association of South East Asian Nations 2016). The One Health Network South Asia, initiated by Massey University, comprises a network of hubs in different South Asian countries; each hub is a national network led by a government institution and together they form the 'Hubnet' with all hubs connected by a secure online platform (One Health Network South Asia 2014). In 2018 most nations are developing or have already developed their own action plans and coordinated approaches instigated by public health and veterinarian groups, governments or universities. In the Asia–Pacific region, a wide range of national activities, networks and national organisations operate with particular emphasis on the importance of the animal–human interface, and of the need for a strong cross-sectorial response (Coghlan and Hall 2013; Gongal 2013).

One Health organisations concerned with governance, information and educational activities

The following organisations promote and coordinate One Health activities:

One Health Commission

The OHC is a global organisation dedicated to promoting the improved health of people, domestic animals, wildlife, plants and the environment (OHC 2016). The organisation was chartered in Washington DC in 2009 as a not-for-profit entity with eight founding institutional members and is headquartered in the Research Triangle Park region of central North Carolina. Its primary aim is to inform audiences about the need to transcend institutional and disciplinary boundaries, and transform the way that human, animal, plant and ecosystem health professionals, and their related disciplines, work together to improve the health of all living things and the environment. The OHC seeks to connect One Health advocates, to create networks and teams that work together across disciplines, and to educate about One Health and One Health issues. Its charter informs professionals and students from all disciplines, the lay public, policy- and law-makers, healthcare providers from human and animal domains, and those in the agricultural and food production sectors, about the One Health approach. It aims to train and prepare the next generation of One Health leaders and professionals.

One Health Initiative

The OHI is a worldwide strategy for expanding interdisciplinary collaboration and communication in all aspects of healthcare for humans, animals and the environment. This synergism advances healthcare by accelerating biomedical research discoveries, enhancing public health efficacy, expeditiously expanding the scientific knowledge base, and improving medical education and clinical care.

The OHI autonomous team was co-founded by physician Laura H. Kahn, veterinarian Bruce Kaplan and physician Thomas P. Monath in 2007 with the sole purpose of promoting One Health concepts nationally and internationally (OHI 2016). An Honorary Advisory Board was established in 2010, and now consists of One Health advocates worldwide.

The OHI team's purpose and goals centre on educating international multidisciplinary scientific communities, political and government leaders, the news media and people everywhere about One Health. They promote One Health worldwide by their website and national and international publications, including the journal *One Health*. For the last decade, the OHI team has worked closely with the widely read online *One Health Newsletter* produced by the University of Florida's Emerging Pathogens Institute. All reputable One Health organisations, and individuals worldwide, are welcomed as supporters and advocates. The OHI team works pro bono and requires no fees from participating organisations and individuals.

One Health Platform

The OHP was established in 2015 in Belgium as a charitable foundation (OHP 2015). It provides a strategic forum for researchers, early-career investigators, governmental and non-governmental institutions, international organisations and companies to foster cross-sectoral collaborations. Its major objectives are to:

- Provide a strategic forum for researchers, early-career investigators, governmental and non-governmental institutions, international organisations, and companies to foster cross-sectoral collaborations;
- Identify and prioritise research gaps in the fields of zoonoses, emerging infectious diseases and antimicrobial resistance, including the ecological and environmental factors that impact on these diseases, and advocate the resulting scientific research agenda – on both a scientific and policy level;
- Create synergies and facilitate the sharing of data between researchers and research groups to fill the research gaps, and translate the data to anyone who might benefit;
- Disseminate the results and insights of existing and new research projects on zoonoses, emerging infectious diseases and antimicrobial resistance, including the ecological and environmental factors which impact on these diseases;
- Establish an information reference centre for the One Health community; and
- Enhance awareness of the value of the One Health approach through communication, facilitation of interactions between stakeholder groups, education and training, and specific efforts to convince 'non-believers', in both the research community and in the policy arena (OHP 2015).

The platform publishes an occasional newsletter, *One Health Communicator*, and supports the electronic journal, *One Health*, published by Elsevier. From 2018, the platform has organised future One Health Congresses, with the 5th Congress held in 2018 in

Saskatoon, Canada, with the next meeting being held in Edinburgh in 2020. The Platform is also now organizing biennial One Health Forums, the first being a Forum in 2019 in collaboration with the Africa CDC to develop strategies for zoonosis surveillance.

One Health Foundation

The One Health Foundation (OHF), established in 2010 in Zurich, focuses on improving human and livestock health by addressing issues including zoonotic diseases, food safety, and environmental pollution. It remains a small entity in this increasingly crowded space (OHF 2015).

One Health Global Network

In recognition of the number of One Health groups and networks established around the world, and others in the process of development, the One Health Global Network was created – following the CDC Stone Mountain meeting in 2010 – to act as a 'network of networks' facilitating coordination and offering linkages that provide a global geographic dimension and optimal complementarity between initiatives. It became inactive in 2015.

One Health conferences and congresses

One Health conferences and congresses are now commonplace, both regionally and globally. One Health conferences in Africa organised by the Southern African Centre for Infectious Disease Surveillance, the OHCEA One Health conferences, and the 2016 One Health European Interregional Conference in Bucharest, Romania, are some regional examples.

Since 2011 five 'International One Health Congresses' have been held (Melbourne in 2011, Bangkok in 2013, Amsterdam in 2015, Melbourne in 2016 and Saskatoon in 2018). Other international meetings include the 'Global Conferences in One Health', organised by the World Veterinary Association and World Medical Association (the first meeting was held in Madrid in 2015 and the second in Fukuoka in 2016), and the Global Risk Forums on One Health in Davos, Switzerland (2012, 2013 and 2015).

Educational developments in support of One Health

An essential aspect of One Health development is educating professionals – veterinarians, medical practitioners, biomedical scientists, wildlife biologists, and others – to better understand a One Health approach through improved communication and co-operation across the disciplines and across a wide range of subjects, such as responding to known or new zoonotic diseases, detecting and tracking the origins of antibiotic resistance, ensuring food security and food safety, and mitigating the effects of climate change. Breaking down the disciplinary silos is an essential component of One Health education. The One Health Masters course for students in the Asia–Pacific region, established with the support of the World Bank, the European Commission and Massey University in New Zealand (One Health at Massey 2016; Vink et al. 2013), is a good example of multidisciplinary learning. Other examples include the One Health Institute at the University of California at Davis, the One Health Center of Excellence at the University of Florida, the Center of One Health Research at the University of Washington, and the One Health Center Illinois at the University of Illinois. The University of Edinburgh, the Royal Veterinary College in London, Ross University School of Veterinary Medicine, the University of Hokkaido, Duke University and the University of Saskatchewan have all established graduate courses in One Health. There are others.

The most important and sustainable training developments occur when medical and veterinary programs introduce One Health concepts into their undergraduate as well as postgraduate degree courses. Many universities do this, with many more planning to do it, especially those with faculties of veterinary medicine, but the effects of this may not be visible until future clinicians and veterinarians enter their professional careers.

'One Health' has become a *lingua franca* in global terms. Nevertheless, while it professes to be the intersection of human, animal and ecosystems health, it is understood by many to focus mainly on the animal–human interface, irrespective of whether the subject is disease emergence, zoonoses, food safety, AMR, or climate change. In the past, environmental factors were seen only in relation to human or animal health rather than as substantial components of the health of our environment. This is where EcoHealth has been preeminent and filled the void.

The EcoHealth world: what is it and where did it come from?

EcoHealth and One Health share a holistic approach but EcoHealth is broader, incorporating the earth's ecosystems and their impact on human health. EcoHealth examines changes in the biological, physical, social and economic environments and relates these changes to human health. The modern EcoHealth concept emerged with the founding of the EcoHealth Alliance in 1971 by British naturalist Gerard Durrell, in collaboration with local and international conservation partners. With close links to conservation medicine, EcoHealth grew during the 1990s, supported by the International Development Research Centre of Canada (IDRC) (Lebel 2003). At its core is an appreciation that environmental health, human and animal health, and the social and political context in which they exist, make up a complex system – the ecosystem. EcoHealth supports a systems approach to tackling complex problems, rather than the more reductionist approach taken by scientists working in individual health specialties or 'silos' (i.e. human health, veterinary medicine, ecology, social science, politics).

The ecosystem approach to human health is a union of ecological approaches to public health and ecosystem health from environmental management. The IDRC, a long-time advocate of ecosystem health, first introduced the EcoHealth research program in 1996. In 2004, the IDRC founded the *EcoHealth* journal, merging two previous journals – *Ecosystem Health* and *Global Change and Human Health*. The IDRC established the International Association for Ecology and Health (IAEH) in 2006, in part to fill the *EcoHealth* publisher's need to have the financial backing of a society; but more relevantly to address the need to organise the EcoHealth movement globally as well as to curate the journal.

EcoHealth was shaped by the sustainable development movement of the 1980s espousing the principles in the seminal Brundtland Report of 1987 (United Nations 1987), which articulated the movement's goals in terms of social justice, participation, and equity across and between generations. These principles, and the holistic spirit of the Brundtland Report, continue to inform current EcoHealth thinking and practice, and are evident in global and local initiatives that give primacy to the health and wellbeing of humans in healthy environments and systems.

The IAEH is a scholarly organisation that supports EcoHealth activities, with members from all continents (IAEH 2015). Committed to fostering the health of humans, animals and ecosystems, IAEH members conduct research and help scholars and field-based practitioners to recognise the inextricable linkages between the health of all species and their environments. A basic tenet in EcoHealth is that health and wellbeing cannot be sustained in a resource-depleted, polluted and socially unstable planet. EcoHealth members engage in integrated systemic approaches to health by seeking to sustain ecosystem health services, foster social stability and promote the peaceful coexistence of humans, animals and environments.

EcoHealth objectives include serving a diverse international community of scientists, educators, policy makers and practitioners, and providing mechanisms and forums to facilitate international and interdisciplinary discourse. This is achieved through the journal *EcoHealth*, biennial conferences, promotional activities in line with the mission, by encouraging the development of transdisciplinary teaching, research and problem solving that cuts across many fields of scholarship (including natural, social and health sciences and the humanities), and by fostering intercultural knowledge exchange, validating holistic knowledge and creating conditions that sponsor creativity among diverse groups of people.

EcoHealth focuses on interdisciplinary, transdisciplinary and collective social learning processes in which the environment is regarded in the broadest sense. Maintaining healthy environments in which all members of a system can flourish is a primary goal.

Conservation and equity (of gender, resources and opportunity) are critical issues, coupled with a strong appreciation of the need to engage with everyone about problems and solutions. EcoHealth scholars are conscious of the limitations in the way that we think, and recognise that solutions can emerge not only from compartmentalised interests, but also from collaborative contributions. EcoHealth is engaged with factors affecting health and wellbeing in their own right, and as interconnected, making this approach multidimensional, complex and reflective of the diversity within the ecosystems of concern.

Originally, the IDRC EcoHealth program was based on three methodological pillars of transdisciplinarity, participation, and equity. These were subsequently expanded to six key principles: systems thinking, knowledge to action, transdisciplinarity, participation, equity and sustainability (Parkes 2011). These principles are dependent on, and fully expressed through, the four interacting areas of society, economics, politics and ecology. This appreciation for complex systems underpins the ecosystems approach to achieving health and wellbeing for people, animals and environments. Those working under the banner of EcoHealth are ethically driven to make positive long-lasting changes, leading to sustainability through environmentally sound processes and the promotion of durable and equitable social change.

EcoHealth studies differ from traditional, single-discipline studies. A traditional epidemiological study, for example, may show increasing rates of malaria in a region, but not address how or why those rates are increasing. An environmental health study may recommend spraying a pesticide in certain areas to reduce spread, while an economic analysis may calculate the cost and effectiveness of every dollar spent on such a program.

An EcoHealth study brings multiple specialist disciplines together with members of the affected community *before* the study begins. Through pre-study meetings, the group shares knowledge, adopts a common language and develops a shared vision for the outcome of their work. These pre-study meetings often lead to creative and novel approaches and more 'socially robust' solutions.

Transdisciplinarity differentiates this field from other multidisciplinary studies. EcoHealth studies value the participation of all groups, even those with radically different and sometimes opposing views. Transdisciplinarity values and harnesses the knowledge of all the disciplines, placing equal value on contributions from decision makers, artists, philosophers, scientists, inventors, citizen activists and community leaders. It recognises all elements such as good quality air and waterways, healthy wetlands and river systems, nutrient-rich, fertile topsoil and native flora and fauna.

The principle of equality of diversity underpins EcoHealth: everything is different but equal. Equity (between genders, socioeconomic classes, age brackets and even species) is not a desired outcome in itself; rather it is a field of practice, a part of the process and a way of comprehending and contributing to the problem being studied, and the consequences that might come from resolving it.

After a decade of international conferences in North America and Australia, under the more contentious umbrella of ecosystem health, the first 'ecosystem approach to human health' forum was held in Montreal in 2003. This was followed by conferences and forums in Wisconsin, US, and Mérida, Mexico – all with major support from the IDRC. Since then the IAEH and the linked journal *EcoHealth* confirm the field as a legitimate scholarly and development activity. The EcoHealth movement is aligned with the Ottawa Charter, Rio Declaration, International Panel on Climate Change, and the Millennium Ecosystem Assessment, with new initiatives such as the Resilience Alliance continually emerging and gaining traction.

Planetary Health Alliance

The Planetary Health Alliance (PHA), formed in December 2015, is an alliance of universities, NGOs and other organisations dedicated to increasing understanding of the human health impacts of accelerating global environmental change; to building an educational platform that enables the teaching of planetary health topics in classrooms around the world, and to ensuring growing understanding of these topics is applied to real-world natural resource management and policy making. Ultimately, it envisages a global public educated about the connection between human health and our management of earth's natural systems, and policy makers who are able to calculate the human health costs and benefits of their resource management decisions. Planetary health is 'the health of human civilization and the state of the natural systems on which it depends' (PHA 2016).

The PHA is hosted by Harvard University's Center for the Environment and the T.H. Chan School of Public Health, and seeks to draw together like-minded organisations and individuals. The alliance's products are publicly accessible, with the intention that Harvard's faculty will be housed in universities and other organisations around the world. The steering committee includes international senior faculty, scientists and policy makers. The PHA aims to be a unifying and integrating force by engaging with other organisations, groups, and individuals around the world to support them in developing a robust field of planetary health.

The PHA also aims to establish a community of practice across a variety of disciplines by generating common ground and stimulating the growth of the field through educational materials, shared literature, common sources of communication about new scientific findings, alerts regarding job opportunities and meetings, shared methodologies, protocols and datasets, and an online journal club. A robust research effort investigating and quantifying the human health impacts of global environmental change is the engine at the heart of building a discipline of planetary health and policy. Although the PHA does not carry out research itself, it exists within a rich research environment where numerous planetary health-related research activities are ongoing.

The PHA supports training in planetary health topics, using relevant datasets and research methodologies. It also makes announcements about new research and job opportunities and sponsors an annual research meeting with the ambition of providing a cadre of young investigators with the capacity and motivation to break new ground in this field. In addition, the PHA awards full-time research positions to postdoctoral candidates with outstanding track records within their disciplines and strong capacity to step out of their disciplinary experience, and engage in transdisciplinary, planetary health research with the PHA-associated faculty.

Although the PHA recognises that funding for this approach is limited, it plans to stimulate growth in the planetary health field through its support of US government agencies – such as the National Institutes of Health, National Science Foundation, and USAID – to create programs focused on planetary health. Without funding sources, universities will be unable to develop and promote faculty work, and civil society and other stakeholders will be unable to take action based upon the science and evidence-based policies.

The commissioners on the Rockefeller Foundation–Lancet Commission on Planetary Health believe that degradation of ecosystems can lead to negative public health impacts. Until these impacts are proven and quantified in actionable ways, they remain vague externalities that are not factored into decisions about public health or natural resource management. The emergent field of planetary health is poised to deliver powerful new and convincing arguments that demonstrate the range of critical relationships between the state of natural systems and health.

Where are we currently?

The 'all-inclusive' view of health, or One Health, is the systematic understanding and management of health within a sociopolitical and ecological framework (Zinsstag et al. 2011). There are social and ecological drivers for the emergence of disease in humans, animals and plants. Impaired human, animal and plant health has social and ecological consequences, which create new socioecological drivers. Effective intervention strategies require an understanding of the socioecological drivers of disease, along with the sociopolitical and ecological factors determining intervention (equity) effectiveness and consequences.

Although One Health is the accepted term that represents all this, and the organisations under this umbrella seek to take a multidisciplinary and cross-sectorial (health, environment, agriculture) approach, they each have varying degrees of focus on particular aspects. EcoHealth has an emphasis on the health of the environment with an ecosystems approach, while the One Health Platform highlights infectious diseases with a focus on the health both of humans and animals as well as issues around food security and safety. This diversity may be valuable and provide a rich tapestry of approaches to global health, but it may also have drawbacks, and a range of issues within this context need to be considered (Zinsstag 2012).

Organisational issues

The following five structured organisations purport to represent the new order of One Health: EcoHealth, the One Health Platform, One Health Foundation, One Health Initiative, and the One Health Commission. They each have mandates and missions linked to objectives and outcomes, and varying membership arrangements and management or governance approaches. Most seek funding through these arrangements and have a call out for membership. While this provides choice, it is also confusing, competitive and divisive. This fragmentation sends a message to governments and funding bodies of complexity and uncertainty about the organisations' longevity, which impedes serious investment or attention by traditional groups or silos that have dominated health in the past. The essence of the problem – a lack of cross-sectorial collaboration and thinking – is hardly helped by this multi-organisational approach to One Health concepts and solutions. Nevertheless, working together, the One Health Commission, One Health Initiative and the One Health Platform initiated an annual One Health day, starting in 2015. Held on 3 November each year, it promotes the One Health concept with a particular focus on students research activities for which they compete for monetary prizes.

But organisation and structure are essential building blocks. For a time One Health advocates believed that by sharing ideas, encouraging collaboration and expounding multidisciplinary approaches to complex issues, the desired One Health approach would be successful (Gibbs and Gibbs 2013). It was not, and many examples are testimony to this. At the national level and international levels, One Health entities within the Mongolian and Laotian governments and within regions such as Asia–Pacific Economic Cooperation and the African Union are the only ones demonstrating progress.

Would not a single international One Health organisation be better? One established through a union of these existing bodies? Each entity has its own organisational culture, which has both refined its thinking and contributions but at the same time compartmentalised shared interests, resulting in intense competition for resources. Each entity understands its capacity to solve real-life threats to global security, but to the exclusion of others. Taken together, these factors have created within each of these agencies a sense of legitimacy, singularity and purpose. This development has created conditions for competition rather than convergence, resulting in divisions that have crept into our accepted understanding of the nature of the world, even though they are humanly constructed (Brown 2008). While solutions can emerge from within these separate knowledge systems, little consideration is given to how these different contributions fit together, even though each has made, or could make, a major contribution in its own right. It appears that unifying under a single entity may be easier said than done.

Financial issues

Two major financial problems beset the One Health arena. First, none of the organisations are financially secure, having to rely upon subscriptions and donations. Only relatively small cohorts of researchers and advocates work in this space, making it unlikely to have sufficient capacity to sustain current engagement. While each of the entities described has a favoured funding or resource base, a better and more sustainable solution would be to unify competing cells into a single entity representing One Health.

Secondly, One Health research has no identified champion or patron. Most national or international bodies fund through a specific One Health sector, for example, human health, agriculture, the environment. Finding a single financial source for a One Health project is still a substantial challenge – with the exception of the Bill and Melinda Gates Foundation and the Wellcome Trust, which support One Health. Progress is slow and much of One Health research exists within a sector that should only be partially funding the work. Having a single international One Health organisation might provide an opportunity to seek serious funding specifically for One Health research.

Communication and publishing issues

The journal *EcoHealth,* now more than nine years old, has an impact factor of 2.48. It publishes on a broad range of topics, including the environment, ecology, diseases and health. Editorials and forum pieces provide views on a range of One Health and EcoHealth issues as well as a reading focus for EcoHealth and One Health researchers and advocates. A further three journals have begun publishing in the One Health area including the One Health Platform–linked *One Health* journal and the One Health Outlook. This diversity of publishing opportunities is valuable, but is not without challenges, such as identifying the most appropriate journal to publish research. The journals face simultaneous demands to maintain their impact factor, readership and subscription figures.

Congresses and conferences

The first EcoHealth conference was held in Madison, Wisconsin, in 2006. A legacy of this conference, and all future ones, has been the Conference Statement, outlining an agenda for EcoHealth around the world. Since the first One Health International Congress in Australia in 2011, a plethora of One Health conferences and meetings have been held, leaving a confusing set of agendas. Most noticeable was the attempt by the city of Davos in Switzerland to establish an annual One Health Conference along similar lines to the Davos Economic Forum. Despite diminishing attendees and presentations in the last five years, it continues to compete with other One Health conferences.

In 2016 a joint congress between EcoHealth (6th Biennial Conference) and One Health (4th International Congress) was held in Melbourne. But the challenges of finance, membership and scope experienced in organising this conference make it unlikely to be repeated in two years. These conferences are vital for boosting the One Health agenda, sharing research and ideas across disciplines and sectors, continents and cultures, and for social and political advocacy beyond that of the scientific papers. The plethora of meetings and conferences dilutes the trans-sectorial and multidisciplinary approaches One Health strives for and weakens the opportunities for messaging and lobbying for resources and attention.

What should the future be?

The scientific approach for the past 200 years has been primarily reductionist in nature and increasingly specialised, driven largely by complexities in understanding the basics and developing workable solutions to scientific problems. This is also the case in healthcare. Specialisation in human health, agriculture, and environmental management, has created sub-specialties with a large number of disciplines, with their own methods, modes of inquiry, languages, professional bodies, qualifications, and professional support in the form of journals, conferences and educational initiatives.

The start of this century, with so many intractable global and local concerns, casts doubt on whether conventional approaches will work. Rittel and Webber (1973) termed a class of issues facing our current planetary dilemmas as 'wicked problems': that defy complete definition and for which there is unlikely to be a final solution. Brown (OHP 2015) saw wicked problems as part of the community that generates them, meaning that any resolution requires changes in that society (governance or way of living), or changes in the 'thought' community (novel approaches to research methods and to actions and decisions based on that research). The authors cautioned against rejecting the powerful tools that enabled reductions in diseases or increased world food production (Brown 2010). They suggested that an alternative to a limited focus on any single avenue of enquiry is a requirement that current and future researchers and decision makers be receptive to new ideas and directions – matching that of the times.

Today, the deleterious manner in which centuries of human activity have devastated the natural systems on Earth is acknowledged and recognised. The disruption of the functional integrity of the planet by human activity, and at the same time accepting that the processes underlying this integrity are intrinsically linked, is in itself a difficult problem for scientists and thought leaders. Although we are yet to fully understand these links, a viable future founded on life-sustaining solutions cannot be achieved without a more holistic and systems-oriented approach to local and global matters.

One Health viewpoints recognise the imperative of whole-of-system and ecosystem analyses, noting that the social and political changes required are beyond discipline-based approaches. However, these disciplines remain powerful, and fragmentation and diversification continues. People engaged in these disciplinary traditions have strong membership identities; the power of those identities is a significant motivating factor for maintaining the status quo. Identification as a member of a particular group is narrow, and often too socially or politically exclusionary to facilitate finding the solutions required. The benefits that these entities might bring are often lost due to the narrowness of the allegiance they inspire.

The multiple shared views of these specialty and sub-specialty groups could inspire a shared identity – offering both motivation and universality – sharing effort, resources and support. In this way, we could maintain identity through a singular entity (EcoHealth practitioner, One Health scientist, parks ranger) as well as participate in a shared identity that includes other voices. The new generations of scholars, scientists, decision makers and policy advisers will need to facilitate shared platforms.

The issue of scale: is a regional rather than global approach more realistic?

While these issues of identity vex global efforts to come together, the future of One Health entities might be better approached using a regional model – one that makes sense ecologically. Regionalisation is an effective spatial framework for systems research and protects the biological, linguistic and cultural diversity specific to each region. Regional initiatives may provide the greatest opportunity for engagement, knowledge exchange and the development of integrative practices that draw on all the knowledge domains.

In 2012, EcoHealth scholars based in Oceania discussed regional initiatives at the 4th Biennial Conference of the International Association for Ecology and Health (IAEH) in Kunming, China, and made a commitment to ensure voices, concerns and ideas of the region would be heard in global forums. The IAEH can establish regional chapters using a constitutional trigger. (This was activated at an Oceania-focused forum in December 2013.) The specific mandate of the Oceania EcoHealth Chapter is to consult and engage with IAEH members and advocate for local and regional issues that represent the diversity of the region and the mission of the international organisation (Arabena and Kingsley 2016). With foundational principles of co-creation, collaboration and relationship building, the chapter has facilitated regional activities, demonstrations, short courses, student activities, and social media and place-based strategic engagement across institutions, entity representatives and Indigenous communities. However, as inspiring as this might be, the viability of this initiative depends on the enthusiasm of its members and leadership.

A missing link: custodianship

Despite treaties, statements, manifestos and congresses, billions of people have not been convinced that environmental issues are serious and myriad, and that co-operative action is essential to survive. We have failed to unite people to act. Communication strategies have either failed to engage at an individual level and/or do not provide information about how to get from point A (the problem) to point B (a sensible alternative or different code to live by). People invested in modern societies are left with a sense of inevitability about the destruction left for future generations.

The Oceania Chapter's path mentioned above examines the historical knowledge of local and Indigenous peoples in various regions and, in particular, draws on their knowledge about 'how to live in place'. Knowledge systems have sustained populations over thousands of years without destroying the integrity of their environments. Evidence from studies on hunting, herding, fishing and gathering from across Australia, Micronesia, and the Pacific Islands demonstrates that local communities are able to 'marshal powerful emotional resources' (Anderson 2014), and societal strength from their cultures, which are closely linked to, and informed by, their connection to land and sea.

These studies critically highlight connection to Country, working from the premise that ecosystem approaches are far more than a biophysical focus on health. Rather, they incorporate a holistic way of understanding environmental issues by drawing on interconnections between culture, identity and wellbeing, and a deep appreciation for environments as a life-source – a non-negotiable foundation for all life (Parkes 2010). This theme, explored in a special issue of *EcoHealth*, coincided with the adoption of the United Nations Declaration on the Rights of Indigenous Peoples (Stephens, Parkes and Chang 2007; United Nations 2007). These traditional and local cultures and societies show us how to devise practical strategies for environmental management, in the context of land being a non-negotiable life-source, and uniting people to act on these strategies. Custodianship of the environment and the biological systems it supports has been embraced by Aboriginal and Torres Strait Islander peoples for over 60,000 years, and supported with irreversible frameworks of cultural obligations that underpin this sustainable approach (Arabena 2015).

Combining united disciplinary knowledge with a custodianship framework has the potential to refocus learning and knowledge, in a way that includes the views of people whose knowledge systems have been linked for thousands of years. This will require all knowledge, ideologies and future initiatives to adopt, in a real sense, the principles of tolerance, diversity, reciprocity and solidarity. These must be at the core of all custodial relationships and are essential for the future of One Health and EcoHealth platforms.

Works cited

Anderson, E.N. (2014). *Caring for place: ecology, ideology and emotion in traditional landscape management.* Walnut Creek, CA: Left Coast Press.

Arabena, K. (2015). *Becoming Indigenous to the universe: reflections on living systems, indigeneity and citizenship.* Melbourne: Australian Scholarly Publishing.

Arabena, K., and J. Kingsley (2016). Oceania. *EcoHealth.* 13(4): 615–7.

Association of South East Asian Nations (2016). The ASEAN Coordinating Centre for Animal Health and Zoonoses (ACCAHZ). https://bit.ly/2EgAF1y.

Atlas, R.M. (2013). One Health: its origins and future. *Current Topics in Microbiology & Immunology* 365: 1–13.

Beato, M.S., and I. Capua (2011). Transboundary spread of highly pathogenic avian influenza through poultry commodities and wild birds: a review. *Revue Scientifique et Technique* 30(1): 51–61.

Brown, V.A. (2008). *Leonardo's vision: a guide to collective thinking and action.* Rotterdam, NL: Sense.

Brown, V.A., P.M. Deane, J.A. Harris, and J.Y. Russell (2010). Towards a just and sustainable future. In *Tackling wicked problems through the transdisciplinary imagination*, V.A. Brown, J.A. Harris, and J.Y. Russell, eds., 2–9. London: Earthscan.

Centers for Disease Control and Prevention (2010). Operationalizing 'One Health': a policy perspective – taking stock and shaping an implementation road map. Stone Mountain, Georgia, USA, May 4–6. https://bit.ly/2AUBsRn.

Coghlan, B., and D. Hall (2013). The development of One Health approaches in the Western Pacific. *Current Topics in Microbiology & Immunology* 366: 93–111.

Cook, R.A., W.B. Karesh, and S.A. Osofsky (2004).One World, One Health: Building Interdisciplinary Bridges to Health in a Globalized World. New York: Wildlife Conservation Society.Accessed 18 April 2016. https://bit.ly/2MSCTp9.

Cook, R.A., W.B. Karesh, and S.A. Osofsky (2004b). *The Manhattan principles on 'one world one health'. One World, One Health: building interdisciplinary bridges to health in a globalized world.* New York: Wildlife Conservation Society. http://bit.ly/2Qup7gw.

Direction Générale de la Mondialisation, du Développement et des Partenariats (2011). Position française sur le concept One Health/Une seule santé. https://bit.ly/2E3Tggj.

European Union (2016). EEAS content. https://bit.ly/2SyVLLF.

Field, H., P. Young, J.M. Yob, J. Mills, L. Hall, and J. Mackenzie (2001). The natural history of Hendra and Nipah viruses. *Microbes and Infection* 3(4): 307–14.

Forum on Microbial Threats, Board on Global Health, and Institute of Medicine. (2004). *Learning from SARS: preparing for the next disease outbreak: workshop summary.* Washington, DC: National Academies Press.

Forum on Microbial Threats, Board on Global Health, and Institute of Medicine. (2015). *Emerging viral diseases: the One Health connection: workshop summary.* Washington, DC: National Academies Press.

Gibbs, S.E., and E.P. Gibbs (2013). The historical, present, and future role of veterinarians in One Health. In *One Health: the human–animal–environment interfaces in emerging infectious diseases*, J.S. Mackenzie, M. Jeggo, P. Dazsak, and J.A. Richt, eds., 41–4. Berlin: Springer.

Gongal, G. (2013). One Health approach in the South East Asia region: opportunities and challenges. *Current Topics in Microbiology & Immunology* 366: 113–22.

Institute of Medicine (2012). *Improving food safety through a One Health approach.* Washington, DC: National Academies Press.

Institute of Medicine (US) Committee on Emerging Microbial Threats to Health in the 21st Century (2003). *Microbial threats to health: emergence, detection, and response.* Washington, DC: National Academies Press.

International Association for Ecology and Health (2015). Mission and objectives. https://bit.ly/2G27ec3.

International Ministerial Conference on Animal and Pandemic Influenza (2008). Contributing to One World, One Health. A strategic framework for reducing risks of infectious diseases at the human–animal–ecosystems interface. http://ftp.fao.org/docrep/fao/011/aj137e/aj137e00.pdf.

International Ministerial Conference on Animal and Pandemic Influenza (2010). Hanoi Declaration. Animal and pandemic influenza: the way forward. https://uni.cf/2RDfCJk.

Lafferty, K.D., and E.A. Mordecai (2016). The rise and fall of infectious disease in a warmer world. *F-1000 Faculty Rev-2040* 5. doi: 10.12688/f1000research.8766.1.

Lammie, S.L., and J.M. Hughes (2016). Antimicrobial resistance, food safety, and One Health: the need for convergence. *Annual Review of Food Science & Technology* 7: 287–312.

Lebel, J. (2003). Health: an ecosystem approach. *Canada: International Development Research Centre* Ottawa: IDRC. https://bit.ly/2GceeeC

Mackenzie, J.S., D.J. Gubler, and L.R. Petersen (2004). Emerging flaviviruses: the spread and resurgence of dengue, Japanese encephalitis and West Nile viruses. *Nature Medicine* 10: S98–S109.

Mackenzie, Jeggo, Daszak, Richt (2013). One Health: the human–animal–environment interfaces in emerging infectious diseases: Food safety and security, and international and national plans for implementation of One Health activities. *Curr. Top. Microbiol. Immunolo.,* 366: 1–255.

Mackenzie, J.S., M. McKinnon, and M. Jeggo (2014). One Health: from concept to practice. In *Confronting emerging zoonoses: the One Health paradigm,* A. Yamada, L.H. Khan, B. Kaplan, T.P. Monath, J. Woodall, and L. Conti, eds., 163–89. Berlin: Springer.

McMichael, A.J. (2015). Extreme weather events and infectious disease outbreaks. *Virulence* 6(6): 543–7.

One Health at Massey (2016). Building human and institutional capability throughout South Asia to detect and respond to emerging disease threats. https://bit.ly/2UiYb2x.

One Health Central and Eastern Africa (OHCEA) (2016). One Health Central and East Africa; a regional network of public health and veterinary institutions. https://bit.ly/2Swyl9r.

One Health Commission (2016). www.onehealthcommission.org.

One Health Foundation (2015). www.onehealthfoundation.org.

One Health Initiative (2016). www.onehealthinitiative.com/.

One Health Network South Asia (2014) www.onehealthnetwork.asia/.

One Health Platform (2015). http://onehealthplatform.com/.

Parkes, M.W. (2010). *EcoHealth and Aboriginal health: a review of common ground.* Prince George, BC: National Collaborating Centre for Aboriginal Health.

Parkes, M.W. (2011). Diversity, emergence, resilience: guides for a new generation of EcoHealth research and practice. *EcoHealth* 8(2): 137–9.

Planetary Health Alliance (2016). http://planetaryhealthalliance.com/.

Prime Minister's Science, Engineering, and Innovation Council (2009). Epidemics in a changing world: Expert Working Group on Epidemics in a Changing World. https://bit.ly/2KWlwCR.

Public Health Agency of Canada (2009). One World One Health: from ideas to action. www.phac-aspc.gc.ca/owoh-umus/index-eng.php.

Review on Antimicrobial Resistance (2015). *Antimicrobials in agriculture and the environment: reducing unnecessary use and waste.* London: Wellcome Trust.

Rittel, H.W.J., and M.W. Webber (1973). Dilemmas in a general theory of planning. *Policy Sciences* 4(2): 155–69.

Rweyemamu, M., et al. (2013). Development of a One Health national capacity in Africa: the Southern African Centre for Infectious Disease Surveillance (SACIDS) One Health virtual centre model. *Current Topics in Microbiology & Immunology* 366: 73–91.

Schwabe, C. (1984). *Veterinary medicine and human health,* 3rd edn. Baltimore: Williams & Wilkins.

Silva, C., E. Calva, and S. Maloy (2014). One Health and food-borne disease: Salmonella transmission between humans, animals, and plants. *Microbiology Spectrum* 2(1): 20.

Stephens, C., M.W. Parkes, and H. Chang (2007). Indigenous perspectives on ecosystem sustainability and health. *EcoHealth* 4(4): 369–70.

United Nations (1987). *Report of the World Commission on Environment and Development: our common future (The Brundtland Report).* Geneva: United Nations.

United Nations General Assembly. Resolution 61/295. *Declaration on the Rights of Indigenous Peoples,* A/RES/61/295 (13 September 2007).

Vallat, B. (2009). One World, One Health (Editorial). *OIE Bulletin* 2: 1–2.

Vink, W.D., J.S. McKenzie, N. Cogger, B. Borman, and P. Muellner (2013). Building a foundation for 'One Health': an education strategy for enhancing and sustaining national and regional capacity in endemic and emerging zoonotic disease management. *Current Topics in Microbiology & Immunology* 366: 185–205.

World Bank (2010). *People, pathogens, and our planet. Volume 1: towards a One Health approach for controlling zoonotic diseases.* Washington, DC: International Bank for Reconstruction & Development/World Bank.

World Health Organization (2010). The FAO-OIE-WHO collaboration. Sharing responsibilities and coordinating global activities to address health risks at the animal–human–ecosystems interfaces. A tripartite concept note. https://bit.ly/1AeLcT7.

World Health Organization (2014). *Antimicrobial resistance: global report on surveillance.* Geneva: World Health Organisation.

Zinsstag, J. (2012). Convergence of EcoHealth and One Health. *EcoHealth* 9(4): 371–3.

Zinsstag, J., E. Schelling, D. Waltner-Toews, and M. Tanner (2011). From 'one medicine' to 'one health' and systemic approaches to health and well-being. *Preventive Veterinary Medicine* 101(3–4): 148–56.

Zinsstag, J., E. Schelling, K. Wyss, and M.B. Mahamat (2005). Potential of cooperation between human and animal health to strengthen health systems. *Lancet* 366(9503): 2142–5.

Zinsstag, J., D. Waltner-Toews, and M. Tanner (2015). Theoretical issues of One Health. In *One Health: the theory and practice of integrated health approaches,* J. Zinsstag, E. Schelling, D. Waltner-Toews, M. Whittaker, and M. Tanner, eds., 18–24. Wallingford, UK: CABI.

3
Global governance approaches to Planetary Health: new ideas for a globalised world

Obijiofor Aginam

> To be on earth is to live within a finite and restricted environment … The life-support system based on air, earth, and water is delicate, subtly intertwined, and remarkably intricate … The tendencies toward the destruction of life cannot be dealt with until there emerges a much stronger sense of the reality of wholeness and oneness, of the wholeness of the earth and of the oneness of the human family.
>
> Richard Falk, 1971

> The challenge of space exploration has joined with the depletion and degradation of the earth's environment … to entice or compel individuals and governments to think in terms of our common destiny: to counter humanity as a single gifted but greedy species, sharing a common, finite and endangered speck of the universe.
>
> Thomas Franck, 1995

Two decades ago, Richard Falk (1971) and Thomas Franck (1995) – influential scholars of our time – challenged regulatory stakeholders and global governance to be proactive and pragmatic in saving our endangered planet. Despite these clarion calls, the (global) governance architecture of transnational health and environmental problems, or what one influential school of thought has termed 'earth system governance'[1] (Biermann 2014; Nicholson and Jinnah 2016; Young 2010) has not been built on a pedestal that recognises the 'wholeness of the earth' and 'oneness of the human family'. Why? The human family, categorised by Falk and Franck as a greedy species, is composed of approximately 7.5 billion people who inhabit planet Earth and plunder its resources within the territorial boundaries of over 190 political entities currently recognised as nation-states by the contemporary international system. The International Human Dimensions Programme on Global Environmental Change observed that 'humans now influence all biological and physical systems of the planet. Almost no species, no land area, no part of the oceans has remained unaffected by the expansion of the human species' (International Human Dimensions Programme on Global Environmental Change [IHDP] 2009, 13).

Since 1648 when the Peace of Westphalia was signed, issues transcending national boundaries have been largely regulated and governed through a multilateral system dominated by nation-states.[2] The classic notion of sovereignty postulates that nation-states enter into treaties, agreements and other regulatory and governance arrangements with one another either bilaterally, regionally or multilaterally; and exercise legitimacy and control over their geopolitical territories including regulating human behaviour through laws, regulations, and coercive sanctions. Since 1972 (when the United Nations convened the Stockholm Conference on Human

---

1   The Earth System Governance Project is a long-term interdisciplinary research initiative involving scholars across all continents asserting that 'since prehistoric times, humans have altered their local environment. Beginning about a century ago, they are altering their planet. More and more parameters of the earth system are changing due to human influences. The scientific knowledge about the earth system and its current transformation becomes more confident every day.' (Earth System Governance website)

2   The Treaty of Westphalia 1648, also known as the Peace of Westphalia, ended 30 years of war and conflict in Europe and led to the emergence of nation-states as the primary and dominant actors in international relations.

Environment), international environmental governance has largely proceeded on this Westphalian governance model, recognising nation-states as the dominant actors in global affairs (Birnie and Boyle 1992; Kiss and Shelton 1991). Global health governance, on the other hand, has evolved almost exclusively through multilateral interstate agreements since the adoption of the World Health Organization (WHO) Constitution at the International Health Conference in New York in 1946 (Aginam 2005; Burci and Vignes 2003; Fidler 1999; Fidler 2004; Gostin 2014; WHO 2001).

This chapter explores the challenges of adapting global governance regulatory frameworks, processes and outcomes beyond the traditional confines of nation-state interests to address the emergent concept of planetary health that recognises the oneness and wholeness of human and planetary health. The chapter builds on the key governance recommendations of the 2015 Report of the Rockefeller Foundation–Lancet Commission on Planetary Health (Rockefeller Foundation–Lancet Commission 2015) which are largely in tandem with the inexorable linkages of people, places and the planet highlighted by the science and implementation plan of the Earth System Governance Project (IHDP 2009).

Transiting from 'international' to 'global' governance: implications for One Planet, One Health

Governance is a much-contested term in policy literature for two main reasons. First, the word is a fairly recent invention that didn't exist in some of the world's leading languages such as German, and second, governance is often erroneously construed as being synonymous with government (Rosenau 2000). Notwithstanding this misconception, there is consensus about the emergence and involvement of multiple actors in the international policy arena who, along with nation-states as the dominant actors, now influence institutional outcomes on a range of health and environmental issues that transcend the territories and geopolitical boundaries of nation-states. Thus global governance actors now include nation-states, regional and international organisations, charitable foundations, civil society and non-governmental organisations (NGOs), and private and corporate sector interests – business enterprises, and transnational corporations (Lee and Kamradt-Scott 2014). While many definitions exist, the commonly accepted definition of global governance is from the widely referenced Report of the Commission on Global Governance:

> The sum of the many ways individuals and institutions, public and private, manage their common affairs. It is a continuing process through which conflicting or diverse interests may be accommodated and co-operative action may be taken. It includes formal institutions and regimes empowered to enforce compliance, as well as informal arrangements that people and institutions either have agreed to or perceive to be in their interest. (Commission on Global Governance 1995, 2)

Nearly two decades ago, Lee and Dodgson argued that:

> The emergence of global governance as a central concept in international relations responds to a perceived change in the nature of world politics. In contrast to international governance, the defining feature of global governance is its comprehensiveness. Global governance views the globe as a single place within which the boundaries of the interstate system and nation-state have been eroded. Although the nation-state remains an important actor, processes and mechanisms of global governance are growing to encompass the structures of international governance that manage the system of nation-states ... The processes and mechanisms of global governance are diverse, as are the actors and structures that participate in them. (Lee and Dodgson 2000, 227–8)

Global governance derives its impetus from the density and outcomes of 'international and transnational regimes' (Young 1999), and the complex interconnectedness of the world's human systems across many sectors (Whitman 2002). Governance frameworks, no matter how efficient, are not synonymous with government (Keohane and Nye 2000; Rosenau 2000). Government and governance rule systems differ markedly. While sovereignty and constitutional legitimacy legitimise government rule systems, the effectiveness of governance rule systems also derives from 'traditional norms and habits, informal agreements, shared premises, and a host of other practices' (Rosenau 2000, 225).

The demand for governance is increasing due to rapidly evolving, complex relationships and interdependencies found in organisations, corporations, professional and business associations, and advocacy and other non-government entities (Rosenau 2000). Governance processes and institutions – both formal and informal – that guide and restrain collective action by a group are not the exclusive domain of governments or delegated international organisations. Numerous NGOs and their associations as well as private entities with or without government permission create governance (Keohane and Nye 2000, 12). Rosenau sees *governance* and *government* as purposive and goal-oriented activities complying with systems of rule. However, he distinguishes government activities as ones backed by formal authority, including powers to implement policies, whereas governance is more about activities underpinned by shared goals, which may not have legally prescribed responsibilities and do not rely on police powers to overcome defiance and attain compliance (Rosenau 1992).

Given the complex interactions between nations and peoples, and humanity and the planet, the dynamics of the increasingly borderless character of emerging and re-emerging global health issues – ones that defy the territorial boundaries of sovereign countries – makes global governance necessary. The classic and still maintained global governance architecture that was 'designed and constructed' by nation-states more than three centuries ago is no longer capable of addressing all the emerging and re-emerging global issues of our time (Aginam 2007; Fidler 2004; Zacher 1992).

States and intergovernmental organisations have dominated international decision-making for most of the last century; this is often referred to as 'the Westphalian international order' (Zacher and Keefe 2008, 138). With no world government, global governance fills a void by describing systems of rule-making, political advocacy, co-ordination and problem solving that transcend sovereign states and societies (Held and McGrew 2002, 8). In this post-Industrial age, humans have altered the planetary systems in search of development. Emergent planetary health issues – climate change, biodiversity loss, desertification, emerging and re-emerging diseases and pandemics, and sustainability crises generally – can only be effectively managed through what Rosenau called 'a bifurcated system' (one based on the state-centric system driven largely by governments) and a 'multi-centric system' driven by non-state actors (Rosenau 2000, 225). He further observes that 'the proliferating centers of authority on the global stage is thus dense with actors, large and small, formal and informal, economic and social, political and cultural, liberal and authoritarian, who collectively form a highly complex system of global governance' (Rosenau 2000, 225).

The cumulative effect of the interaction of the bifurcated and multi-centric systems is that global governance has emerged as a pragmatic framework that complements the Westphalian inter-state system. Distinguished from international governance, global governance involves multiple actors (nation-states and non-state actors), with better prospects to address pandemic diseases, climate change, biodiversity loss, transboundary pollution, and other global health issues – nearly all of which defy the geopolitical boundaries of nation-states.

The embedded orthodoxy of international governance processes relies upon treaties and agreements between nation-sates, and, while relevant, offers limited opportunities for *One Planet, One Health* strategies. Conversely, global governance underscores the linkages between nation-states and non-state actors, and offers a more holistic approach to planet Earth and health. While the idea of governance without government, sovereignty or supranational authority can be confusing, it is important to note that global governance refers to efforts to bring orderly responses to social and political issues that elude state action (Gordenker and Weiss 1995).

Key governance challenges

Tasked with the mission of assessing the potential implications for human health of the multiple changes in the earth's natural systems, the Rockefeller Foundation–Lancet Commission on Planetary Health

Report of July 2015 observed that humans have mortgaged the health of future generations for economic and development gains in the present:

By unsustainably exploiting nature's resources, human civilisation has flourished but now risks substantial health effects from the degradation of nature's life support systems in the future. Health effects from changes to the environment including climate change, ocean acidification, land degradation, water scarcity, over-exploitation of fisheries, and biodiversity loss pose serious challenges to the global health gains of the past several decades and are likely to become increasingly dominant during the second half of this century and beyond.

This timely report demonstrates the link between human health and environmental change (Clark 2015). Anchoring the discussion in the Anthropocene epoch, the report provides evidence that the current trajectory of human activity is unsustainable (Sachs 2008, 57); technological and other innovative successes over past two centuries have brought vast benefits but at a great cost (Sachs 2008, 57–66). Although the Anthropocene has been intensely debated in academic literature in recent times, Sachs reminds us that

We have reached the beginning of the twenty-first century with a very crowded planet: 6.6 billion people living in an interconnected global economy producing an astounding $60 trillion of output each year. Human beings fill every ecological niche on the planet, from the icy tundras to the tropical rain forests to the deserts. In some locations, societies have out-stripped the carrying capacity of the land, at least with the technologies they deploy, resulting in chronic hunger, environmental degradation, and large-scale exodus of desperate populations. We are, in short, in one another's faces as never before, crowded into an interconnected society of global trade, migration and ideas, but also risks of pandemic diseases, terror, refugee movements, and conflict. (Sachs 2008, 17)

The paradox of vast benefits and significant risks confronting humanity in the Anthropocene epoch is a clarion call to reassess the governance model to safeguard our endangered planet. The Rockefeller Foundation–Lancet Commission identified implementation failures (governance challenges) such as governments' and institutions' tardiness in recognising and responding to threats, especially when faced with uncertainties. Pooled common resources and time lags between action and effect are major impediments. These challenges require improved governance at global, national, and subnational levels before irreversible changes in key earth systems occur (Rockefeller Foundation–Lancet Commission 2015). The commission proposed that planetary heath governance frameworks should 'engage civil society and community organisations by promoting public discourse, participation, and transparency of data and systems models to allow monitoring of trends and to encourage polycentric governance building on local capabilities to steward environmental resources and protect health' (Rockefeller Foundation–Lancet Commission on Planetary Health, July 2015).

Postscript: governance parameters of One Planet One Health

An underpinning value of the Rockefeller Foundation–Lancet Commission was the belief that human health and human civilisation depend on thriving natural systems and judicious stewardship. Therefore, it follows that governance must go beyond the capacities of the Westphalian state-centric model to a range of governance paradigm shifts (Horton 2013). Horton went further than the commission report, saying that a failure to recognise the interdependencies of human and natural systems could be catastrophic due to diminished potential of the planet to sustain our species.

The idea that global sustainability is a precondition for human health, survival, and prosperity underpins the development of the 17 Sustainable Development Goals (SDGs) and offers the opportunity to establish new governance networks. The 2030 Agenda for Sustainable Development anticipates a surge in the proliferation of new public–private partnerships and other governance networks. These partnerships and networks will need creative strategies to advance and catalyse new ideas for reconstructing the governance architecture of

One Planet One Health. In this discourse, one certain fact is the uncertain promise of the Westphalian governance model. As mechanisms, principles and norms currently guiding global health governance are found wanting, new ones will be redefined and reinvented to adapt to this instantaneously interconnected, complex world. They will be needed in the realm of institutions, where new rules, decision-making procedures, resources, and participants are required if the expectations and behaviour of the world's countries and citizens are to realise the reality, rather than just the ideal, of health for all.

Looking beyond the Westphalian (state-centric model), the successor system will be crafted to accommodate all relevant stakeholders including states and non-state actors locally, nationally and globally.

Works cited

Aginam, O. (2005). Conceptual Framework and Methodology. In *Global Health Governance: International Law and Public Health in a Divided World* (pp. 12-26). Toronto: University of Toronto Press. DOI: 10.3138/9781442675377

Aginam, O. (2007). Global governance. In *Macrosocial determinants of population health*, S. Galea, ed., 159–68. New York: Springer.

Biermann, F. (2014). *Earth system governance: world politics in the Anthropocene.* Cambridge, MA: MIT Press.

Birnie, P.W., and A.E. Boyle (1992). *International law and the environment.* New York: Oxford University Press.

Burci, G.L., and C. Vignes (2004). *World Health Organization.* The Hague: Kluwer.

Clark, H. (2015). Governance for planetary health and sustainable development. *Lancet* 386(10007): e39–e41.

Commission on Global Governance (1995). *Our global neighborhood: the report of the Commission on Global Governance.* New York: Oxford University Press.

Cooper, A.F., J.J. Kirton, and T. Schrecker (2007). Governing global health in the twenty-first century. In *Governing global health: challenge, response, innovation*, A.F. Cooper, J.J. Kirton, and T. Schrecker, eds. Aldershot, UK: Ashgate.

Falk, R. (1971). *This endangered planet: prospects and proposals for human survival.* New York: Random House.

Fidler, D.P. (1999). *International law and infectious diseases*. Oxford: Clarendon Press.

Fidler, D.P. (2004). Constitutional outlines of public health's "new world order". *Temple Law Review* 77(2): 247–72.

Franck, T. (1995). *Fairness in international law and institutions*. New York: Oxford University Press.

Gordenker, L., and T. Weiss (1995). Pluralising global governance: analytical approaches and dimensions. *Third World Quarterly* 16(3): 357–87.

Gostin, L.O. (2014). *Global health law*. Cambridge, MA: Harvard University Press.

Held, D., and A. McGrew (2002). Introduction. In *Governing globalization: power, authority and global governance*, D. Held and A. McGrew, eds. Cambridge, UK: Polity.

Horton, R. (2013). Planetary health – a new vision for the post-2015 era. *Lancet* 382(9897):1012. https://doi.org/10.1016/S0140-6736(13)61936-4

International Human Dimensions Programme on Global Environmental Change (2009). *Earth system governance: people, places, and the planet. IHDP Report No. 20*. Bonn, DE: The Earth System Governance Project.

Keohane, R.O., and J.S. Nye Jr. (2000). Introduction. In *Governance in a globalizing world*, J.S. Nye and J.D. Donahue, eds. Washington DC: Brookings.

Kiss, A., and D. Shelton (1991). *International environmental law*. New York: Transnational Publishers.

Lee, K., and R. Dodgson (2000). Globalization and cholera: implications for global governance. *Global Governance* 6(2) 213-36.

Lee, K., and A. Kamradt-Scott (2014). The multiple meanings of global health governance: a call for conceptual clarity. *Globalization and Health* 10(28): 1–10.

Nicholson, S., and S. Jinnah (2016). *New earth politics: essays from the Anthropocene*. Cambridge, MA: MIT Press.

Rockefeller Foundation–Lancet Commission on Planetary Health (2015). *Safeguarding human health in the Anthropocene epoch: report of the Rockefeller Foundation–Lancet Commission on Planetary Health. Lancet* 386(10007):1973-2028.

Rosenau, J.N. (1992). Governance, order, and change in world politics. In *Governance without government: order and change in world politics*, J. Rosenau and E. Czempiel, eds. Cambridge, UK: Cambridge University Press.

Rosenau, J.N. (2000). Governance in a new world order. In *The global transformations reader*, D. Held and A. McGrew, eds. Cambridge, UK: Polity.

Sachs, J.D. (2008). *Common wealth: economics for a crowded planet*. New York: Penguin.

Whitman, J. (2002). Global governance as the friendly face of unaccountable power. *Security Dialogue* 33(1): 45–57.

World Health Organization (2001). *Basic documents*, 43rd edition. Geneva: World Health Organization.

Young, O.R. (1999). *Governance in world affairs*. New York: Cornell University Press.

Young, O.R. (2010). *Institutional dynamics: emergent patterns in international environmental governance*. Cambridge, MA.: MIT Press.

Zacher, M.W. (1992). The decaying pillars of the Westphalian temple: implications for international order and governance. In *Governance without government: order and change in world politics*, J. Rosenau and E. Czempiel, eds., 58–101. Cambridge, UK: Cambridge University Press.

Zacher, M.W., and T.J. Keefe (2008). *The politics of global health governance: united by contagion*. New York: Palgrave Macmillan.

4
The ethics of One Health

Chris Degeling, Angus Dawson and Gwendolyn L. Gilbert

The essence of One Health, as described in Chapter 2, is the interdependence of human, animal, and environmental health. Greater recognition of these co-dependencies will ensure that interventions designed to protect health or mitigate disease threats in one sector will not have unintended or disproportionate adverse consequences for others. This interdependence raises ethical questions about how to balance competing values and priorities within and between different sectors.

Science can be described as a set of systematised approaches to understanding and predicting features of the universe, whereas ethics is a systematised approach to normative questions about how we should live our lives, and what we value and consider to be good and right. Science relies on theories to generate testable hypotheses. Ethics, similarly, has well-established theories that allow us to compare, explain and justify different approaches to normative questions, some of which we explore in this chapter. One Health draws on scientific methodologies and evidence, but it also has ethical dimensions. It assumes that health is a good thing and that understanding interactions between humans, animals, and the environment will help us to optimise the health of all, including maintaining and sustaining a flourishing ecology. Ethical and economic issues in One Health overlap but are distinct. Both employ theories of *value* to identify, analyse, and, potentially, justify people's preferences. But, while economics typically *measures* the costs and benefits of different policies and actions in monetary terms, ethics *evaluates* them against normative standards (Anderson 1995). While the economic case for One Health has been repeatedly made (Häsler et al. 2012; World Bank 2010), literature about the urgent need for a One Health approach rarely mentions ethics (Degeling et al. 2015).

In this chapter we argue that One Health is necessarily a normative project. Describing infectious disease risks, such as antimicrobial resistance or the pandemic potential of highly pathogenic avian influenza viruses (HPAI), as One Health 'problems' raises a normative question, since the term implies that these problems should concern us all, and that resolving them will provide a balanced One Health benefit and/or require some form of collective action. Such assertions appeal to community values – our shared beliefs about how the world should be, for us and for future generations. Ideas such as collaboration, sustainability and security are prominent in One Health discourse, but which community values are important to One Health and in which contexts they should apply have yet to be clearly articulated (Rock and Degeling 2015; Verweij and Bovenkerk 2016). One Health is gaining momentum as a global, scientific, and cross-sectoral approach to zoonotic disease, food security, and environmental degradation. The normative dimensions and implications are in urgent need of discussion and debate (Capps et al. 2015; Degeling et al. 2015).

One Health as an ethical project

Early work in One Health was oriented towards developing *clinical* solutions for endemic or emerging zoonotic diseases and risks. Technological responses were favoured because they promised substantial benefits without the need for revisionary thinking or major structural and socioeconomic reforms. Today, One Health (like its conceptual ally EcoHealth) increasingly recognises that zoonotic disease control programs are most effective when the broader socioeconomic and ecological determinants of health are included (Charron 2012; Zinsstag 2012). This greater emphasis on policies and programs enables assessment and mitigation of the risks of pathogen 'spillovers' between non-human and human populations (Dixon, Dar and Heymann 2014; McCloskey et al. 2014). This *preventive* approach to infectious disease control raises different moral concerns from those raised by clinically focused human and animal healthcare practices. The success of One Health interventions (Okello et al. 2014) is likely to be determined by the extent to which they reflect local circumstances and needs (Hinchliffe 2015) and the extent to which the people affected by them can be persuaded to accept the possibility of a personal cost in return for collective benefit. Limitations of freedom necessarily require consultation to determine which specific measures are legitimate in light of perceived conflicts of different interests between individuals, institutions and the broader community (Rock and Degeling 2015). Even if the proposed interventions are ethical, they are likely to be summarily rejected by stakeholders unless they are perceived to be fair, not disproportionately burdensome, and appropriately implemented.

Most human activities, social and physical conditions, policies, and decisions have the potential to impact on human, animal, and/or environmental health. Threats posed by endemic animal diseases and zoonotic risks are complex and driven by socioeconomic and sociopolitical factors; their consequences extend far beyond the immediate disease impact. One Health provides a context in which people, animals and their shared environments create and sustain their shared conditions for health; but this laudable goal might also provide grounds to intervene in almost every facet of human life. Expanding medical, biological, ecological and epidemiological knowledge has increased opportunities to create benefits and avoid harms to humans and non-human others by changing how we use and affect animal populations and ecological systems. How far should our individual and collective responsibility for the health of people, animals and environments extend? If One Health is potentially about everything, it may succumb to paralysis and inertia.

For One Health interventions to succeed they must address fundamental ethical questions about what is valuable, what is to be protected and, ultimately, what is dispensable. Public health ethics, a specialist field developed over the last 15 years, can contribute to answering these questions (Verweij and Bovenkerk 2016). Rather than seeking abstract universal truths, public health ethics is committed to the development of practical and just solutions informed by interdisciplinary research. One Health must be similarly oriented if it is to have substantive impact (Craddock and Hinchliffe 2015; Whittaker et al. 2015). Population health benefits are realised in One Health by focusing on interactions between populations within systems (Rock and Degeling 2016; Zinsstag et al. 2006). Public health ethics sees the health of population groups and communities as central to public policies that mediate individual and collective actions by promoting conditions that sustain human flourishing (Dawson and Verweij 2007). Public health ethics arguments can support and justify the types of sustainable collective action on which the success of a One Health approach depends.

The normative nature of One Health problems

One Health problems are ecological and political (Bardosh 2016; Hinchliffe 2015). Emerging and actual health risks at the human–animal–environment interface often result from human activities, especially changing land use, increasing global trade and travel, and intensifying animal husbandry practices that have adverse effects on biodiversity (Cascio et al. 2011; Greger 2007; Kilpatrick and Randolph 2012; Plowright et al. 2008). The impacts of zoonotic risks and outbreaks typically extend beyond the direct medical effects. Human–animal interdependencies sustain livelihoods for the vast majority of people worldwide who live rurally (Grace 2015; Perry and Grace 2009). Policies designed to protect human populations from zoonotic risks often disrupt fragile ecological systems, destroy livelihoods, and threaten food supplies (Coker et al. 2011; Otte, Nugent and McLeod 2004).

Below we demonstrate the profound social, cultural, and economic impacts of zoonotic disease by giving canonical examples of pandemic, food-borne, and/or endemic diseases. In this context, endemic and emerging zoonotic diseases are on a continuum; their categorisation reflects the microbiological, sociopolitical and geographic influences on disease transmission (Hooker, Degeling and Mason 2016; Wallace et al.

2015). Endemic zoonoses are found throughout the developing world, where they occasionally cause epidemics in human populations (Grace 2015; Maudlin, Eisler and Welburn 2009). Emerging and re-emerging zoonotic diseases, in contrast, are defined as zoonoses that have spilled over and are causing diseases in new locations and/or populations.

The costs and burdens of emerging zoonotic infectious diseases

Severe acute respiratory syndrome (SARS) is a human respiratory infection, caused by a coronavirus carried by Chinese horseshoe bats (Wang et al. 2006). It was first reported in Asia in 2003 and within months had spread to 37 countries in the Americas, Europe, and Asia. More than 8,000 people were affected and 774 died from SARS, before it was eliminated by concerted international effort. The outbreak itself and the response to it, focused in Toronto, Singapore, Vietnam, Hong Kong, and mainland China, are estimated to have cost the Canadian and East-Asian economies more than US$200 billion (World Bank 2010).

Less prominent in the public imagination is variant Creutzfeld Jakob disease (vCJD)/ bovine spongiform encephalopathy (BSE) (popularly known as 'mad cow disease'). vCJD is a rare but fatal human neurodegenerative condition, caused by consumption of bovine products contaminated with the prions (proteinaceous infectious particles) that cause BSE. Person-to-person transmission can occur by blood transfusion (Davidson et al. 2014) and, potentially, organ/tissue transplantation (Molesworth et al. 2014). Since vCJD was first identified in 1996, 175 cases have been reported in the UK and 49 elsewhere. The World Bank estimates the direct costs of vCJD/BSE by 2018 to be more than US$11 billion, due to trade bans and other measures instituted to mitigate the risks of BSE resulting in losses to small agricultural businesses, rural communities, tourism and the pharmaceutical/blood product industry. With an estimated one in 4,000 UK residents carrying vCJD, the costs and burdens of contamination of human food supplies with BSE prions, will continue (Turner and Ludlam 2009).

Nipah virus (NiV) is spread from the East-Asian flying foxes into domestic pigs, humans, and other animals, causing respiratory disease and severe encephalitis. First recognised in Malaysia in 1998, it has spread to parts of South-East and South Asia (particularly Bangladesh). Of 522 proven human cases, more than 50 per cent have died (Field and Kung 2011). In 1999, NiV control programs devastated Malaysia's pig industry and caused high unemployment and dislocation of rural populations, at a cost of more than US$1 billion to the national economy (Nor and Ong 2001). On top of the economic costs of control, more than 36,000 people in Malaysia lost their jobs because of the outbreak.

Global experience of SARS, vCJD, and NiV outbreaks demonstrates the enormous socioeconomic and cultural costs of controlling real and perceived human health risks from zoonotic pathogens (World Bank 2010; WHO 2004). While One Health approaches to zoonotic disease control appear to offer great promise, international experience shows that the effectiveness of any public policy depends on the effective implementation and alignment of the policy with stakeholder and public values, more than the conceptual frame or developmental process (Donaldson 2008; Selgelid 2005). In the case of BSE, early government decisions were dominated by powerful interests wanting to avoid public controversy and significant economic costs. Even when evidence of the link between BSE and vCJD became clear, feed bans continued to be poorly enforced and communication strategies were driven by the fear of irrational public panic and harm to farmers' interests (Forbes 2004). More than half a million infected animals were estimated to have entered the food chain during this time. The ban on consumption of offal was progressively extended to more species and a broader age-range of animals (at slaughter). But the evidence for these measures was unclear, depriving the public of an accurate risk assessment and leaving them potentially exposed to BSE prions for far longer than necessary (Phillips, Bridgeman and Ferguson-Smith 2000).

The history of vCJD highlights the risk of public harm when there is a failure in policy development or a failure to enforce a policy expeditiously. Alternatively, the experience with the pathogenic avian influenza (HPAI) virus, H5N1, in China and South-East Asia demonstrated that excessively zealous policy responses may also have adverse consequences. H5N1 was first identified in geese flocks in Guangdong Province, China, in 1994, with later outbreaks in poultry and associated human cases in Hong Kong in 1997; the appearance of H5N1 soon followed across Asia. In Vietnam alone, almost 40 million birds were culled in 2004 in an attempt to eradicate it (Rushton et al. 2005). Many of the birds were owned by large commercial operations, but the households of most rural smallholders and villagers in the developing world rely on small poultry flocks as a source of food, income, and insurance against unexpected expenses. The effects of potential HPAI exposure for smallholders were far more than a risk of infection (Sonaiya 2007). Mass culling may appear decisive, but it places an excessive burden on vulnerable 'backyard' farmers and, paradoxically, may promote the spread of the disease by pushing farmers to conceal sick birds (Alders et al. 2014; Sims 2007). It can also have serious, longstanding effects on the social and economic health of communities and on human wellbeing; for example, the increased incidence of childhood stunting in Egypt due to malnutrition following an outbreak of HPAI in 2006 (FAO 2009). These cases demonstrate that ethical policy development requires careful consideration of the potential consequences, rather than a 'knee-jerk' response to an immediate threat or sectional interests.

The costs and burdens of endemic zoonotic diseases

In biology, 'endemic' refers to a condition that remains relatively stable, in a defined geographical region, contrasting with 'emerging', which implies novelty and invasiveness. HPAI H5N1 is now endemic among poultry flocks in at least six countries (Centers for Disease Control and Prevention 2015) and has caused epidemics in others, including the USA. Newer strains of HPAI are creating havoc in the poultry industry in North America (Nonthabenjawan et al. 2016). Global health authorities have committed significant resources to monitoring avian influenza, because of its pandemic potential, but there have been only 852 confirmed cases and 456 deaths in humans since 2003 (until January 2017) (WHO 2017). Meanwhile, other endemic zoonoses, of far greater significance to human health and wellbeing, are tragically neglected.

Brucellosis is caused by bacterial pathogens belonging to several *Brucella* species that can be transferred to humans from infected cows, sheep, goats, and dogs. Human brucellosis is rarely fatal but causes symptoms, of variable severity, including undulating fever, fatigue, severe joint pain, neurological problems and ongoing debility (Rubach et al. 2013). Infection with *Brucella* spp. in domestic animals causes abortions and adversely affects herd health, agricultural productivity, and human nutrition. Because of this heavy burden of disease, brucellosis is consistently ranked among the most economically important zoonoses globally (Grace and Jones 2011; Perry and Grace 2009). High rates of human and animal brucellosis occur in tropical Africa and Asia. It is consistently under-reported, and there is a lack of effective control in most low-income countries, where its impact is borne largely by impoverished and marginalised communities (Halliday et al. 2015). Successful eradication measures used in high-income countries are not easily transferred to poor communities, where the monetary value of animals and animal products is lower. Livestock owners are less committed to control measures and less likely to be compensated, and the indirect economic impact of animal diseases is less. As a result, the socioeconomic and political focus is on more pressing needs and problems (McDermott, Grace and Zinsstag 2013).

Endemic zoonoses, such as brucellosis, echinococcosis (hydatid disease), cysticercosis, and anthrax, disproportionately affect poor, disadvantaged people in low-income countries by damaging their livelihoods and killing or lowering the productivity of their livestock. Endemic zoonoses also kill people. Rabies has been eradicated or controlled in much of the northern hemisphere, but remains endemic among dogs and is a leading cause of human mortality in Africa and Asia (Anderson and Shwiff 2015). When endemic zoonoses affect poor people they have less access to effective treatments and are less likely to withstand the socioeconomic burdens of serious illness (Maudlin, Eisler and Welburn 2009). The control of endemic zoonoses in low-income countries is essential for economic development and public health, but rarely a priority for international or national healthcare systems.

Against this background of under-reporting and inadequate funding, One Health practitioners focus on improving disease surveillance, risk communication, and public health programs, with the goal of controlling endemic zoonotic diseases in low-income settings (Perry and Grace 2009). The emergence of One Health programs in the last decade has highlighted how little has been done to combat human and animal health risks where longstanding disparities in resource allocation exist. The relatively few cases and deaths from H5N1 infections globally over 10 years, contrast starkly with the estimated 500,000 new cases of brucellosis and 59,000 deaths from rabies annually (Hampson et al. 2015; Pappas et al. 2006). Notwithstanding the evidence of global morbidity and mortality, most One Health policies and research agendas continue to be dominated by *potential* threats to global 'security' and the economy from zoonotic diseases with pandemic potential, while neglecting the *actual* physical, social, and economic burdens on the world's poorest people (Chien 2013; Davies 2008; Halliday et al. 2015).

How can ethics inform One Health policies and practices?

Endemic and emerging zoonotic diseases have major implications for the distribution of resources, access to healthcare, and regulation of health services. The examples described above demonstrate how policy responses to infectious disease threats are politicised and compromised by failure to address their sociocultural determinants and ethical impacts, and highlight the limitations of scientific and technocratic approaches to governance (Hinchliffe 2001; Hinchliffe et al. 2012).

Policy making in health, without reference to the relevant scientific evidence, would be perverse and dangerous; but so would policy making without explicit reference to ethical principles. Choosing one alternative action or policy over another (including doing nothing) is an ethical decision. Either maintaining the status quo or making an alternative decision affects the health of people, animals and their shared environments. The interests of industry and distant populations are often prioritised over vulnerable and less well-resourced communities; there is inadequate consideration of those at immediate risk from disease or those who bear the burden of measures designed to protect them (and, often, distant others) from risk. The incidence of zoonotic diseases in human populations is a key indicator of otherwise covert social structures and hierarchies that have become naturalised in infectious disease discourse and practice (Petersen and Lupton 1996). They show us the patterned effects of poverty, economic development, and environmental degradation (Bardosh 2016; Farmer 1996).

Ethics is a systematic philosophical approach to thinking about what is good and right in general (Kerridge, Lowe and Stewart 2013); applied ethics focuses on what we ought to do in response to specific situations, through systematic analysis of various possible options and their justifications. It is a fundamental tenet of ethical reasoning that, although we may disagree about what we *should* do, or even about what is good and right, it is possible to arrive at a justifiable answer to the question of what, practically, we *can* do. We argue that a modest form of pluralism (committed only to the view that there is more than one morally important value) can couple with common-sense decision-making based on discussion about relevant values (Grill and Dawson 2015). Values in ethics can be construed quite broadly, and can include honouring of duties to others, non-infringement of rights, and development and expression of virtues. In the less individualistic field of public health ethics, other values and goals are also important, such as solidarity, reciprocity, fairness, transparency, trust, community, as well as a complex set of considerations relating to common and public goods, shared resources, and social justice (Dawson 2011).

In the absence of an agreed set of relevant values in the One Health sphere, the values embodied in public health ethics are relevant, also, to One Health, since they are socially embedded, integrated, holistic and expressed as a human–animal–environment paradigm. Articulating relevant values can provoke disagreement or facilitate progress. A first step in reaching agreement is to understand the other's point of view; our own views may change, suggesting new perspectives, situations and issues. The examples described above show that, when faced with a complex One Health problem, favouring or pursuing some values and goals at the expense of others can cause harms and conflicts between stakeholders. The key task of ethical analysis is to articulate these considerations before evaluating them.

Different one health policies will have different impacts on different stakeholders

Stakeholders are likely to be affected differently by any decision about One Health policies and practices because of their different concerns, interests and responsibilities. Consider HPAI in South-East Asia: backyard farmers have different interests from those of large agricultural companies; in the event of human transmission, the interests of local and remote consumers of poultry products and company shareholders will differ again. Enlarging our concerns beyond the health and wellbeing of humans, poultry kept for human use and wild bird populations, arguably, also have ethically relevant, but different, interests. Granting independent legal status to the Whanganui River in New Zealand is another example of the emerging recognition that protection of the interests of non-human entities might be central to the pursuit of environmental health and justice (Hsiao 2012; Vines, Bruce and Faunce 2013).

Externalising factors that cannot be measured in economic terms and relying on economic instruments such as cost-benefit analyses to guide actions does not take into account the stakeholder interests, concerns and responsibilities that need to be considered in decision making. These ethical considerations are often late additions to, or even left out of, the pursuit of policy options. If considered, they are typically conceptualised as constraints on the pursuit of predetermined goals (Grill and Dawson 2015). Ethical issues ought to be at the heart of formulations of what One Health is, what its goals should be, and how they should be pursued (Capps and Lederman 2015; Degeling, Lederman and Rock 2016; Scoones and Forster 2009).

The idea of freedom is central to modern liberal societies; usually understood as the freedom of individuals to do as they please unless there is significant (negative) impact on others. However, such freedom cannot be absolute. Sovereign states are free to pass laws – as part of legitimate democratic processes – that restrict the freedoms of legal persons (people and corporate entities). Such laws are usually justified in terms of public protection, especially of those vulnerable to harm. One Health (or indeed EcoHealth) interventions – such as prohibiting overfishing, stopping the felling of native forest to protect wildlife habitat, or regulating antimicrobial use in animal production systems – may be inconvenient, unwanted, or costly to some people or communities, but are deemed acceptable 'all-things-considered' if they are necessary to protect human or animal health or the essential ecological systems on which they depend. Not all limitations to personal or corporate freedom can be justified just because there is a collective or public interest at stake; the difficult issue is trying to determine which policies, laws, or regulations are justifiable. An appropriate One Health response should not immediately assume that restrictions of freedom are problematic, but should consider, objectively, the burdens and advantages that might arise. While an option may restrict freedom or financial benefit to some parties, it may also bring about greater equity or sustainability overall. One Health ethics requires consideration of the long-term impacts of an intervention on human, animal, and environmental health and their local priorities. It also needs to consider the influence of local and global power dynamics, history, and political economy (Bardosh 2016).

How should we decide what to do?

Such questions can be examined using ethical arguments to formulate goals, motivate action, and effect policy change. How to distribute harms, benefits, and goods of any proposed One Health intervention justly is a key ethical question. What counts as a relevant harm or benefit, and how to weigh one against the other, should be a primary consideration. Relevant harms and benefits are not just financial, but include the non-monetary effects of the disease and of measures to control and prevent it. Because One Health focuses on populations within larger systems, today's actions will have direct effects on future outcomes. Consequently, the relevant harms of One Health policies and practices will include immediate and future costs and the cost of inaction (to lives and finances). Additional interrelated questions that require discussion include how to take into account future generations, whether future costs and benefits are discounted, and if so, by how much. Should we weigh the future health of ecological systems against the health and welfare of people living now? How do we balance the economic advantages of intensive agriculture with the risks of zoonotic disease emergence? People and institutions should not be judged for any apparent failure to act appropriately, without considering the social, economic, environmental and cultural structures that constrain and shape their actions (Giddens 1984; Hooker, Degeling and Mason 2016). One Health ethics requires that human health be placed within a broad ecological context.

Do we need a different type of ethics for One Health?

At the heart of One Health is the recognition of a need to manage the risks of human–animal–environmental interdependencies in a new way. Some One Health challenges are the consequence of ethically problematic practices such as the structural legacies of colonialism, which treated livestock, wildlife, and the natural environment as exclusively economic assets (Anomaly 2015; Verweij and Bovenkerk 2016). The values encompassed by public health ethics will be useful, but their strongly humanist orientation is insufficient to guide ethical thinking about One Health (Verweij and Bovenkerk 2016); this requires a broader perspective, encompassing environmental and animal health and the sociocultural factors that affect them (Rock et al. 2009; Zinsstag et al. 2015). A One Health approach could potentially justify *privileging* non-human interests in some circumstances, with the presumptive aim of promoting mutual benefits to both humans and non-human animals (Capps and Lederman 2014; Rock and Degeling 2015). But significant differences still remain between One Health approaches that prioritise human interests and those seeking to protect the interests of, and distribute benefits to, non-humans. The interdependence of human, animal, and environmental systems means that ethical considerations about more-than-human collectives, logically, can be linked to concern for humans (Verweij and Bovenkerk 2016). Nevertheless, apparent inconsistencies and ambiguities in stated One Health objectives and our ethical concern for non-human others emphasises a need for review of the conditions under which we use and interact with other species – and any obligations that should follow (Capps et al. 2015; Rock and Degeling 2015).

Conclusion

One Health policies and practices require us to balance the needs of human individuals and populations with the health and wellbeing of non-human others and our shared ecological systems. An emerging focus in One Health programs and policies, converging in many ways with EcoHealth and planetary health, is the idea of 'upstream' prevention (Rüegg et al. 2017). In this context 'prevention' means more than reducing threats to human health. It requires conserving a healthy ecological state while maintaining a sustainable, secure food system that inhibits emergence of zoonotic risks and disease burdens, and depends on the co-ordinated activity of individuals and civil or government agencies. Any significant costs to industries, communities, or individuals will raise important justice issues between and within countries. However, the costs of any proposed changes based on One Health principles or broader sets of ecological or planetary concerns must be weighed against the costs of existing, unjust situations; there is no good argument for regarding the status quo as the natural state. Ethics can help to justify change and show that policies designed to reduce the burdens and threats of endemic and emerging zoonotic diseases, locally and internationally, must be part of a coherent global health strategy, for which individuals, populations, nation-states, and international organisations must share responsibility.

In proposing measures to control endemic zoonotic diseases, we must consider the effects of structural disadvantage and avoid the politics of blame. The traditional model of top–down policy making should be inverted so that the interests of those most affected directly influence policy prioritisation, formulation, and implementation. These issues are complex; universally accepted solutions are difficult, but this does not mean they should not be attempted. Public health ethics draws upon the resources of ethical and political theory and relevant empirical issues to formulate policy proposals. While it may be too early to give a full account of what One Health ethics ought to be, we can suggest areas to be explored in future. The core values of One Health and other holistic and ecologically oriented approaches are likely to correspond with those of public health ethics around concepts such as group/community/ population, public goods/common goods, solidarity/reciprocity, welfare/ wellbeing, and justice. This predominantly social focus need not mean ignoring individual concerns, or sacrificing individuals for the sake of human or non-human populations. The way forward is surely a rich, pluralistic account of One Health that eschews such dichotomous thinking and is sensitive to, and grounded in, the reality of social, political, and ecological relationships.

Works cited

Alders R., Adongo Awuni J., Bagnol B., Farrell P., de Haan N. Impact of Avian Influenza on Village Poultry Production Globally. *Ecohealth*. 2013. doi: 10.1007/s10393-013-0867-x

Anderson, A., and S.A. Shwiff (2015). The cost of canine rabies on four continents. *Transboundary and Emerging Diseases* 62: 446–52.

Anderson, E. (1995). *Value in ethics and economics*. Cambridge, MA: Harvard University Press.

Anomaly, J. (2015). What's wrong with factory farming? *Public Health Ethics* 8: 246–54.

Bardosh, K. (2016). *One Health: science, politics and zoonotic disease in Africa*. London: Routledge.

Capps, B., et al. (2015). Introducing One Health to the ethical debate about zoonotic diseases in Southeast Asia. *Bioethics* 29: 588–96.

Capps, B., and Z. Lederman (2015). One Health and paradigms of public biobanking. *Journal of Medical Ethics* 41(3); 258–262.

Capps, B., and Z. Lederman (2015). One Health, vaccines and ebola: the opportunities for shared benefits. *Agriculture & Environmental Ethics*. 28(6): 101-1032.

Cascio, A., M. Bosilkovski, A.J. Rodriguez-Morales, and G. Pappas (2011). The socio-ecology of zoonotic infections. *Clinical Microbiology & Infection* 17: 336–42.

Centers for Disease Control and Prevention (2015). Highly pathogenic avian influenza A (H5N1) in birds and other animals. https://bit.ly/2BSBo6C.

Charron, D.F. (2012). Ecosystem approaches to health for a global sustainability agenda. *EcoHealth* 9: 256–66.

Chien, Y. (2013). How did international agencies perceive the avian influenza problem? The adoption and manufacture of the 'One World, One Health' framework. *Sociology of Health & Illness* 35: 213–26.

Coker, R.J., B.M. Hunter, J.W. Rudge, M. Liverani, and P. Hanvoravongchai (2011). Emerging infectious diseases in Southeast Asia: regional challenges to control. *Lancet* 377: 599–609.

Craddock, S., and S. Hinchliffe (2015). One world, one health? Social science engagements with the one health agenda. *Social Science & Medicine* 129: 1–4.

Davidson, L.R., C.A. Llewelyn, J.M. Mackenzie, P.E. Hewitt, and R.G. Will (2014). Variant CJD and blood transfusion: are there additional cases? *Vox Sanguinis* 107: 220–5.

Davies, S.E. (2008). Securitizing infectious disease. *International Affairs* 84: 295–313.

Dawson, A. (2011). Resetting the parameters. In *Public health ethics: key concepts and issues in policy and practice*, 1–20. Cambridge University Press.

Dawson, A., and M. Verweij (2007). *Ethics, prevention, and public health.* Oxford: Oxford University Press.

Degeling, C., et al. (2015). Implementing a One Health approach to emerging infectious disease: reflections on the socio-political, ethical and legal dimensions. *BMC Public Health* 15: 1–11.

Degeling, C., Z. Lederman, and M. Rock (2016). Culling and the common good: re-evaluating harms and benefits under the One Health paradigm. *Public Health Ethics* 9: 244–54.

Dixon, M.A., O.A. Dar, and D.L. Heymann (2014). Emerging infectious diseases: opportunities at the human–animal–environment interface. *Veterinary Record* 174: 546–51.

Donaldson, A. (2008). Biosecurity after the event: risk politics and animal disease. *Environment & Planning* 40: 1552–67.

Food and Agriculture Organization of the United Nations (2009). *Highly pathogenic avian influenza: a rapid assessment of its socio-economic impact on vulnerable households in Egypt.* Rome: FAO.

Farmer, P. (1996). Social inequalities and emerging infectious diseases. *Emerging Infectious Diseases* 2: 259.

Field, H., and N. Kung (2011). Henipaviruses: unanswered questions of lethal zoonoses. *Current Opinion in Virology* 1: 658–61.

Forbes, I. (2004). Making a crisis out of a drama: the political analysis of BSE policy-making in the UK. *Political Studies* 52: 342–57.

Giddens, A. (1984). *The constitution of society: outline of the theory of structuration.* Berkeley: University of California Press.

Grace, D. (2015). Zoonoses of poverty: measuring and managing the multiple burdens of zoonoses and poverty. In *Zoonoses – infections affecting humans and animals: focus on public health aspects*, A. Sing, ed., 1127–37. Dordrecht: Springer Netherlands.

Grace, D., and B. Jones (2011). *Zoonoses (Project 1): wildlife/domestic livestock interactions. Final project report to DFID submitted by the International Livestock Research Institute (ILRI) and Royal Veterinary College.* London: International Livestock Research Institute.

Greger, M. (2007). The human/animal interface: emergence and resurgence of zoonotic infectious diseases. *Critical Reviews in Microbiology* 33: 243–99.

Grill, K., and A. Dawson (2017). Ethical frameworks in public health decision-making: defending a value-based and pluralist approach. *Health Care Analysis* 25(4): 291–307.

Halliday, J., et al. (2015). Endemic zoonoses in the tropics: a public health problem hiding in plain sight. *The Veterinary Record* 176: 220–5.

Hampson, K., et al. (2015) Estimating the global burden of endemic canine rabies. *PLOS Neglected Tropical Diseases* 9(4): e0003709.

Häsler, B., et al. (2012). The economic value of One Health in relation to the mitigation of zoonotic disease risks. In *One Health: the human–animal–environment interfaces in emerging infectious diseases*, 127–51. Mackenzie, J., Jeggo, M., Dazak, P., Richt, J. eds., 127–51. Berlin: Springer.

Hinchliffe, S. (2001). Indeterminacy in-decisions – science, policy and politics in the BSE (bovine spongiform encephalopathy) crisis. *Transactions of the Institute of British Geographers* 26: 182–204.

Hinchliffe, S. (2015). More than one world, more than one health: re-configuring interspecies health. *Social Science & Medicine* 129: 28–35.

Hinchliffe, S., J. Allen, S. Lavau, N. Bingham, and S. Carter (2012). Biosecurity and the topologies of infected life: from borderlines to borderlands. *Transactions of the Institute of British Geographers* 38: 531–43.

Hooker, C., C. Degeling, and P. Mason (2016). Dying a natural death: ethics and political activism for endemic infectious disease. In *Endemic: essays in contagion theory*, K. Nixon and L. Servitje, eds., 265–90. London: Palgrave Macmillan.

Hsiao, E.C. (2012). Whanganui River Agreement. *Environmental Policy & Law* 42: 371–5.

Kerridge, I., M. Lowe, and C. Stewart (2013). *Ethics and law for the health professions*. Sydney: The Federation Press.

Kilpatrick, A.M., and S.E. Randolph (2012). Drivers, dynamics, and control of emerging vector-borne zoonotic diseases. *Lancet* 380: 1946–55.

Maudlin, I., M.C. Eisler, and S.C. Welburn (2009). Neglected and endemic zoonoses. *Philosophical Transactions of the Royal Society B: Biological Sciences* 364: 2777–87.

McCloskey, B., O. Dar, A. Zumla, and D.L. Heymann (2014). Emerging infectious diseases and pandemic potential: status quo and reducing risk of global spread. *The Lancet Infectious Diseases* 14: 1001–10.

McDermott, J., D. Grace, and J. Zinsstag (2013). Economics of brucellosis impact and control in low-income countries. *Revue Scientifique et Technique* 32: 249–61.

Molesworth, A., et al. (2014). Investigation of variant Creutzfeldt-Jakob disease implicated organ or tissue transplantation in the United Kingdom. *Transplantation* 98: 585–9.

Nonthabenjawan, N., C. Cardona, A. Amonsin, and S. Sreevatsan (2016). Time-space analysis of highly pathogenic avian influenza H5N2 outbreak in the US. *Virology Journal* 13: 1–8.

Nor, M.N., and B.L. Ong (2001). The Nipah virus outbreak and the effect on the pig industry in Malaysia. In *JE/Nipah Outbreak in Malaysia*, 128–33. Kuala Lumpur: Ministry of Health, Malaysia.

Okello, A.L., K. Bardosh, J. Smith, and S.C. Welburn (2014). One Health: past successes and future challenges in three African contexts. *PLOS Neglected Tropical Diseases* 8: e2884.

Otte, M.J., R. Nugent, and A. McLeod (2004). *Transboundary animal diseases: assessment of socio-economic impacts and institutional responses*. Rome: Food & Agriculture Organization of the United Nations.

Pappas, G., P. Papadimitriou, N. Akritidis, L. Christou, and E.V. Tsianos (2006). The new global map of human brucellosis. *The Lancet Infectious Diseases* 6: 91–9.

Perry, B., and D. Grace (2009). The impacts of livestock diseases and their control on growth and development processes that are pro-poor. *Philosophical Transactions of the Royal Society of London B: Biological Sciences* 364: 2643–55.

Petersen, A., and D. Lupton (1996). *The new public health: health and self in the age of risk*. Thousand Oaks, CA: Sage Publications.

Phillips, N., J. Bridgeman, and M.A. Ferguson-Smith (2000). The BSE Inquiry. Stationary Office, London UK Government.

Plowright, R.K., S.H. Sokolow, M.E. Gorman, P. Daszak and J.E. Foley (2008). Causal inference in disease ecology: investigating ecological drivers of disease emergence. *Frontiers in Ecology & the Environment* 6: 420–9.

Rock, M., B.J. Buntain, J.M. Hatfield, and B. Hallgrímsson (2009). Animal–human connections, 'one health', and the syndemic approach to prevention. *Social Science & Medicine* 68: 991–5.

Rock, M., and C. Degeling (2015). Public health ethics and more-than-human solidarity. *Social Science & Medicine* 129: 61–7.

Rock, M., and C. Degeling (2016). Towards 'One Health' promotion. In *A companion to the anthropology of environmental health*, M. Singer, ed., 68–82. Hoboken, NJ: Wiley.

Rubach, M.P., J. Halliday, S. Cleaveland, and J.A. Crump (2013). Brucellosis in low-income and middle-income countries. *Current Opinion in Infectious Diseases* 26: 404–12.

Rüegg, S.R., et al. (2017). Expectations for a new WHO Director General: health in a rapidly changing environment. *The Lancet Planetary Health* 1: e44-e45.

Rushton, J., R. Viscarra, E. Guerne Bleich, and A. McLeod (2005). Regional report: impact of avian influenza outbreaks in the poultry sectors of five South East Asian countries (Cambodia, Indonesia, Lao PDR, Thailand, Viet Nam) outbreak costs, responses and potential long term control. *World's Poultry Science Journal* 61: 491–514.

Scoones, I., and P. Forster (2009). One World, One Health? *Rural 21* 43: 22–4.

Selgelid, M.J. (2005). Ethics and infectious disease. *Bioethics* 19: 272–89.

Sims, L.D. (2007). Lessons learned from Asian H5N1 outbreak control. *Avian Diseases* 51: 174–81.

Sonaiya, E.B. (2007). Family poultry, food security and the impact of HPAI. *World's Poultry Science Journal* 63: 132–8.

Turner, M.L., and C.A. Ludlam (2009). An update on the assessment and management of the risk of transmission of variant Creutzfeldt-Jakob disease by blood and plasma products. *British Journal of Haematology* 144: 14–23.

Verweij, M., and B. Bovenkerk (2016). Ethical promises and pitfalls of One Health. *Public Health Ethics* 9: 1–4.

Vines, T., V. Bruce, and T.A. Faunce (2013). Planetary medicine and the Waitangi Tribunal Whanganui River Report: global health law embracing ecosystems as patients. *Journal of Law & Medicine* 20: 528–41.

Wallace, R.G., et al. (2015). The dawn of Structural One Health: a new science tracking disease emergence along circuits of capital. *Social Science & Medicine* 129: 68–77.

Wang, L., et al. (2006). Review of bats and SARS. *Emerging Infectious Diseases* 12: 1834–40.

Whittaker, M., J. Zinsstag, E. Schelling, D. Waltner-Toews, and M. Tanner (2015). The role of social sciences in One Health-reciprocal benefits. In *One Health: the theory and practice of integrated health approaches*, J. Zinsstag, E. Schelling, D. Waltner-Toews, M. Whittaker, and M. Tanner, eds., 60. Wallingford, UK: CABI.

World Bank (2010). *People, pathogens, and our planet. Volume 1: towards a One Health approach for controlling zoonotic disease*. Washington, DC: International Bank for Reconstruction & Development/World Bank.

World Health Organization (2004). *Report of the WHO/FAO/OIE joint consultation on emerging zoonotic diseases*. Geneva: Food & Agriculture Organization of the United Nations, World Health Organization, and World Organisation for Animal Health.

World Health Organization (2017). Cumulative number of confirmed human cases for avian influenza A(H5N1) reported to World Health Organization.

Zinsstag, J. (2012). Convergence of EcoHealth and One Health. *EcoHealth* 9: 371–3.

Zinsstag, J., E. Schelling, D. Waltner-Toews, M. Whittaker, and M. Tanner (2015). *One Health: the theory and practice of integrated health approaches.* Wallingford, UK: CABI.

Zinsstag, J., E. Schelling, K. Wyss, and M.B. Mahamat (2005). Potential of cooperation between human and animal health to strengthen health systems. *Lancet* 366(9503): 2142–5.

5

Interdisciplinary health research

Darryl Stellmach, Brigitte Bagnol, David Guest, Ben Marais and Robyn Alders

Interdisciplinary research focusing on the intersection of human, animal and environmental health has risen to prominence in response to a range of issues articulated in the preceding chapters.

An editorial in *Nature* stressed that the 'best interdisciplinary science comes from the realization that there are pressing questions or problems that cannot be adequately addressed by people from just one discipline'. It also emphasised that interdisciplinary research takes longer than conventional projects, making it more expensive in time and money. It takes time for all involved to become confident that colleagues from other disciplines use equal academic rigour, even if the methods in rival fields seem alien. When interdisciplinary research deals with problems associated with the lives and livelihoods of communities, the challenge of removing disciplinary hierarchies between researchers is just the first step. The researchers are also confronted by the need to acknowledge the importance of community knowledge, perspectives and priorities and so break down perceived hierarchies between 'researchers' and those who are 'researched'.

The first part of this chapter gives a brief introduction to the foundational concepts of social research – its epistemology and methods – and highlights the central influence that gender plays in research. The remainder of the chapter is composed of four examples, small case studies, of mixed research methods in the context of applied planetary health research. The case studies provide insight into how interdisciplinary research is tackling some of the world's most significant and complex problems and sharing lessons learned along the way.

Mixed methods research: natural and social science approaches to health

This section is a short primer on social research for natural scientists. It discusses social research in the context of planetary health initiatives. Social research is taken to include social sciences (such as anthropology, political science, and sociology) and humanities (such as history, cultural studies, media studies, and legal scholarship), as well as qualitative methods undertaken in the context of health research and the natural sciences.

It is important to note that social research is not synonymous with qualitative research. Not all social research is qualitative, just as not all natural science research is quantitative. Very broadly speaking, qualitative research is enquiry primarily conducted at the level of individuals, while quantitative research focuses on aggregates. There is quantitative social research (the predominant method in economics, also extensively used in psychology, sociology and human geography) and there are qualitative methods in the natural sciences (e.g. in descriptive studies of animal behaviour or plant forms).

What makes social research distinct, unsurprisingly, is its focus on the social: interactions between people within a specific context. These interactions are complex and occur in multiple registers at once (e.g. the briefest greeting between two people simultaneously relies on registers of speech, body language, historic memory, shared assumptions and emotion). Any attempt to understand, interpret, predict or react to human behaviour must account for this complexity, both in method and analysis. The importance of context obliges social scientists to work with other disciplines and to account for factors such as environment, religion, class, education and so on.

There is a long tradition of social research into health. One of the first and most insightful proponents of social science in medical research was pathologist Rudolph Virchow. A pioneer of pathology and public health, Virchow worked both as a physician and a social scientist. In his study of the spread of disease in 19th-century Europe, Virchow recognised that virological and social factors worked in tandem to propagate disease. Living conditions, workplace exposures, food and hygiene practices, social interactions – all have a role to play in the spread of disease. Pathogenicity is a factor both of biological virulence and social condition. This is encapsulated in Virchow's famous dictum: 'medicine is a social science'.

From the late 19th century through to the mid-20th century, rapid advances in the sciences enabled vast strides against infectious disease and malnutrition. Developments in parasitology, virology, dietetics, botany, engineering and other disciplines led to rapid progress in sanitation, agriculture, nutrition, and human and animal medicine. Public enthusiasm for science was echoed in government funding for bold, visionary scientific enterprise. The hope of scientific solutions to age-old scourges temporarily eclipsed the role of social factors in health behaviour. Vaccines promised to wipe out polio, measles, mumps and rubella, while effective prophylaxis contained malaria.

However, the late 20th century and early years of the new millennium brought a renewed focus on the role of social factors in health. Attempts at disease eradication faltered, not on scientific grounds, but social and political ones. International vaccination campaigns were damaged by inadequate health infrastructure, corruption and deeply rooted historical suspicions. It might be tempting to think such rejections are characteristic of remote regions at the periphery of globalisation, yet the rise of anti-vaccination movements in Euro-America demonstrates this is not the case. Social research can help explain how and why such phenomena emerge.

Social and natural research share some fundamental similarities in how they view the world. However, there are also philosophical differences. It is important to be aware of these similarities and differences in order to correctly read and interpret the results of social research. Most social researchers and natural scientists share the same basic starting points for understanding the material world: we are individuals, endowed with consciousness (a sense of self) able to act upon and be acted upon by an external world. The external world is apprehended through the senses, can be interpreted, and inferences drawn from past experience. This is a theory of being (an ontology) that allows the possibility of empirical research: knowledge derived from observation and experience (for a more detailed comparison of ontology in the natural and social sciences, see Moon and Blackman 2014).

With some degree of empiricism as a common starting point, social research and the natural sciences may diverge in their conception of method, verifiability and the nature of evidence itself. The vast majority of social researchers will argue that pure observer neutrality and objectivity are impossible – more so when the object of study is human social interaction. They will maintain, however, that rigorous empirical accounts of human behaviour are nevertheless epistemologically reliable and valid. Pure objectivity may be impossible, but well-reasoned, logical interpretations from empirical observation represent a robust form of evidence.

Quantitative social research uses mathematical and statistical methods familiar to the natural sciences, while methods of qualitative social research include document analysis, interview, survey and observation. Qualitative evidence, among other forms, may be documentary (e.g. archival studies of history), oral (such as information solicited from interview), or observational (noted from direct observation of a practice or behaviour). In each case, the researcher is the primary research instrument: evidence is collected by and filtered through the critical faculties of the researcher. Qualitative researchers must be highly disciplined, alert to the possibility of error, bias or misreading. This means much social research is interpretative in character, meaning that, despite rigorous observation and analysis, it remains up to the individual researcher, and the peer community, to draw meaning out of the data. This motivates the scepticism of some natural scientists that qualitative research is inherently subjective and therefore biased. However, qualitative research can provide deep and well-contextualised insight that is impossible to capture with quantitative approaches. Qualitative research can in some cases integrate quantitative information to help describe the local context and compare or contrast it to findings in other settings. Often in these cases a large amount of quantitative information can be collected.

Social research must take account of a wide variety of influences, and this changes the nature and generalisability of the conclusions. Individual human behaviour cannot be isolated from social relations, biology or the environment. Further, social research is often performed in some degree of open setting – public spaces, workplaces or the home – where random or confounding influences cannot be isolated or controlled for. Quantitative social research attempts to smooth some of these differences through the use of aggregates, and can make reasonably definitive statements about the general composition or characteristics of a given population. However, it is more difficult to draw inferences about individuals; there are no laws of society that parallel the laws of physics. Thus, social research generally yields insight rather than certainty.

Positionality, gender and research

One of the foundational social research insights of the last 50 years is the central importance that positionality – the inescapable perspective of one's gender, age, ethnicity, class, sexual orientation – plays in research findings in both the natural and the social sciences. For example, when arriving in a community to carry out a research survey, it is not uncommon to have a group of male researchers and enumerators introduced to the male local authorities and male resource persons. Such research is often conducted at the level of households, and usually the research team takes extreme care to ensure that the selection of the households is statistically random and representative of the area. This, it is believed, makes the data representative of the reality of the area under survey. Yet most studies still interview the head of the household without analysing the consequences of this choice. As a result, researchers end up interviewing a majority of male informants.

This is clearly problematic. In most countries (industrialised and industrialising) men and women do not have access to the same resources. Women still carry out most of the unpaid work such as caring for children, the sick and the old. They produce, keep and prepare the food. They work longer hours than men and get little benefit from this extra effort. On the contrary, they have fewer economic resources and less access to decision making than men (World Economic Forum).[1] At the household level, women eat less nutritious food, such as meat, than their male partner.

Women are more likely to be among the malnourished as a result of pregnancy and breastfeeding and because of unequal distribution of resources in society and within the household. Discriminatory access to input, knowledge, land, credit, technologies, innovation, markets, etc., and unequal intra-household decision-making power all serve to exacerbate gender inequalities and vulnerability. This means that men and women do not have the same position, do not have the same views of the world they live in and do not have the same needs. Socioeconomic reasons, sociocultural attitudes, and group and class-based obligations influence men and women's roles, responsibilities and decision-making functions. Cultural beliefs and practices limit women's mobility, social contact, access to resources, and the types of activities they can pursue. Institutional arrangements can also create and reinforce gender-based constraints or, conversely, foster an environment in which gender disparities can be reduced. Risks and vulnerabilities, many of which are gendered, create poverty.

All these aspects affect the way women and men are impacted by disease and their environment. It also influences their ability to adapt; to adopt new measures, for example, to scale-up agricultural production or participate in community decision-making.

Thus, it is clear how the notion of a single household head introduces a gender bias and supports the idea that leadership is a male privilege. It assumes that when there is a couple, the man is designated as the head, no matter the degree to which responsibilities are shared within the household. It assumes that there is a need to have a head, that the head is a single person, that decisions cannot be taken by two or more persons, that the head represents and works in the best interest of the household. These unspoken assumptions do not conform to observed reality. On the contrary, focusing enquiry on a single head of household is highly problematic. Many women around the world have fought, and continue to fight, to give women domestic equality by changing national constitutions, family law or the definition of head of household. For

---

1   http://bit.ly/2W9muRy

Box 5.1: Key recommendations to ensure more accurate gender representation in research

- Carry out a gender analysis of the social context.
- Analyse how men and women (of different age, class, race, sexual orientation, etc.) are impacted specifically by a situation and impact the same situation (this includes the analysis of roles, access, control and benefit related to all relevant resources).
- When dealing with local authority, stress the importance of women's voice and point of view and ask to meet female leaders.
- 50 per cent of research staff should be women.
- Interview 50 per cent of women individually or in a same-gender group.

---

example, in Mozambique after years of struggle by women, academics and civil society, the New Family Law (2004) defined that men and women act together as head of the household and have the same rights and obligation to ensure the wellbeing of the household. In the same way that women have managed to change it in law in some jurisdictions, it is important as researchers that we change it in our practices. In reality, what is called in research 'male-headed household' should be 'male- and female-headed household' or 'joint-headed household'.

Ensuring consideration of both male and female points of view is both a human right and a practical development issue. For researchers, it is incumbent to ensure that data collected represent some of the 51 per cent of women in the world. Addressing gender issues is both holistic and transdisciplinary. It offers a unique transversal lens through which to understand EcoHealth, One Health and Planetary Health. Gender is an essential element to be addressed if these unifying paradigms are to realise their potentials.

Case studies

The remainder of this chapter explores ways in which interdisciplinary methods can be used to gain insight on problems of central importance to planetary health. The first example explores infectious disease through the lens of One Health, and illustrates how historical and evolutionary approaches can complement our biological understanding of disease. The second case study gives an example of interdisciplinary applied research, with the goal of bettering livelihoods for rural cocoa-growing farmers in Sulawesi, Indonesia, and Bougainville, Papua New Guinea. The third case study examines the gendered impacts of avian influenza on poor rural households in Indonesia. It highlights the importance of interdisciplinary approaches to understanding how power dynamics influence experience, identity and livelihoods. This topic is further explored in Chapter 10. The final case study highlights the importance of enrolling communities as partners in interdisciplinary research when tackling issues intimately associated with their lives and livelihoods.

1. One/Eco/Planetary Health approach to infectious diseases

The medical discipline of infectious diseases concerns itself with the causes of cellular dysfunction resulting from infection by another living organism or virus. Following the medical community's acceptance of the germ theory of disease in the early 20th century it took the field nearly a century to appreciate that most human infectious diseases have an animal or environmental origin. Pathogens that are able to infect humans, but have their major reservoir in an animal host are called zoonoses. It is now recognised that the transition from a predominantly animal to a predominantly human pathogen is a dynamic two-way process and that a variety of organisms have different levels of host-specific adaptation. This led to a greater appreciation of the need to study the interrelationship between humans and their environment, including wild, domestic or companion animals. A recent example of the devastating effect that a new pathogen can have on the human population is the human immunodeficiency virus (HIV) type-1, which evolved from the simian immune deficiency virus affecting chimpanzees in central Africa. Other examples include the largest ever outbreak of Ebola virus in West Africa in 2013–16 and the notorious influenza pandemic of 1917–18.

Tuberculosis remains the top infectious disease killer on the planet, responsible for nearly 1.5 million premature deaths in 2015. Described as 'the captain of all these men of death', tuberculosis was considered to be the archetypical example of an animal disease that became adapted to the human host. However, with the advancement of genome sequencing and detailed evolutionary analysis it became apparent that *Mycobacterium tuberculosis* has ancient origins and that humans are probably the primary reservoir of the ancestral *M. tuberculosis* complex. It remains intriguing to consider how a relatively harmless environmental mycobacterium could evolve to become a major pathogen and why humans became the primary reservoir. Of all species on the planet only *Homo sapiens* have successfully controlled fire. The available evidence suggests that this created the environmental niche necessary for *M. tuberculosis* to evolve and flourish as a respiratory pathogen. Excessive smoke exposure in cave dwellings and poorly ventilated built shelters may have increased vulnerability through lung and airway inflammation. The cooking of food and the ability to manipulate the environment with fire increased human population density, while campfires also increased socialisation and close human interaction. All of these changes created the environment for a respiratory pathogen to evolve and sustain epidemic spread through aerosol transmission.

The example of tuberculosis illustrates how the human species has been able to influence its environment to such as degree that it creates new ecological niches for pathogens to fill. It provides a prescient example that environmental manipulation may bring benefits, which the taming of fire undoubtedly did, but it also exposes us to new risks. Recent environmental changes provide major opportunities for pathogens to emerge and spread. These changes include a dramatic increase in human population density, reduced genetic diversity among domesticated animals and plants, intensified farming practices, as well as our global connectedness through trade and travel. Wildlife and plant habitats are threatened by increased deforestation and expanded agriculture, resulting in more frequent interaction of wild species with domesticated animals and rural villagers. Human-induced ecosystem changes may disrupt ecological pyramids or introduce new species without natural predators, resulting in uncontrolled multiplication of lower level organisms.

Such a changed environment requires new ways of thinking and more sophisticated tools to predict risk and rapidly respond to outbreaks. It also requires a far deeper understanding of the interconnectedness of things, since all life on the planet ultimately depends on a functional ecosystem. Maintaining the integrity of ecological systems may provide the best form of disease prevention. This would require multidisciplinary teams who can assess a whole variety of risks from an ecosystem perspective using complex systems analyses. A vertical silo-approach has supported great gains in HIV care and malaria control, but narrowly focusing on single disease entities has fractured integrated primary care and may blind us to emerging threats and unintended social or environmental consequences. Sustaining life on our small blue planet, where 'health' is ultimately dependent on life-sustaining ecosystem services, requires careful assessment of ecological impacts with detailed risk mapping to identify key priorities for infectious disease prevention.

2. Linking agricultural production and human health

While the impacts of agriculture on food quality, nutrition and environmental and human health ('agri-health') are widely recognised, health also affects the capacity of smallholder farmers to increase productivity and alleviate poverty. Poor health and nutrition trap smallholder farmers in cycles of poverty, as they are unable to implement changes that improve crop yields and income. Poverty, in turn, limits their access to improved nutrition and healthcare.

Cocoa farming is a valuable source of income in many wet tropical countries. Well-managed cocoa trees have the potential to yield several tonnes of dry beans per hectare but the global average yield for smallholder producers remains around 300 kg/ha. Yields remain low because of a combination of poor crop, soil and water management, inadequate infrastructure, inefficient supply chains, financial constraints, pest and disease losses, the inappropriate use of pesticides and fertilisers, unsafe food storage, and low returns to labour.

Technologies to reduce crop losses and increase cocoa yields, based around regular weekly pod harvesting, canopy pruning, sanitation and fertiliser application, have been demonstrated to cocoa farmers in many countries. An analysis of the benefits to labour in Vanuatu showed that investing 52 extra hours of labour per month to improve the management of smallholder cocoa crops increased yields by 238 per cent and gave a return to labour of 150 per cent.

Despite this investment in farmer training, yields remain at low levels because, while farmers are conscious of the potential benefits, they choose not to invest in increasing cocoa yields. Evidence from Sub-Saharan Africa shows that poor adoption may result from the lack of a clear economic incentive because of global cocoa price uncertainty, pest and disease losses, climate uncertainty, poor infrastructure, inadequate technical and financial support, and the limited availability of labour. Our research in PNG and Indonesia shows that the wealthiest smallholder cocoa farmer families are well educated, have diversified incomes and have good health.

The limited pool of labour prioritises food gathering and customary obligations, and is further depleted by the migration of youth to urban centres for education and employment, by alternative employment opportunities, and is constrained by poor health and nutrition. If farmers suffer physical or mental illness, or if they have to take their children to clinics and hospitals and are absent for extended periods, they may be unable to apply essential crop management interventions. In many areas of Indonesia and Papua New Guinea these factors have encouraged farmers to shift to lower-input but less rewarding crops such as oil palm and maize.

Understanding how malnutrition and ill health compound labour shortages would facilitate the development of strategies to holistically address rural poverty. Technologies and communication networks could be tailored to better engage women and youth, foster entrepreneurship, address limited capital availability, and improve health. Such approaches require closely integrating agricultural, health and community interventions from the early planning stages. In two current projects, interdisciplinary teams, including agricultural scientists, health and nutrition researchers, community development specialists, entrepreneurship trainers, marketing experts and human geographers, work together with farmers and stakeholders to identify and address key constraints. The core proposition in this approach is that higher yields of cocoa beans can be achieved when farm families make moderate progress with more intensified management, including rehabilitation of existing cocoa, replanting with improved genotypes, improved cocoa agronomy, soil management and integrated pest and disease management. Whole family extension approaches supporting intensified cocoa production releases land for supplementary activities generating incomes for women and youth – including food crops and small livestock – that lead to diversified incomes and improved nutritional outcomes. Furthermore, implementing better fermentation and drying procedures will produce higher quality beans that will, when linked through more efficient value chains to niche markets, return significantly higher prices.

A suite of projects aim to diversify and improve the sustainability and profitability of cocoa-based farming, develop opportunities for women and youth, understand the opportunities for improved community health and nutrition, foster innovation and community enterprise development, and strengthen cocoa value chains. Project elements include support to communities by trained primary crop, livestock and healthcare advisers using mobile technologies and apps to access wider expertise. This initiative entails deep engagement with farming communities, particularly women and youth, who are involved in the design, inception and implementation of the project. Communities will be enabled to celebrate their achievements in annual chocolate festivals.

3. Gender, health and agriculture

The first outbreak of highly pathogenic avian influenza H5N1 (HPAI) in Indonesia was reported in 2003. HPAI has since established as an endemic zoonotic disease in certain provinces of the country. This case study is an economic analysis of the gendered impact of HPAI on poor rural households in Indonesia.

An estimated 295 million indigenous chickens and 45 million ducks were kept by small-scale producers in Indonesia. Family poultry provide a valuable source of meat and eggs, particularly important in childhood nutrition. Poultry are also an important source of income for women, especially in poor rural households with more children and less access to education.

At the height of the HPAI outbreak, interventions aimed at preventing the impacts of HPAI included the death and culling of over 10 million birds between August 2003 and September 2005. Simultaneously, demand for poultry feed dropped 45 per cent and export volumes dropped 97 per cent. The cull and sharp drop in consumption had the effect of bankrupting poultry producers (an industry that employs over one million in Indonesia). The consequences of decreased poultry consumption on childhood nutrition have not been quantified.

The specific impact on small-scale poultry producers has not been studied. Village poultry contribute to income and food security, and, as these flocks are usually owned or managed by women, contribute to intra-household gender equality. They also provide insurance against income and nutrition shocks. Household poultry-keeping is, by nature, decentralised, and characterised by low levels of management, including minimal biosecurity practices, which can contribute to a high risk of losses to diseases such as HPAI should an incursion take place. Despite these risks, direct financial losses to small-scale poultry farmers were probably minimised where household income was diversified. For the reasons outlined above, however, it is almost certain those losses were disproportionately greater for women and poor rural households.

These facts have important implications for training and compensation programs. Such programs need to be focused on the rural poor, who rely on poultry for income and nutrition. Given their role in raising poultry, women must be actively involved in training and compensation programs.

4. Interdisciplinary community-based food and nutrition security research

The preceding case studies have highlighted the benefits of and lessons learned implementing interdisciplinary health research. The third case study emphasised the crucial importance of ensuring gender-sensitive research methodology to give voice to the knowledge and perspectives of women.

This fourth case study relates to interdisciplinary research addressing complex problems that are bound up with the lives and livelihoods of communities. It builds on the 'Village chickens and their contributions to mixed farming households in resource-poor settings' section in Chapter 8 of this book. In that section we advocate for longer term, mixed-methodology research based on the active involvement of communities, governments, the private sector and researchers that facilitates joint learning and problem solving. Similar issues will be found in research that seeks to tackle complex problems.

To recap, sustainable food and nutrition security is a global priority requiring a multi-pronged approach based on nutrition-sensitive landscapes and value chains. In Tanzania and Zambia, the prevalence of undernutrition in children under five years (U5) remains high – with the levels of stunting (low height for age, an indicator of chronic undernutrition) averaging 42 per cent and 40 per cent respectively. Both countries are seeking sustainable solutions to the food security challenge that will improve human nutrition through increased household income and dietary diversification. The 'Strengthening food and nutrition security project through family poultry and crop integration in Tanzania and Zambia' (Nkuku4U) project was designed in response to this situation.

Nkuku4U is a mixed-methods, five-year, cluster-randomised controlled trial implemented across the two countries involving four communities in each of five wards. Project sites were recommended by the Country Coordinating Committees (a group of national project team members, from a range of disciplinary backgrounds/institutions, who oversee project activities in each country). Suitable sites were based on: 1) the level of child undernutrition; 2) an absence of existing human nutrition interventions, and 3) a willingness of leaders at the regional, district and ward level to be involved. In each ward, households per community were selected on the basis of having one child under the age of two years at the time of enrolment following a ward-wide census. The enrolled households are followed longitudinally. Male and female community members trained as enumerators administer questionnaires in local languages, to obtain data on maternal and child health and nutrition from mothers/carers of enrolled children, and on livelihood strategies, livestock ownership and poultry-keeping practices from a mix (approximately 50:50) of male and female adult respondents in enrolled households. Children's length/height measurements are recorded at six-monthly intervals. Qualitative data has also been gathered through annual participatory rural appraisals and impact assessments using male and female focus group discussions with representatives from four socioeconomic groups. The number of social groups and their characteristics were developed by the community participants during the baseline and varied slightly in each ward.

Human subject research ethics approval for this project was obtained from the relevant institutions in Tanzania and Zambia with approval subsequently granted by the University of Sydney's Human Research Ethics Committee. Animal ethics approval was obtained from the University of Sydney's Animal Ethics Committee only, as counterpart committees have not yet been established in Tanzania or Zambia.

Vaccination of village chickens against Newcastle disease (ND) by community vaccinators administering the I-2 ND vaccine via eye drop every four months on a fee-for-service basis was introduced in each ward in the first year of implementation. Cost-sharing through farmers making a payment to community vaccinators increases the likelihood that the ND control program will be sustained beyond the end of the project. Crop interventions were determined through participatory workshops in each project ward involving male and female participants, with an emphasis on the involvement of representatives from households enrolled in the project. The selected crop interventions were implemented the year after the introduction of the ND vaccination campaigns.

Communication plays a crucial role in interdisciplinary approaches, and sharing of results, problems and solutions and managing planning is of extreme importance. A Senior Advisory Board known as the Project Coordinating Committee (PCC) has been established to assist with broad long-term oversight and cross-sectoral co-ordination. The PCC meets every six months, alternating between Tanzania and Zambia. The involvement of government agencies enables research findings to contribute to positive impacts within the regulatory, financial and policy environment in which the findings are to be applied. The Country Coordinating Committee meets every 3–4 months in each country with community meetings held in participating wards on a monthly basis in association with data collection activities. We emphasised the importance of gender equity in terms of the project team composition from the community to the project management level.

This is a large, complex project, complicated further by poor rainfall during two of the three wet seasons since the project commenced. Collecting and analysing the data is a huge task with team members spread across the globe. In addition, the development of viable solutions during a time of significant weather variability has further increased the degree of difficulty.

Conclusion

As stated in *Nature* (2015) interdisciplinary research cannot be rushed. It takes time for researchers from different disciplines to appreciate the perspectives of other disciplines and non-academic research partners. Part of the solution is assembling a research team that is inclusive of all key partners and that is clearly focused on problem solving. Such teams form over years and are to be nurtured and highly prized. Other parts of the solution include funding bodies committing to longer-term projects that facilitate learning by doing and research institutions recognising that the conduct and publication of high quality, mixed-methods interdisciplinary research requires longer horizons.

Acknowledgements

Funding provided by the Australian government, especially the Australian Centre for International Agricultural Research (ACIAR) (HORT/2014/094 and FSC/2012/023) and the Australia–Indonesia Centre, the Food and Agriculture Organization of the Unite Nations and the Crawford Fund in support of research on disease prevention and improved food and nutrition security is gratefully acknowledged.

Works cited

Alders, R.G., et al. (2003). Controlling Newcastle disease in village chickens: a training manual. https://bit.ly/2QBuV81.

Alders, R.G., et al. (2014). Using a One Health approach to promote food and nutrition security in Tanzania and Zambia. *Planet@Risk* 2(3): 187–90. https://bit.ly/2BU0Rwo.

Alders, R.G., et al. (2016). Approaches to fixing broken food systems. In *Good nutrition: perspectives for the 21st century*, K. Kraemer, et al., eds., 132–44. Basel, CH: Karger. https://bit.ly/2E2DH8x.

Australian Centre for International Agricultural Research (2014). Developing the cocoa value chain in Bougainville. https://bit.ly/2dBfhqd.

Bagnol, B. (2009a). Gender issues in small-scale family poultry production: experiences with Newcastle disease and highly pathogenic avian influenza control. *World's Poultry Science Journal* 65(2): 231–40.

Bagnol, B. (2009b). Improving village chicken production by employing effective gender-sensitive methodologies. In *Village chickens, poverty alleviation and the sustainable control of Newcastle disease*, ACIAR Proceedings 131, R.G. Alders, P.B. Spradbrow, and M.P. Young, eds., 35–42. Canberra: Australian Centre for International Agricultural Research. https://bit.ly/2H6AR5w.

Bagnol, B. (2012). *Advocate gender issues: a sustainable way to control Newcastle disease in village chickens*. Good Practices for Family Poultry Production Note No. 03. Rome: International Network for Family Poultry Development, International Fund for Agricultural Development, and Food & Agriculture Organization of the United Nations. https://bit.ly/2zGa89O.

Bagnol, B., R. Alders, and R. McConchie (2015). Gender issues in human, animal and plant health using an EcoHealth perspective. *Environment & Natural Resources Research* 5(1): 62–76.

Bagnol, B., et al. (2016). Transdisciplinary project communication and knowledge-sharing experiences in Tanzania and Zambia through a One Health lens. *Frontiers in Public Health* 4: 10.

Bernard, H.R. (2012). *Research methods in anthropology: qualitative and quantitative approaches*. Lanham, MD: Rowman Altamira.

Birn, A. (2009). The stages of international (global) health: histories of success or successes of history? *Global Public Health* 4(1): 50–68.

Bloom, B.R., and C.J. L. Murray (1992). Tuberculosis: commentary on a reemergent killer. *Science* 257(5073): 1055–64.

Catley, A., J. Burns, D. Abebe, and O. Suji (2008). *Participatory impact assessment: a guide for practitioners*. Somerville, MA: Feinstein International Center, Tufts University. https://bit.ly/2zEpFqL.

Central Statistical Office (Zambia), Ministry of Health (Zambia), and ICF International (2014). *Zambia demographic and health survey 2013–14*. Rockville, MD: Central Statistical Office, Ministry of Health, and ICF International. https://bit.ly/2GeuqNB.

Chisholm, R.H., J.M. Trauer, D. Curnoe, and M.M. Tanaka (2016). Controlled fire use in early humans might have triggered the evolutionary emergence of

tuberculosis. *Proceedings of the National Academy of Sciences* 113(32):
9051–6. doi: 10.1073/pnas.1603224113.

Collier, E. (2007). *Um perfil das relações de género*. Edição actualizada de 2006.
Maputo, MZ: Agência Sueca para o Desenvolvimento Internacional (ASDI).

Crooks, D.L., L. Cliggett, and S.M. Cole (2007). Child growth as a measure of
livelihood security: the case of the Gwembe Tonga. *American Journal of
Human Biology* 19(5): 669–75.

Daniel, R., et al. (2011). Knowledge through participation: the triumphs and
challenges of transferring Integrated Pest and Disease Management (IPDM)
technology to cocoa farmers in Papua New Guinea. *Food Security* 3(1):
65–79.

de Bruyn, J., J. Wong, B. Bagnol, B. Pengelly, and R.G. Alders (2015). Family
poultry and food and nutrition security. *CAB Reviews* 10(013): 1–9.

Díaz Bordenave, J. (1998). Relation of communication with community
mobilization processes for health. In *Community mobilization for health:
multidisciplinary dialogue*, L.R. Beltrán and G.S. Fernando, eds., 94–8. John
Hopkins University and SAVE.

Donni, O., and S. Ponthieux (2011). Approches économiques du ménage: du
modèle unitaire aux décisions collectives. *Travail, Genre et Sociétés* 26(2):
67–83.

Iannotti, L.L., M. Barron, and D. Roy (2009). Nutrition impacts of highly
pathogenic avian influenza (HPAI). *The FASEB Journal* 23(1 Supplement):
918.3.

Janes, C.R., K.K. Corbett, J.H. Jones, and J. Trostle (2012). Emerging infectious
diseases: the role of social sciences. *Lancet* 380(9857): 1884–6.

Kirk, J., and M.L. Miller (1986). *Reliability and validity in qualitative research*.
Newbury Park, CA: SAGE Publications.

Leatherman, T. (2005). A space of vulnerability in poverty and health:
political-ecology and biocultural analysis. *Ethos* 33(1): 46–70.

Leonardo, W.J., et al. (2015). Labour not land constrains agricultural production
and food self-sufficiency in maize-based smallholder farming systems in
Mozambique. *Food Security* 7(4): 857–74.

Mackenbach, J.P. (2009) Politics is nothing but medicine at a larger scale:
reflections on public health's biggest idea. *Journal of Epidemiology &
Community Health* 63(3): 181–4.

Moon, K., and D. Blackman (2014). A guide to understanding social science
research for natural scientists: social science for natural scientists.
Conservation Biology 28(5): 1167–77.

Muzari, W., W. Gatsi, and S. Muvhunzi (2012). The impacts of technology adoption on smallholder agricultural productivity in sub-Saharan Africa: a review. *Journal of Sustainable Development* 5(8): 69.

Naipospos, T.S.P. (2009). Current situation with highly pathogenic avian influenza (HPAI) in Indonesia, with special emphasis on control at village level. In *Village chickens, poverty alleviation and the sustainable control of Newcastle disease*, ACIAR Proceedings 131, R.G. Alders, P.B. Spradbrow, and M.P. Young, eds., 141–6. Canberra: Australian Centre for International Agricultural Research. https://bit.ly/2H6AR5w.

National Bureau of Statistics (Tanzania) (2011). Tanzania: demographic and health survey 2010. https://bit.ly/2KX4FQo.

Nature Editorial (2015). Mind meld: interdisciplinary science must break down barriers between fields to build common ground. *Nature News* 525(7569): 289.

Ottersen, O.P., et al. (2014) The political origins of health inequity: prospects for change. *Lancet* 383(9917): 630–67.

Padmawati, S., and M. Nichter (2008). Community response to avian flu in central Java, Indonesia. *Anthropology & Medicine* 15(1): 31–51.

Picchioni, F., et al. (2017). Roads to interdisciplinarity – working at the nexus among food systems, nutrition and health. *Food Security* 9(1): 181–9.

Sumiarto, B., and B. Arifin (2008). *Overview on poultry sector and HPAI situation for Indonesia with special emphasis on the Island of Java*. Washington, DC: International Food Policy Research Institute. https://bit.ly/2SukXCP.

United Nations Development Program (2001). *Gender in Development Program learning and information pack: gender analysis*. New York: United Nations Development Program. https://bit.ly/28JpY3K.

Virchow, R. (1848). Der armenarzt. *Medicinische Reform* 18:125-7.

Viseu, A. (2015). Integration of social science into research is crucial. *Nature* 525(7569): 291.

Wong, J.T., et al. (2017). Small-scale poultry and food security in resource-poor settings: a review. *Global Food Security* 15: 43–52. https://bit.ly/2RIjRDK.

World Health Organization (2016). *Global health estimates 2015: deaths by cause, age, sex, by country and by region, 2000–2015*. Geneva: World Health Organization. https://bit.ly/1zAaIAK.

World Organisation for Animal Health (2016). Indonesia animal health situation: OIE World Animal Health Information System. https://bit.ly/19kEuOn.

6

Gender, health and smallholder farming

Kirsten Black, David Guest, Brigitte Bagnol, Yngve Bråten Braaten and Anna Laven

Over the last decade governments and others have come to recognise that sustainable development requires gender equality (Box 6.1) (Sweetman 2002; United Nations 2014). The United Nation's Sustainable Development Goals (SDGs) for gender equality (Goal 5) acknowledge that achieving gender parity will require nations to address gender-based violence, equality of employment opportunities for women, sexual and reproductive health and rights, as well as implementing legislative changes that support women's empowerment and their access to economic resources and technology (United Nations Development Program [UNDP] 2016). Gender issues are also reflected in other SDGs relating to health and poverty alleviation. Target 1.B under SDG 1 urges countries to 'Create sound policy frameworks at the national, regional and international levels, based on pro-poor and gender-sensitive development strategies, to support accelerated investment in poverty eradication actions.'

Linking gender equality with sustainable development is critical because any vision of a just and sustainable world must include the rights of women and acknowledge that, compared to male counterparts, women and girls in certain settings are disproportionally affected by economic, social and environmental stresses (Leach, Mehta and Prabhakaran 2016). According to the United Nations, women's active involvement in decision-making has enormous potential 'to improve resource productivity, enhance ecosystem conservation and promote

---

Box 6.1: Gender

'Gender refers to culturally and socially constructed differences between men and women, boys and girls. The perspectives of women and men are different simply because their experience and perception of the fundamental agencies, structures and relationships involved is different. Gender equality recognises the different behaviours, roles, aspirations, values and needs of women and men in the pursuit of equal opportunities. This pursuit is more effective when both women and men are engaged. Gender equity is the fair and just distribution of responsibilities and benefits between women and men, in agriculture involves a committed focus on impact pathways that are inclusive and respect the role of women.' (B. Chambers. Working paper on gender in agriculture. ACIAR, 24 June 2014)

---

sustainable use of natural resources, and to create more sustainable, low-carbon food, energy, water and health systems' (United Nations 2014).

Gender inequalities are persistent and reinforced

In most countries (from low to high income) men and women do not have equal access to the same natural, human and capital resources. The 2016 Global Gender Gap Report by the World Economic Forum (2017) includes the 11th edition of the Global Gender Gap Index, which quantifies the magnitude of gender-based disparities, and measures the relative gaps between women and men across four key areas: health, education, economy and politics. The index was developed in part to address the need for a consistent and comprehensive measure for gender equality that tracks a country's progress. The data reported in the index, while incomplete, identifies countries, irrespective of wealth, that divide resources more equitably between women and men. This report concludes that progress is still too slow, concluding that economic gender equality will not be achieved for another 170 years.

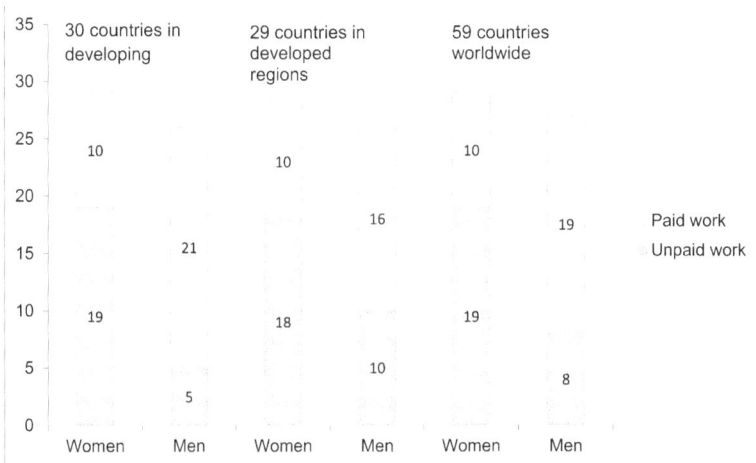

Figure 6.1 Proportion of time spent on unpaid and paid work in selected countries, women and men, 2000–2014 (percentage of time spent per day). Source: https://bit.ly/2RXssq2

The 2016 Global Gender Gap Report also highlights the 'triple burden of women', who still undertake unpaid reproductive and domestic work such as caring for children, the sick and the old, and producing, keeping and preparing water and food. They also contribute significantly to production, particularly in smallholder agriculture. Yet, while women in many countries work longer hours than men, they receive no additional benefit. At the household level, international data shows women, when compared to male partners, eat less nutritious food such as meat, and are more likely to be malnourished because of pregnancy and breastfeeding. The unequal distribution of resources in society is reflected within the household (Sen 1983).

The roles, responsibilities and decision-making functions for males and females are generally influenced by socioeconomic factors, sociocultural attitudes, and group and class-based obligations (Bagnol 2012). Such cultural beliefs and practices limit women's mobility, social contact, access to resources, and the types of activities they can pursue.

Institutional arrangements – formal and informal – also create and reinforce gender-based constraints or, conversely, foster an environment in which gender disparities are reduced (Bagnol 2009a; 2009b).

Gender is also expressed through technology. Frances Bray writes:

> Men are viewed as having a natural affinity with technology, whereas women supposedly fear or dislike it. Men actively engage with machines, making, using, tinkering with, and loving them. Women may have to use machines, in the workplace or in the home, but they neither love nor seek to understand them: They are considered passive beneficiaries of the inventive flame. (Bray 2007)

As such, technologies and institutions are not 'gender-neutral', as gender relations impact on the way they are embedded in communities and other settings. This is relevant to smallholder agriculture where technology is used. Understanding how gender relations interlink and interlock underpins the design, implementation and monitoring of technologies. The same applies to research in technologies and policies. Research is often gender-blind, which creates biased outcomes and detrimental effects. A range of reasons explaining why research has failed to account for women's contributions to agriculture have surfaced including applying a narrow definition of work and economic activity, stereotypes and sex biases among those who design the research tools and the enumerators who collect the data at the field level (Food and Agriculture Organization of the United Nations [FAO] 1994).

Making the links between gender, agriculture and health

In developing countries, where the majority of the population (>80 per cent) are involved in smallholder farming, men and women play important, but distinct, roles. Overall, the roles of women are steadily expanding (Box 6.2). The gendered division of labour in agriculture differs both between and within countries. Women comprise about 43 per cent of the agricultural labour force in developing countries and up to 60–80 per cent in some African countries (CARE 2013). The health and nutrition of women therefore can significantly impact

---

Box 6.2: The feminisation of agriculture

Studies have shown that since the 1960s, men have migrated from rural to urban areas in many developing countries in search of better income opportunities. Women's share in agriculture has, as a result, steadily increased over time, leading women to take on agricultural 'roles' that have historically been in the hands of men. However, it is important to note that the feminisation of agriculture does not mean that women farmers necessarily are better off from engaging in agriculture as women are often denied the benefits of their labour (see Box 6.4).

---

on agricultural productivity because they are restricted in their access to productive resources, opportunities and healthcare, and as a result produce less than male farmers.

In this chapter, we make the case for interlinking and establishing relationships between gender and agriculture and health research and development programs. We examine how these linkages play out in practice, using a gender lens, and identify the research gaps in understanding the full potential of how these Eco/One Health/gender linkages impact on development programs.

A gender lens countenances a gender analysis of the interplay between the *division of labour,*[1] *access to/control over resources, norms and values,* and *intra-household dynamics.* Key to understanding gender dynamics in agriculture and health is to examine the way these separate dimensions and factors influence each other and interlock (Eerdewijk and Danielsen 2015).

The interlinkages between gender are well documented (CARE 2013; FAO 2011; International Bank for Reconstruction and Development/ World Bank 2009; Royal Tropical Institute [KIT], Agri-ProFocus and International Institute of Rural Reconstruction [IIRR] 2012); particularly so for the gendered division of labour, and access to and control over resources.

Studies demonstrate that a 'gender gap in agriculture' exists where women farmers experience inequalities compared with men for productivity, wages, time-use, access to information, social protection,

---

1 Both productive and reproductive work.

extension advice, control over resources and access to decision making (FAO 2011; KIT, Agri-ProFocus and IIRR 2012). Every global gender and development indicator for which data are available reveals that women in rural areas do worse than rural men and urban women, and that they disproportionately suffer poverty, exclusion, poor access to healthcare and poorer nutrition.

Traditionally men in rural areas focus their agricultural activities on cash crops, while women's labour is focused on food crop production, primarily for domestic consumption, with any surpluses sold at local markets. Women are at the forefront of feeding families, making their contribution to household food production paramount for the intake of essential micronutrients by children and the elderly (Sanyang et al. 2014).

Women's role in cash crop production in many low- and middle-resource countries is often invisible or undervalued. Cocoa production is a sector identified as 'man's business' because men traditionally dominate decision-making process and in some countries also the commercial transactions. When women work on cocoa farms, they often do so as unpaid family or casual labour whose contribution does not count (Barrientos 2013) despite substantive research showing women perform half of the tasks on the cocoa farms. Better understanding and recognition of the labour contributions made by women to the production process is the first step towards improving cocoa production.

This illustrates how women working as 'free family labour' are often not counted as farmers in research studies and agricultural value chains because their main responsibility is domestic work (FAO 2011). Evidence suggests that, in addition to work on cocoa, women are involved in most of the household tasks and other 'domestic' work (such as food crop farming and trading). A Ghana study of cocoa farmers, showed that, with all tasks combined, men worked 49 hours per week on average, of which around 10 hours related to household tasks and 39 hours on the farm, while women with an average working week of 63 hours spend around 26 hours on household tasks and 37 hours on the farm (Hill and Vigneri 2011).

A woman's 'reproductive role' has traditionally not been seen as 'economic employment', notwithstanding women farmers are often essential contributors to the wellbeing and health of rural households (FAO 2011). The toolbox on gender and cocoa livelihoods, developed

---

Box 6.3: Intersectionality

'Intersectionality refers to overlapping and intersecting social identities that a person inhabits in relation to oppression and domination'. (Pyburn et al 2015)

A lot of the literature on intersectionality refers to social categories (e.g. 'race'/ethnicity, gender, class, sexuality and ability) as being constructed and dynamic. Hence, the concept of intersectionality allows for a closer investigation of how power dynamics in different agricultural contexts impact on the health of women farmers of different social groupings. For example, in the same farming community, does a young divorced woman have the same access to high-quality fertilisers as a married elderly woman?

---

by KIT (an institute in the Netherlands) and the World Cocoa Foundation (http://bit.ly/2CanI7b), presents evidence that women, more than men, spend their income on health, education and nutrition of their family members. Included in the toolbox are facts about how the lack of female empowerment correlates with childhood malnourishment on cocoa plantations in West Africa (de Boer and Sergay 2012; Schubert 2013). Conversely, when women are empowered chronic child malnutrition is reduced (International Fund for Agricultural Development 2016).

A growing body of literature is critical of research and development programs that group women farmers together as unitary subjects, opposed to men (Ravera et al. 2016). Better understanding is needed about the way women and men with different social identities (age, ethnicity, class, caste and so on) are positioned within agricultural value chains, and how this 'intersectionality' (see Box 6.3) affects productivity and the health of women and men. Women do not necessarily produce food separately from men. Food production is often a collaborative process among family members and other labourers (FAO 2011).

Generally women in agriculture have less access to better quality seeds, fertilisers and equipment, resulting in lower crop yields than those of men (FAO 2017). They also have poorer access to export markets but good access to local markets where they can buy and sell produce, and seek information and establish networks (FAO 2011). Access to training programs is often difficult for women due to household duties (see section on division of labour), lack of agency and their sometimes limited ability to apply new knowledge due to financial and cultural constraints. Staying with the cocoa sector, women tend to benefit less from technical training, extension services, credit and production inputs than men (Chan and Barrientos 2010). Explanations for this include extension services that have biased selection criteria, such as minimum land size, literacy and ability to purchase inputs, which (often unintentionally) excludes many women (Manfre et al. 2013).

Another explanation is found in institutional structures that hinder women's access to vocational organisations such as farmer groups.

Although cocoa farmer organizations are essential for sharing knowledge, providing services and boosting productivity, they are often dominated by men. Those who are members, who are officers, who get trained and who are served by these farmer organizations are predominantly male farmers. (Velyvis, Murray and Fortson 2011)

Membership of a cocoa cooperative is often limited to the person selling the cocoa (usually male), or it requires land ownership or registration of minimum production or harvest volumes. These requirements exclude the majority of women involved in cocoa production from accessing beneficial services available to men (Chan and Barrientos 2010).

If these gender inequalities were addressed, estimates suggest that yields on women's farms could increase by 20–30 per cent, which could raise total agricultural output in developing countries by 2.5–4 per cent (FAO 2011). Women's roles in food crops plus increased yields combined with more decision-making power could reduce the number of malnourished people in the world by 100 to 150 million or 12–17 per cent (FAO 2017).

Why is it so difficult to close this gender gap? One reason is the gap in Official Development Assistance (ODA) showing women receive less aid in agriculture, forestry and fisheries. A multitude of barriers mean women in many settings are less visible because support programs are mainly designed for men by men with leadership roles. Only 15 per cent of agricultural extension workers globally are women. Only 10 per cent of agricultural aid goes to women (FAO website) and women

---

Box 6.4: Social norms and gender relations

Gender relations are produced and reproduced through social norms and values, and influence the various activities that women and men do, what decisions they can make and which resources they have access to. Understanding the dynamic relations between men and women in various institutional settings (household, community, political forums and so on) can contribute to food security and increased health by going beyond addressing the symptoms of gender inequality (i.e. gaps in access to resources) to addressing the causes of these inequalities (Pyburn et al 2015).

---

receive only 5 per cent of extension services. Not well documented are the groups of women who benefit least (or most) from ODA.

Agricultural development programs have historically paid little attention to the differential access to assets and knowledge between men and women in agriculture (Johnson et al. 2016; Meinzen-Dick et al. 2011). Many donor-funded activities seek to improve cash crop productivity to boost incomes, and consequently men, traditionally responsible for this activity, have been the primary recipients of training. Understanding gender relations in agricultural settings is key to whether development programs and interventions can successfully promote gender equality and women's empowerment, especially in regards to access and control over resources and intra-household decision-making (see Box 6.4).

The impacts of agriculture on food quality, nutrition and environmental and human health are well recognised. Poor human health affects the capacity of smallholder farmers to improve production. When compared to Australia, countries in the Asia–Pacific region typically lose between five and 24 times the potential labour due to communicable disease, inadequate maternal and perinatal care, and nutritional conditions (World Health Organization 2008).[2] Poor health and nutrition trap smallholder farmers in cycles of poverty, with little scope to improve crop yields and income. Poverty, in turn, limits their access to improved nutrition and healthcare.

---

2   The World Health Organization compiles data on disability-adjusted life years (DALY).

Health inequalities between men and women likely reflect biological sex and societal gender differences (Denton, Prus and Walters 2004). Women have lower mortality rates across many settings but higher levels of chronic illness and poor mental health (Baum and Grunberg 1991; McDonough and Walters 2001). Women with restricted access to cash and limited control over resources are less autonomous in caring for their own health and deciding on their children's health. Due to geographical, cultural and economic constraints, many women cannot travel alone to a clinic without the authorisation of a male partner or male family member. Thus, while some diseases or afflictions can be gender specific, gender roles and religious, cultural and economic characteristics explain gender differences in health perception and reporting. A 2016 study in Nigeria found women with symptoms of TB and other chronic illnesses did not access healthcare because they were unable to travel to clinics without their husbands' approval, as well as being hampered by unhelpful clinic hours which did not take into consideration their income-generating activities (Oshi et al. 2016).

Women's sexual and reproductive health is also adversely affected by unequal gender relations. Gender inequity results in sexual coercion and physical violence (Fulu et al. 2013) with the consequence that safe sexual practices are impossible to initiate and maintain (Courtenay 2000; Duggal and Ramachandran 2004). These women are more vulnerable to HIV (UNAIDS 2009), other sexual diseases, unwanted pregnancies and have limited access to health services for treatments not directly related to pregnancy (Esplen 2009a). Lack of control over sexual and reproductive health compromises young women's access to education and a productive life and limits participation in community initiatives and leisure time. Women's and girls' sexual and reproductive health and rights are further challenged in many Central, South-East Asian and Pacific Island communities where they tend to marry before 18, either because their right to choose is non-existent or where marriage is the only alternative presented to them (Corrêa and Rosalind 1996; Girls Not Brides 2017).

That most cocoa farmers live below the poverty line (Oomes et al. 2016) refocuses the link between cocoa farming and health. Well-managed cocoa trees have the potential to yield several tonnes of dry beans per hectare, yet the global average yield for smallholder producers remains around 300 kg/ha. Low yields persist because of a combination of poor crop, soil and water management, inadequate infrastructure, inefficient supply chains, financial constraints, pest and disease losses, the inappropriate use of pesticides and fertilisers, unsafe food storage, and low returns to labour.

Technologies to reduce disease losses and increase cocoa yields, based around regular weekly pod harvesting, canopy pruning, sanitation and fertiliser application, have been widely demonstrated to cocoa farmers in many countries (Daniel et al. 2011). An analysis of the benefits to labour in Vanuatu showed that investing 56 hours of labour per month to improve the management of one hectare of cocoa increased yields by 131 per cent and gave an economic return on investment of 150 per cent (Martyn 2013). However, the limited pool of labour is already committed to food gathering and customary obligations (Box 6.5). Labour is further depleted by the migration of youth to urban centres for education and employment, alternative employment opportunities, and constrained by poor health and nutrition (Leonardo et al. 2015).

An alternative approach for improving the livelihoods of cocoa-farming communities involves the close integration of agricultural, health and community interventions. In 2016, the Australian Centre for International Agriculture Research (ACIAR) project, in the Autonomous Region of Bougainville (PNG), involved interdisciplinary project teams[3] working together with cocoa farmers and stakeholders to address key constraints to improving their livelihoods. The core proposition is that higher yields of cocoa beans can be achieved when farm families make moderate progress with more intensified management, including rehabilitation of existing cocoa, replanting with improved genotypes, improved cocoa agronomy, soil management and integrated pest and disease management (Daniel et al. 2011; Simitab 2007). Gender-sensitive family extension approaches supporting intensified cocoa production recognise the complementary roles of men and women in smallholder cocoa production. Intensified cocoa production through improved

---

3   Including agricultural scientists, health and nutrition researchers, community development specialists, entrepreneurship trainers, marketing experts and human geographers.

management potentially frees land for supplementary activities, diversifying incomes for women and youth – including food crops and small livestock – that could improve nutritional outcomes.

This project aims to develop opportunities for women and youth, improve community health and nutrition, foster community enterprise development, and strengthen cocoa value chains. Communities are supported by trained community-based primary crop, livestock and healthcare advisers using mobile technologies and apps to access wider expertise. This initiative entails deep engagement with farming communities, particularly women and youth, who are involved in the design, inception and implementation of the project. Communities celebrate their achievements in an annual chocolate festival that promotes income diversification, improved health and equity.

Interconnections between gender, farming system and health

While the relation between gender and agriculture, gender and health, and health and agriculture are well documented, the interlinkage between gender, agriculture and health is less researched; it has the potential to address women's lack of agency around their sexual and reproductive lives and their ability to participate in domestic and agriculture activities. Understanding how malnutrition and ill health compound labour shortages requires a multidisciplinary strategic approach – one which addresses the deployment of technologies and communication networks to better engage women and youth, foster entrepreneurship, address limited capital availability, and improve health.

Interaction between women and men and their physical and social environments diverge as they have different experience of the same environmental niche with different access to, control over and benefit from resources. Different cultural and ecological settings give rise to differentiated needs, interests, rights and responsibilities over natural resources as well as in relation to plant, animal and human health issues. Crops, animals and natural resources are thus 'gendered' (FAO 2011). Similar inequalities exist in managing natural resources where women play a key role in the organisation and use of natural resources yet they are frequently excluded from making decisions about resources because of their educational, economic, social, political and cultural status (United Nations Environment Programme et al. 2013).

The primary role of women in caring for the young, elderly and sick and in food preparation devalues their important role in food production (Tallis 2002). This responsibility for providing nutrition for adults and children is not accompanied by any power to make decisions, nor the knowledge that can improve nutritional and health outcomes (Asian Development Bank 2013). The unequal distribution of resources and gender discrimination within households often lead to disparities related to health status. In some cultural settings in Africa and elsewhere boys and men traditionally eat first, and girls and women eat the leftovers (Nube and Van Den Boom 2003). When food is short, females eat very little or nothing at all (United Nations International Children's Emergency Fund nd).

Women have different nutritional needs to men and change over a woman's lifecycle: as adolescents, pregnant women and breastfeeding women. In countries such as India (Sivakumar 2008), Tanzania (Bagnol 2015), Sudan (Paul et al. 2014) and South Africa (Oxfam 2014) women have less food than males and the food may also be of lower quality, leading to increased risk of health problems and malnutrition. Widespread nutritional deprivation among women perpetuates an inter-generational cycle of nutrition deprivation in children. Women are also more affected by anaemia (De Benoist et al. 2008) and obesity than men (Kanter and Caballero 2012).

Data from the last Demographic Health Survey carried out in Tanzania and Zambia show women, when compared to men, are less educated and have less access to print and electronic media (Table 6.1). Women in these two countries carry most of the emotional and physical burden of caring for children, the sick and old without preparation and psychological support. Due to the social, cultural and economic discrimination against women and girls, they have no autonomy in relation to their health; only 15.8 per cent of women in Tanzania and 31.7 per cent in Zambia make decisions about their own healthcare (see Table 6.2) (Central Statistical Office and Macro International Inc. 2009; National Bureau of Statistics [Tanzania] and ICF Macro 2011).

	Tanzania		Zambia	
	Women	Men	Women	Men
Women and men aged 15 to 49 who cannot read (%)	27.4	17.6	36.1	18.3
Women and men aged 15 to 49 who are not regularly exposed to any media (TV, radio, or written press) at least once a week (%)	36.0	18.8	33.1	19.1

Table 6.1. Indicators related to gender issues. Source: Central Statistical Office and Macro International Inc. 2009; National Bureau of Statistic [Tanzania] and ICF Macro 2011.

	Mainly wife		Wife and husband jointly		Mainly husband	
	Tanz.	Zambia	Tanz.	Zambia	Tanz.	Zambia
Own healthcare	15.8	31.7	45.0	33.0	38.1	34.0

Table 6.2. Decision making about women's healthcare amongst couples in Tanzania and Zambia. Source: Central Statistical Office and Macro International Inc. 2009; National Bureau of Statistics [Tanzania] and ICF Macro 2011.

Emerging strategies

Strategies to address the impacts of gender inequity once focused on empowering women but today positive changes result when both sexes, together, question how traditional gender norms, cultural practices and social norms impact on livelihoods. This is an essential step to improving equity and access to productive resources in rural smallholder communities.[4]

In view of the need for better evidence about gender equality including the need to involve men in health, development and gender

---

4   WorldFish has published a book on 'Gender Transformative Approaches' (see http://bit.ly/2Q4XZoY).

equality issues, the International Center for Research on Women (ICRW) and Instituto Promundo (Brazil) have been conducting research across a range of countries (ICRW 2012). This multifaceted research aims to develop evidence-based, practical strategies for engaging men in gender equality, particularly in sexual and reproductive health and gender-based violence. A tool to help civil society organisations engage with men and boys in gender equality was published in 2016 to build awareness (Promundo and United Nations Population Fund 2016).

Programs for men and boys developed by Promundo and South African organisations (Sonke Gender Justice Network and EngenderHealth) cover gender roles and masculinity. Promundo's Mencare+ program engages men aged 15–35 as partners in maternal and child health and in sexual and reproductive health and rights (Promundo 2017). The Sonke Gender Justice Network works with young men and women in communities in Africa to strengthen individual knowledge and skills around gender equality and how it links with sexual and reproductive health and rights and prevention of HIV and gender-based violence (Sonke Gender Justice 2016). Both Promundo and the Sonke Gender Justice organisations involve men and women in transformative programs (Greene and Levack 2010) which encourage critical awareness among men and women of gender roles and norms, support greater participation of women as leaders, challenge the roles and responsibilities and the distribution of resources between men and women and/or draw attention to the power relationships between women and men in the community (Rottach, Schuler and Hardee 2009).

Conclusion

In this chapter, we discussed the linkages between gender, agriculture and health, showing how a reduction in maternal illness, childhood death and gender violence would significantly improve agricultural productivity.

Given a significant proportion of women and men in low-income countries work in agriculture, scrutinising the links between agriculture, gender and health makes sense if the Sustainable Development Goals (SDGs) are to be achieved.

All areas – research, policies and interventions – require the engagement of both sexes, but in a way that recognises their social and identity differences. The risk of development aid, research and institutions reinforcing existing gender inequalities is ever present. Health programs that emphasise women's role in caring responsibilities reinforce gender stereotypes and unintentionally maintain women in a gender-constrained world with limited access to information and resources. How to increase men's role in domestic work, caring for the sick and the old and sharing the responsibilities of caring for babies and children (Sweetman 2002) are questions for researchers.

Better integration and co-ordination of health and agriculture programs could address the constraints imposed by poor health on agricultural production and, conversely, by poor agricultural production on health. This can help improve food security and nutrition-sensitive agriculture.

Approaches that examine, question, and change rigid gender norms and address power imbalances can benefit agricultural productivity and improve the health and nutrition of men, women and children by better understanding and co-ordination of the gender, agriculture and health nexus.

If we continue to fragment development aid into silos of discrete uni-disciplinary programs, we ignore the interlinkages and potential synergies between gender, agriculture and health that underpin the benefits of Eco/One Health approaches. Embracing these linkages will improve the effectiveness and impacts of programs designed to benefit everyone involved in smallholder agriculture. Improved livelihoods will inevitably lead to better outcomes in community health and education, which will in turn further improve livelihoods and reduce poverty.

Works cited

Asian Development Bank (2013). *Gender equality and food security. Women's empowerment as a tool against hunger*. Philippines: Asian Development Bank.

Bagnol, B. (2009a). Gender issues in small-scale family poultry production: experiences with Newcastle disease and highly pathogenic avian influenza control. *World's Poultry Science Journal* 65(2): 231–40.

Bagnol, B. (2009b). Improving village chicken production by employing effective gender-sensitive methodologies. In *Village chickens, poverty alleviation and the sustainable control of Newcastle disease*, ACIAR Proceedings 131, R.G. Alders, P.B. Spradbrow and M.P. Young, eds., 35–42. Canberra: Australian Centre for International Agricultural Research.

Bagnol, B. (2012). *Advocate gender issues: a sustainable way to control Newcastle disease in village chickens*. INFPD Good Practices for Family Poultry Production Note 03. International Network for Family Poultry Development, International Fund for Agricultural Development, and Food & Agriculture Organization of the United Nations.

Barrientos, S. (2013). *Gender production networks: sustaining cocoa-chocolate sourcing in Ghana and India*, Working Paper No. 186. Manchester: Brooks World Poverty Institute. http://dx.doi.org/10.2139/ssrn.2278193

Baum, A., and N.E. Grunberg (1991). Gender, stress and health. *Health Psychology* 10(2): 80–5.

Bray, F. (2007). Gender and technology. *Annual Review of Anthropology* 36: 37–53.

de Bruyn, J., Wong, J., Bagnol, B. Alders, R. (2015). Family poultry and food and nutrition security. *CAB Reviews Perspectives in Agriculture Veterinary Science Nutrition and Natural Resources* 10(13):1-9. doi: 10.1079/PAVSNNR201510013

CARE (2013). The picture of both opportunity and hunger is decidedly female. https://bit.ly/2SvHv6d.

Central Statistical Office (CSO), Ministry of Health (MOH), Tropical Diseases Research Centre (TDRC), University of Zambia, and Macro International Inc. (2009). *Zambia Demographic and Health Survey 2007*. Calverton, Maryland, USA: CSO and Macro International Inc.

Chan, M., and S. Barrientos (2010). *Improving opportunities for women in smallholder-based supply chains: business case and practical guidance for international food companies*. Seattle: Gates Foundation.

Corrêa, S., and P. Rosalind (1996). Direitos sexuais e reprodutivos: uma perspectiva feminista. *Physis* 6(1–2): 147–77.

Courtenay, W. (2000). Constructions of masculinity and their influence on men's well-being: a theory of gender and health. *Social Science & Medicine* 50(10): 1385–401.

Daniel, R., et al. (2011). Knowledge through participation: the triumphs and challenges of transferring Integrated Pest and Disease Management (IPDM) technology to cocoa farmers in Papua New Guinea. *Food Security* 3(1): 65–79.

De Benoist, B., E. McLean, I. Egli, and M.E. Cogswell (2008). *Worldwide prevalence of anemia 1993–2005. Global Database on Anemia*. Geneva: World Health Organization.

de Boer, F., and N. Sergay (2012). *Increasing cocoa productivity through improved nutrition. A call to action*. Global Alliance for Improved Nutrition, Centre for Development Innovation, and Wageningen University & Research Centre.

Denton, M., S. Prus, and V. Walters (2004). Gender differences in health: a Canadian study of the psychosocial, structural and behavioural determinants of health. *Social Science & Medicine* 58(12): 2585–600.

Djoudi, H., et al. (2016). Beyond dichotomies: gender and intersecting inequalities in climate change studies. *Ambio* 45(Supplement 3): 248–62.

Duggal, R., and V. Ramachandran (2004). The abortion assessment project – India: key findings and recommendations. *Reproductive Health Matters* 12(24 Suppl):122–9.

Esplen, E. (2009a). *Gender and care: overview report*. Brighton: Bridge.

Esplen, E. (2009b). *Gender and care: supporting resource collection*. Brighton: Bridge.

Food and Agriculture Organization of the United Nations (1994) *Alternative data sources for women's work in agriculture*. Asia and Pacific Commission on Agriculture Statistics, 15th Session, Manila, Philippines, 24–28 October 1994, Agenda Item 9. Rome: Food & Agriculture Organization of the United Nations.

Food and Agriculture Organization of the United Nations (2011). *Women in agriculture: closing the gender gap for development*. Rome: Food & Agriculture Organization of the United Nations.

Food and Agriculture Organization of the United Nations (2017). Gender. https://bit.ly/2wiSgQ1.

Fulu, E., et al. (2013). *Why do some men use violence against women and how can we prevent it? Quantitative findings from the United Nations Multi-Country Study on Men and Violence in Asia and the Pacific*. Bangkok: United Nations Development Program, United Nations Population Fund, United Nations Entity for Gender Equality and the Empowerment of Women, and United Nations Volunteers.

Girls Not Brides (2017). Child marriage around the world: Papua New Guinea. https://bit.ly/2spOXX9.

Greene, M., and A. Levack (2010). *Synchronizing gender strategies: a cooperative model for improving reproductive health and transforming gender relations*. Washington, DC: Population Reference Bureau.

Hill, R., and M. Vigneri (2011). *Mainstreaming gender sensitivity in cash crop market supply chains*. ESA Working Paper No. 11-08. Rome: Agricultural

Development Economics Division, Food & Agriculture Organization of the United Nations.

International Bank for Reconstruction and Development/World Bank (2009). *Gender in agriculture sourcebook*. Washington, DC: World Bank.

International Center for Research on Women (2012). Men and gender equality policy project. https://bit.ly/2E41One.

International Fund for Agricultural Development (2017). What works for gender equality and women's empowerment - a review of practices and results. http://bit.ly/2rnRM8X.

Johnson, N.L., C. Kovarik, R. Meinzen-Dick, J. Njuki, and A. Quisumbing (2016). Gender, assets, and agricultural development: lessons from eight projects. *World Development* 83: 295–311.

Kanter, R., and B. Caballero (2012). Global gender disparities in obesity: a review. *Advances in Nutrition* 3(4): 491–8.

Leach, M., ed. (2016). *Gender equality and sustainable development*. London: Taylor & Francis.

Leach, M., L. Mehta, and P. Prabhakaran (2016). Sustainable development: a gendered pathways approach. In *Gender equality and sustainable development*, M. Leach., ed., 1–33. London: Routledge.

Leonardo, W.J., et al. (2015). Labour not land constrains agricultural production and food self-sufficiency in maize-based smallholder farming systems in Mozambique. *Food Security* 7(1): 857–74

Manfre, C., et al. (2013). *Reducing the gender gap in agriculture extension and advisory services: how to find the best fit for men and women farmers*. MEAS Discussion Paper No. 2. Champaign-Urbana: United States Agency for International Development.

Martyn, T. (2013). *Barriers to smallholder adoption of cocoa IPDM: a case study from Malekula, Vanuatu*. Canberra: Australian Centre for International Agricultural Research.

McDonough, P., and V. Walters (2001). Gender and health: reassessing patterns and explanations. *Social Science & Medicine* 52(4): 547–59.

Meinzen-Dick, R., et al. (2011). *Gender, assets, and agricultural development programs: a conceptual framework*. Paper No. 99. Washington, DC: CAPRi Working.

National Bureau of Statistics (Tanzania) and ICF Macro (2011). *Tanzania demographic and health survey 2010*. Dar es Salaam, TZ: National Bureau of Statistics and ICF Macro.

Nube, M., and G.J. van den Boom (2003). Gender and adult undernutrition in developing countries. *Annals of Human Biology* 30(5): 520–37.

Oliver, D. (1955). *A Solomon Islands society*. Cambridge, MA: Harvard University Press.

Oomes, N., Tieben, B., Laven, A., Ammerlaan, T., Appelman, R., Biesenbeek, C., Buunk, E. (2016). *Market Concentration and Price Formation in the Global Cocoa Value Chain*. Amsterdam: SEO Amsterdam Economics

Oshi, D.C., S.N. Oshi, I.N. Alobu, and K.N. Ukwaja (2016). Gender-related factors influencing women's health seeking for tuberculosis care in Ebonyi State, Nigeria. *Journal of Biosocial Science* 48(1): 37–50.

Oxfam (2014). *Hidden hunger in South Africa. The faces of hunger and malnutrition in a food-secure nation*. Oxford: Oxfam.

Paul, A, Doocy S, Tappis H, Funna Evelyn, S. (2014). Preventing malnutrition in post-conflict, food insecure settings: a case study from South Sudan. *PLOS Currents Disasters* July 7 (Edition 1).

Promundo (2017). *MenCare+*. https://bit.ly/1NH2idO.

Promundo and United Nations Population Fund (2016). *Strengthening CSO–government partnerships to scale up approaches. Engaging men and boys for gender equality and SRHR. A tool for action*. Washington, DC; New York: Promundo and United Nations Population Fund.

Pyburn, R., G. Audet-Bélanger, S. Dido, G. Quiroga, and I. Flink (2015). *Unleashing potential: gender and youth inclusive agri-food chains*. KIT SNV Working Paper Series 7. Amsterdam: Royal Tropical Institute (KIT).

Ravera, F., B. Martin-Lopez, U. Pascual, and A. Drucker (2016). The diversity of gendered adaptation strategies to climate change of Indian farmers: a feminist intersectional approach. *Ambio* 45 (Supplement 3): 335–51.

Rottach, E., S.R. Schuler, and K. Hardee (2009). *Gender perspectives improve reproductive health outcomes: new evidence*. Washington, DC: Population Reference Bureau.

Royal Tropical Institute (KIT), Agri-ProFocus, and International Institute of Rural Reconstruction (2012). *Challenging chains to change: gender equity in agricultural value chain development*. Amsterdam: KIT Publishers, Royal Tropical Institute.

Sanyan, S., Pyburn, R., Mur, R., Audet-Bélanger, G. (2014). Against the grain and to the roots. Dakar: CORAF/WECARD and Royal Tropical Institute (KIT).

Schubert, C. (2013). Using bananas to fight gender imbalances on cocoa plantations. https://bit.ly/2G28vsy.

Sen, A. (1983). Poor, relatively speaking. *Oxford Economic Papers*, New Series 35(2): 153–69.

Simitab, H.J. (2007). Towards a sustainable cocoa economy in PNG: enhancing production through adoption of Integrated Pest and Disease Management

(IPDM) with farmers' participation. In *Roundtable Conference on a Sustainable World Cocoa Economy*. Accra, GH.

Sivakumar, M. (2008). Gender discrimination and women's development in India. http://bit.ly/2RCzb4J.

Sonke Gender Justice (2016). *Annual report March 2015–February 2016. Celebrating 10 years of advancing gender justice*. Cape Town, ZA: Sonke Gender Justice.

Sweetman, C., ed. (2002). *Gender, development and poverty*. Oxford: Oxfam.

Tallis, V. (2002). *Gender and HIV/AIDS*. Brighton: Institute of Development Studies.

United Nations Programme on HIV/AIDS. (2009). *Agenda for accelerated country action for women, girls, gender equality and HIV. Operational plan for the UNAIDS*. Action Framework: Addressing Women, Girls, Gender Equality and HIV. Geneva: UNAIDS.

United Nations (2014). *The world survey on the role of women in development 2014*. Gender equality and sustainable development. New York: UN Women.

United Nations Development Program (2016). Sustainable development goals. https://bit.ly/2csURy2.

United Nations Environment Programme, United Nations Entity for Gender Equality and the Empowerment of Women, United Nations Peacebuilding Support Office, and United Nations Development Programme (2013). *Women and natural resources. Unlocking the peacebuilding potential*. New York: United Nations Environment Programme, United Nations Entity for Gender Equality and the Empowerment of Women, United Nations Peacebuilding Support Office, and United Nations Development Programme.

United Nations International Children's Emergency Fund. Eastern and Southern Africa. Gender and nutrition. https://uni.cf/2QgPYO3.

van Eerdewijk, A., and K. Danielsen (2015). *Gender matters in farm power*. KIT, CIMMYT, CGIAR Research Program on Maize. Amsterdam: Royal Tropical Instiute (KIT).

Velyvis, K., N. Murray, and J. Fortson (2011). *Gender mainstreaming strategy and action plan for the Cocoa Livelihoods Program*. Washington, DC: Mathematica Policy Research.

World Health Organization (2008). *Death estimates for 2008 and disability adjusted life year (DALY) estimates for 2004 by cause for WHO member states*. Geneva: World Health Organization.

7
Case studies

Case study 1: Improving the livelihood of farmers in Bougainville

Merrilyn Walton, David Guest, Grant Vinning, Grant A. Hill-Cawthorne, Kirsten Bluck, Thomas Betitis, Clement Totavun, James Butubu, Jess Hall and Dr Josephine Yaupain Saul-Maora.

Partners

University of Sydney (School of Life and Environmental Sciences, School of Public Health), Autonomous Bougainville Government, University of Natural Resources and Environment, PNG Cocoa Board.

Nearly two-thirds of the population in the Autonomous Region of Bougainville (ARoB) produce cocoa. Before the Bougainville civil war, also referred to as the Bougainville conflict or 'the crisis' (1988–1998), about 28 per cent of the total annual production of 15,600 tonnes of Bougainville cocoa came from large plantations (Scales and Craemer 2008) (Figure 7.1). During the crisis, many of these plantations were abandoned and there was a collapse of smallholder production. When the civil war ended, many farming communities rebuilt their lives by focusing on crops that had the most potential to improve their livelihoods. Despite internal and external efforts, the potential benefits of improved cocoa management have not yet eventuated, due to inadequate extension support, labour shortage and inefficient cocoa supply chains.

The crisis had a similarly profound impact on the health sector with the destruction of hospitals and loss of health workers (AusAID 2012). Since 2010 many key health indicators have improved but a great deal more work is required. Childhood stunting along with maternal health are believed to be a significant problems. Importantly the extent to which poor health and access to health services impacts on the work and activities of daily living of people in Bougainville has not been examined (World Bank 2008).

Aims and objectives

The primary aim of this project, derived from priorities identified by communities in the ARoB, is to improve the profitability and vitality of smallholder cocoa-farming families and communities. The project envisaged public and private sector partnerships and the development of enterprises that enhance productivity and access to premium markets, while promoting gender equity, community health and wellbeing.

The project had the following objectives:

- Improve the productivity, profitability and sustainability of cocoa farming and related enterprises;
- Understand and raise awareness of the opportunities for improved nutrition and health to contribute to agricultural productivity and livelihoods;
- Foster innovation and enterprise development at community level; and
- Strengthen value chains for cocoa and associated horticultural products (ACIAR Project Proposal HORT/2014/094, 2016).

Getting the right team together

Cocoa-farming families were central to this project. While increased cocoa production was a primary goal, past experience suggested a focus on agriculture alone would not bring success. Therefore, a multidisciplinary approach involving agriculture, health, nutrition, animal husbandry and economics was required. Research in most low-resource countries has historically been undertaken using a siloed

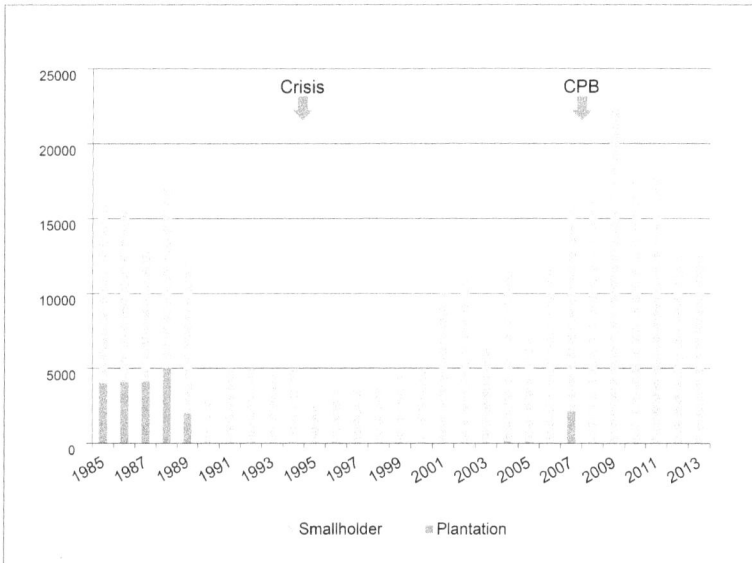

Figure 7.1 Cocoa production in Bougainville (Sources: Scales and Craemer 2008; Cocoa Board of PNG Cocoa Statistics, 2014). The lighter bars indicate the period of the crisis, and the incursion of the Cocoa Pod Borer (CPB) moth.

approach involving just one discipline, with the focus being on a specific area – crop management, or health, or markets. But the experienced lives of people are not neatly compartmentalised – poor health may stop a farmer looking after their crops, a good harvest may rot without an accessible market, and fruit may wither on the vine without attention to climate and pests.

Engaging with communities

Prior to funding, the researchers had a relationship with the communities, having previously worked with them as well as meeting with the communities to explore their health concerns. Once the grant was confirmed, the team met with the ARoB collaborators and visited the communities in Village Assemblies across Bougainville to explain and seek feedback on the aims and approaches of the project, raise awareness of the project and generate community interest.

The community engagement process involved initial meetings with village community members to provide a summary of the project. Separate meetings were held with women and youth to ensure their voices were heard. We collated and analysed the information to ensure that the project incorporated realistic and viable suggestions or comments. During the initial meetings, names of potential community leaders were also obtained. One-on-one meetings were set up with these leaders, who were crucial in preparing for the livelihood surveys.

The project team and the cocoa farmers recognise that intensified farm management – including rehabilitation of existing cocoa, replanting with improved genotypes, improved cocoa agronomy, soil management and integrated pest and disease management (IPDM) – results in higher yields of cocoa beans (Konamet al. 2011). Different extension approaches that support intensified cocoa production will enable supplementary activities, such as food crops and small livestock, and activities to generate incomes for women and youth (Daniel et al. 2011). Diversifying incomes can improve livelihoods, including improved nutritional outcomes.

An annual chocolate festival sponsored by the project in partnership with the Australian High Commission in Papua New Guinea and Autonomous Government of Bougainville (AGB) is now a major community activity with the third festival celebrated in September 2018. Traditional field-day activities include demonstrating new planting materials, fermentation, livestock husbandry, food crops and community health activities. Cocoa buyers and other value-chain stakeholders participate. Music, sports, games and cultural activities are integrated into the festival program. The chocolate competition is a major event, attracting cocoa farmers who supply beans that are processed and made into chocolate samples. Papua New Guinea's largest chocolate maker, Queen Emma in Port Moresby, made the chocolate for judging in the first two festivals according to a standard recipe. In 2018, beans supplied by the growers, were for the first time, prepared for judging at the newly established chocolate processing laboratory built by the Department of Primary Industries and Marine Resources in Buka. Trained chocolate judges and chocolate makers evaluate and rank each sample, with farmers producing the highest quality beans recognised in an awards ceremony at the festival.

Funding

The Australian Centre for International Agricultural Research allocated funding to assist these communities, with a grant being awarded to a multidisciplinary team from the University of Sydney and collaborating partners in the Bougainville (ARoB) Department of Primary Industries, the Cocoa and Coconut Institute of PNG Ltd and the University of Natural Resources and Environment, PNG. Underpinning the funding for this AUD$6 million, six-year project was Australian support for building economic development in the ARoB; one that aimed to support a healthier, better educated, safer and more accessible Bougainville (Australian High Commission 2014).

Methods

Since there were few data available about livelihoods, the first step was to obtain baseline data against which improvements could be measured and priorities established. Survey questions were derived from the following validated questionnaires: the UNICEF Multiple Indicator Cluster Surveys, the USAID Demographic and Health Survey and the WHO World Health Survey, all of which have been used in similar low resource settings. The questions relating to agriculture practices and equipment were developed in a previous ACIAR project (HORT/2012/026) and had content validity.

We used CommCare, a simple mobile data acquisition tool, to collect data about geopolitical factors, economics, populations, livelihood strategies, housing standards, education, healthcare, access to mobile phones, banking, farm sizes and enterprises, details of cocoa activities (number and age of trees, management, yields, fermentation and drying, marketing etc.), and exposure to past training. Data were collected by trained interviewers who were selected from each of the three regions in Bougainville – Buin (South), Arawa (Central) and Tinputz (Northern). Data were

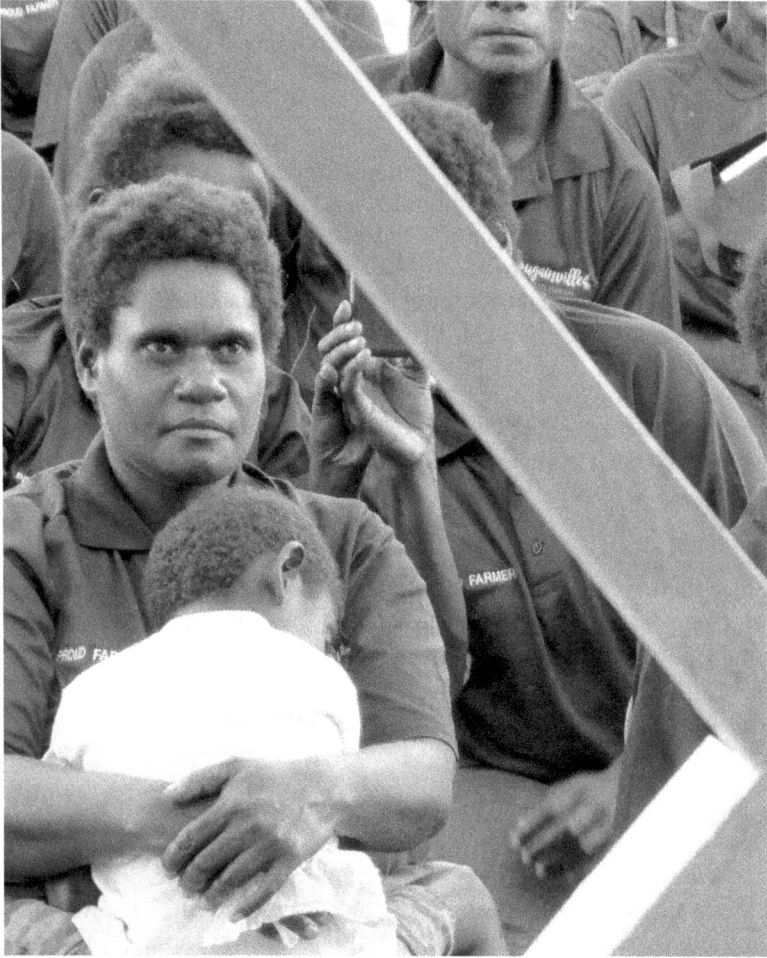

Figure 7.2 Chocolate festival: Arawa, Bougainville, 2016. Photo: Grant Vinning

Box 7.1: Criteria developed with community for selection of villages and Village Assemblies

a. Had to be growing cocoa or identify as a cocoa farmer
b. Motivated and showing leadership
c. Possibility for expansion outside of Village Assembly (VA) with large population group
d. Need to complement existing projects on the ground
e. Balance between villages with good transport access and more remote communities
f. Balance between communities that have and haven't received support before
g. Avoid duplication with other projects
h. Potential for diversification
i. Security of farm ownership and Village Resource Centre security
j. Geographic spread.

collected over a 12-month period and entered into tablets using CommCare; the data was downloaded and compiled centrally.

Results from these surveys have been presented back to communities at meetings held in the three Research and Training Hubs established as part of the project. In addition, the health results have been provided to the ABG Secretary of Health who has used the data to develop the strategic health plan.

The methods for each of the project objectives are summarised below.

Objective 1: To improve the productivity, profitability and sustainability of cocoa farming and related enterprises

Meetings held with Bougainville Government, district government officers, cocoa farmers and village consultations; selection of participating villages

Data on cocoa farming were collected as part of the Baseline Livelihood and Health survey. Thirty-three communities across Bougainville were selected on the basis of transparent criteria and with guidance from the ABG Departments of Primary Industry and Marine Resources and Health and Community Government (see Box 7.1). These communities were surveyed. Village Resource Centres (VRCs) are being established in each Village Assembly (Since the research the name Village Assembly has been changed to Ward.), and Village Extension Workers (VEWs), of whom at least 40 per cent are female, are being selected and trained.

In each of the three regions 11 Village Assemblies (total n = 33 VAs) were selected and all households and villages in the selected VA were included in the study population.

Training of DPI Senior Facilitators, District Officers and selected VEWs

Intensive training was provided for DPI staff to be senior facilitators based at each of the three hubs (a total of 12). Selected participants attended a residential course over two weeks at the Mars Cocoa Academy in Sulawesi, Indonesia. Mars facilitated the training of facilitators with follow-up training delivered at the Kairak Training Centre by CCI and the University of Natural Resources and the Environment (UNRE) staff.

Establish baseline data about cocoa and other farming activities

Basic data were collected on the size and number of cocoa blocks, genotype, age and source of cocoa trees, farming equipment, land ownership, labour, food crops, livestock and incomes.

Establish village budwood gardens and nurseries

The availability of new planting materials limits cocoa rehabilitation. Nurseries are also seen as an alternative source of income for male and female farmers with restricted access to land.

Evaluate soils and compost and fertiliser requirements

Intensification of cocoa production requires improved soil management to sustain higher yields. Farmers have limited access to synthetic fertilisers, and previous research has shown the benefits of on-farm composts, that recycle waste and improve soil fertility. Soils vary, so local trials are to be established to determine optimum soil management.

Establish IPDM demonstration plots

Demonstration plots show the impacts of improved cocoa management, and also serve as training sites ('classrooms in the cocoa block' Guest et al. 2010).

Establish mobile support networks

Very few trained extension staff are available and their travel to remote villages is rare. Establishing mobile networks based on the tablets used in the CommCare surveys enables better access to their skills and advice.

Farmer training

Villages also requested training in cocoa management and processing, supplementary crops, food crops, livestock, budgeting, market access and family teams.

Objective 2: To understand and raise awareness of the opportunities for improved nutrition and health to contribute to agricultural productivity and livelihoods

Establish the extent to which health (including nutrition) and disease impacts on farming activities and workforce availability

This objective had six parts (health includes nutrition):

- Conduct livelihood survey in the 33 Village Assemblies
- Establish baseline data about the health of cocoa-farming families
- Establish the extent to which health and disease impacts upon farming activities
- Establish the health priorities of each community
- Develop an evidence-based cocoa-health framework (Cocoa Farmers Health Framework) that describes best practice in healthcare for communities
- Link with the Department of Health to facilitate community access to and use of existing healthcare services in VRCs.

Establish Advisory Committees

Each participating community has an advisory committee to oversee and guide the studies on the adoption of intensified and diversified cocoa-farming systems and the impacts of health on agricultural labour productivity. This committee is chaired by an appropriate village leader and includes women, youth and cocoa farmers along with the project team.

Terms of reference include oversight of the following activities:

- Approval of the research objectives
- Scope of the health research, including data collection
- Opting out of the health surveys and data collection
- Development and approval of mobile-based tools for collecting data
- Development of educational and training material and technological aids
- Identification of locations for data repositories
- Management of VRCs.

ARoB, district, cocoa farmers and village-level consultations

The impetus for the health component was initiated by cocoa-farming families. This invitation led to initial, but extensive, community consultations and observational visits. We held interactive discussion groups with some of the intervention communities to identify their specific needs and agree upon a realistic focus for the next steps. In order to expand upon this initial work, we conducted additional consultations at all levels (village, district and governmental) to ensure that this project integrating health and agriculture is sustainable and locally relevant to the communities and stakeholders.

The questions posed were:

- What are the main health concerns for the community?
- How are the health needs of the community currently being met?
- Can community members access relevant information via a spoken web application on basic mobile phones?
- Is the Cocoa Farming Health Framework a useful framework for identifying best practice in meeting a community's healthcare priorities?
- Will this be a sustainable model?

By answering these questions, we anticipate we will be able to:

- estimate the extent to which poor family health is impacting on productivity
- estimate the extent to which communities have access and can utilise primary healthcare facilities
- estimate the impact of health educational strategies (written and telephone aids)
- estimate immunisation coverage.

Link health information to rollout of satellite farmer training

In this stage, we plan to link Department of Health programs to the rollout of satellite farmer training centres in remote villages across Bougainville – Village Health Volunteers based alongside Village Extension Workers in Village Resource Centres.

Objective 3: To foster innovation and enterprise development at community level

Support the establishment of DPI regional research hubs in Bougainville

During the decade-long crisis most government and public infrastructure was destroyed. The Department of Primary Industry and Marine Resources (DPI) is the Autonomous Bougainville Government (ABG) department responsible for supporting the redevelopment of agricultural livelihoods. This project is assisting the department to build three regional hubs for applied research and training of village extension staff and farmers.

Establish Village Resource Centres linking CCI, UNRE, AVRDC with DPI and DoH

Trained Village Extension Workers (VEWs), supported by the ABG, the PNG Cocoa Board, PNG University of Natural Resources and Environment and World Vegetable Centre, will establish village resource centres (VRCs) in targeted Village Assemblies. These VRCs will focus community activities in agriculture, health and community development, and will provide feedback on local requirements for future activities.

Develop supplementary food crop and livestock enterprises

While cocoa is a potentially profitable and rewarding cash crop, farmers need to build resilience to buffer radical shifts in world cocoa commodity markets. Supplementary enterprises, including nuts, fruits and food crops as well as small livestock, not only diversify family income, but provide additional income earning opportunities for women and youth and valuable sources of family nutrition.

Support economic development through enterprise development

Intensifying cocoa production requires land, labour and resources that may not be available to all farmers. On the other hand, intensification also supports specialisation so that new business opportunities open up for farmers choosing not to invest in cocoa production, such as establishing nurseries, fermenteries, composting facilities, trading posts and small livestock husbandry. These new enterprises contribute to the resilience of farming communities.

Monitor farming systems

These developments in village activities will be monitored using the Livelihood and Health surveys to evaluate the social and economic impacts they have on village communities.

Objective 4: To strengthen value chains for cocoa and associated horticultural products

- Improve quality through better post-harvest handling, fermentation and drying
- Develop cocoa value chains and market access
- Extension, education and capacity building
- Link resource centres with schools/technical colleges to facilitate technology/skills training and transfer
- Chocolate festivals.

Outcomes

At the time of publication this project had reached the three-year milestone. In that time, the Chocolate Festival has become an annual event celebrating chocolate and the role of cocoa farmers, and linking farmers to buyers and chocolate makers. The livelihood survey has been completed for all three regions and is being analysed. A total of 5,172 respondents completed individual surveys with information available on 12,397 registered household members. A report on the Livelihood Survey has been presented to the Government of Bougainville. The survey findings are summarised below:

- Most farmers either own their land or use clan lands.
- The wealthiest farmers were the healthiest, better-educated and had diversified incomes, independent of other biological, geographical or socioeconomic factors.

- The strongest negative correlations with cocoa production were low levels of education, chronic ill health and physical afflictions and these families tended to live in relative poverty.
- Intensification of cocoa farming makes diversification possible.
- Wealthier farmers grew an average of 2.8 other crops while poorer farmers grew an average of only 2.0 other crops.
- Regardless of wealth many farmers grew coconuts, bananas and betel nut but these crops did not obviously contribute to wealth, perhaps suggesting they are consumed rather than sold.
- A strong correlation exists between ownership of livestock (pigs and chickens) and wealth.

These data support our recommendation to integrate farmer health service delivery with agronomic and family farm teams training. We now have strong evidence that improving farmer health will also increase cocoa production in Bougainville, and the wealth of rural smallholder communities. Cocoa farming communities face hardships in a number of areas, particularly in access to safe water sources and sanitation. While a majority of the population attended a community school only 14 per cent received a high school education and only four per cent attained tertiary education. Only one third have a bank account but over half owned a mobile phone. Around 42 per cent of the population reported moderate to severe food insecurity.

The report to the government separately reports on men's and women's health.

- More than a quarter of the male population and 14 per cent of women had been treated for malaria in hospital within the last six months.
- Both men and women reported that the main reasons for seeking health care in the last six months related to symptoms of cough and fever.
- Both sexes reported symptoms of a range of chronic conditions that were undiagnosed and untreated.
- While nearly all women received antenatal care from a nurse, most did not present for their first appointment until after the first trimester.

- Routine antenatal tests were variable, with over half being tested for HIV during pregnancy.
- One-quarter of women described their last pregnancy as unwanted; 11 per cent were currently using family planning methods.
- Sixty per cent of children were reported to have a registered birth certificate.
- Nearly 100 per cent of mothers reported breastfeeding their baby in the first day.
- Almost one quarter of children in the age group 12–23 months had not received any vaccinations.
- Over one-third of the children in our survey under the age of five years needed to access health care in the 12 months before the survey.
- A significant 58 per cent of children under five years were found to have stunting, with 19 per cent being severely stunted.
- Over a third of children under the age of five years were found to be underweight (513) and almost a fifth wasted (237).

The prevalence levels reported for stunting, wasting and being underweight are considered to be very high, based on the World Health Organization cut off values for public health significance.[1] While a large proportion of stunting is across all regions, the South bears a slightly higher burden.

The data are continuing to be analysed and priority areas identified in consultation with the Bougainville government. Anthropometric data were collected for under-fives including weight, height and circumference of the middle arm and head. Similar data were obtained for mothers.

The survey provides vital information about livelihoods, including demographics, socioeconomic factors, cocoa markets, health, nutritional status, agriculture and more. Hubs are being established with hub managers employed in each of the three regions.

The main challenge facing the project related to combining health and agriculture. Agricultural aid projects, until this one, did not include

---

1   WHO. Nutrition Landscape Information System (NLIS) Country Profile Indicators. Available at http://bit.ly/2Aw3sKU.

a health component. Careful explanation of One Health concepts and the relationship between nutrition, health and productivity as well as strong support from the research team for maintaining the health and nutrition components eventually saw the funding authority embrace the benefits of such a multidisciplinary approach.

In 2019 The Australia Indonesia Centre funded a pilot study of the Village Livelihood Program.

Acknowledgements

This six-year, 6-million-dollar project is funded by the Australian Centre for International Agricultural Research (2016–22).

Case study 2: Sustainability and profitability of cocoa-based farming systems in Indonesia

Merrilyn Walton, David Guest, Peter McMahon, Nunung Nuryartono, Grant Vinning, Jenny-Ann Toribio, Kim-Yen Phan-Thien, Sudirman Nasir, Andiimam Arundhana and Dian Sidik Arsyad

Partners

University of Sydney (School of Life and Environmental Sciences & School of Public Health)

Institut Pertanian Bogor (International Center for Applied Finance and Economics)

Hasanuddin University Faculty of Public Health

The problem being addressed

Improving the productivity of the Indonesian cocoa industry is a high priority within the national agricultural policy portfolio. The multiple causes of the significant drop in production since 2011 include price volatility and uncertainty, limited financial literacy, labour shortages resulting from outside employment, poor farmer health and nutrition,

Decade	Average % growth of cocoa planting area	Average % growth of productivity
1967–1975	0.045	0.138
1976–1985	0.192	0.055
1985–1995	0.222	0.038
1996–2005	0.073	0.037
2005–2015	0.040	-0.041

Table 7.1. Per cent increases in cocoa planting area and productivity for each decade between 1967 and 2015. Source: Unpublished data from Nuryartono and Khumaida (2016)

outmoded farm management (over 85 per cent of farmers are smallholders utilising non-intensive and poor management practices), ageing cocoa trees and the depletion of soil nutrients (forest rent). Because these farmers harvest cocoa worth only around US$600 annually at current prices (IPB survey data, Neilson, Palinrungi, Muhammad and Fauziah 2011), farmers often supplement their income by undertaking work off-farm, and cultivate crops with higher short-term returns.

Indonesian cocoa production since the 1980s has been dominated by an unsustainable boom in smallholder plantings in Sulawesi and a parallel decline in productivity as forest rent becomes exhausted (Table 7.1; Ruf 1987; Akiyama and Nishio 1996).

Aims and objectives

This 18-month project examined opportunities to improve the profitability of cocoa farming in Indonesia and was funded by the Australia–Indonesia Centre (AIC). Included in the project was a critical evaluation of existing and past activities, such as the US$450 million GERNAS-Kakao program (2009–2014), constraints to technology adoption and opportunities for diversification, value chain development, and de-commoditised marketing.

Objective 1

- A comparative analysis between Australia, PNG and Indonesia to understand the constraints and opportunities facing cocoa-based value chains in order to support management and policy recommendations to lift farmer and value chain productivity and profitability.
- A comprehensive review of the literature on farmer livelihoods, diets and health, incomes from crops and livestock, inclusion of women and youth, local and global industry trends, government policy impacts (including GERNAS and the cocoa export tax), and opportunities for adding value through processing and diversification, and improving the efficiency of value chains. Similar data from other countries in the region (Australia and PNG) was obtained to enable comparative analysis, particularly in relation to the impacts of health and diet on agricultural productivity.
- Baseline livelihood surveys and interviews of cocoa farmers and stakeholders to identify constraints and opportunities for diversified value chains to improve the sustainability and profitability of cocoa-based farming systems. Profitability, wellbeing and resilience of communities participating in the following can be compared:
  - diversification programs, e.g. cocoa and goat mixed farming
  - agricultural improvement programs, e.g. cocoa fertiliser trials
  - professionalisation programs, e.g. Mars Cocoa Development Centre program and Mondelez International Cocoa Life program.

Objective 2

- Investigate constraints and opportunities to incorporating small livestock such as goats for compost production, meat, kids and milk at the Mapili demonstration site
- Compare the economic viability of fermented vs unfermented cocoa
- Compare the economic viability of the industrialisation of cocoa production in Indonesia and Australia
- Identify opportunities for satellite businesses and micro-entrepreneurship resulting from diversification

- Identify opportunities for the employment of youth and women resulting from diversification.

Objective 3

- Conduct a baseline survey of health status in cocoa-producing villages
- Develop programs to improve access to better nutrition and maternal health
- Develop a training package for Village Healthy Living Advocates.

Getting the right team together

The team comprised agricultural, food and veterinary scientists, economists and public health practitioners. The team members had each worked previously with at least one member of the team, but this was the first time they all worked together on the same interdisciplinary project.

Engaging with communities

Prior to the study several members of the team held community consultations with the cocoa-farming communities in Sulawesi to ascertain their concerns about cocoa production and health. The study site at Polewali Mandar was chosen because farmers in this area have been exposed to over 30 government and NGO development projects over the past decade, including a series of ACIAR projects involving members of the current team (Hafid and McKenzie 2012). The main healthcare concerns villagers experienced included: respiratory tract infections, tuberculosis diagnosis and management, type 2 diabetes, lack of antenatal services, lack of women's health services, and poor understanding of sanitation and public health.

In addition, the late presentation of children with fever to a health service is not uncommon as parents typically treat their children with traditional medicines. They seek healthcare when there are signs of severe fever (dehydration and reduced consciousness) but the delayed treatment often impacts on the effectiveness of medical interventions.

Healthcare facilities include the Pustu (Puskesmas *Pembantu*; village level health centre), which provides perinatal and midwifery services free of charge. The Pustu is also equipped to treat fevers with paracetamol and respiratory infections with co-trimoxazole. Vaccination of the population using the national PPI program is also coordinated by the Pustu. The *Puskemas* (*Pusat Kesehatan Masyarakat*; sub-district level health centre) provide more advanced services including reviews by medical staff, basic emergency care, dentistry and basic laboratory facilities. First-line TB treatment is coordinated by the Puskesmas. Both facilities identify training as a significant issue.

Funding

Prior to receiving funding from the Australia–Indonesia Centre in 2016 the research team had previously applied for funding from many national and international funding bodies (2013–2015) unsuccessfully. The most common response was that our holistic approach extended beyond the disciplinary mandate of the funding agency, and may overlap with other programs.

Method

Our mixed methods project provided quantitative data as well as contextual information (qualitative) as both are necessary to address the concerns of local communities. The objectives were:

1. A literature review to highlight issues affecting the cocoa value chain within Indonesia, including export relations with key importers and strategies adopted by other cocoa producers.
2. Key informant interviews (KII) with government health, livestock and agricultural extension staff, international cocoa companies and other stakeholders concerned with cocoa sustainability in Indonesia using semi-structured guidelines.
3. An analysis of the impact of the cocoa export tax on the value chain and farmer prices based on published reports and interviews with local cocoa processors and government staff.
4. Two village surveys based on household interviews, which provided baseline data on health and economic livelihood in

communities dependent on cocoa in Polewali Mandar District, a major centre of cocoa production.

5. Development of a Livelihood Curriculum based on survey data and KII to provide guidelines for training village health volunteers and cocoa/farm management volunteers.

6. A cost-benefit analysis of a working mixed farm in a case study of farm diversification, including a trial to reduce kid pre-weaning deaths (by a Sydney Masters candidate).

7. Further project studies based on the village surveys on financial knowledge, technical efficiency, effect of consumption and farming practice on rural carbon footprints and nutritional awareness and behaviour (by Masters and fourth-year students).

8. Two studies on consumer perceptions of niche chocolate and the possibilities for a market for single origin chocolate using sensory flavour evaluation and chemical analysis (by a Sydney-based Honours student).

9. Workshop presentations on project findings to government stakeholders and the Cocoa Sustainability Partnership to obtain feedback and develop recommendations arising from the project.

Village surveys

The Livelihood questionnaire developed for the ARoB (previous case study) was used to capture baseline data for this project. Baseline data were collected from four cocoa-farming villages in the subdistricts of Mapilli and Anreapi, Polewali Mandar District, West Sulawesi Province. Villages dependent on raw cocoa bean sales for community livelihoods were selected for purposive sampling. Half were regarded as either relatively remote while the remainder had easier access to nearby town centres. Households were selected randomly but were excluded if their main income source was not cocoa. Household members were interviewed to elucidate their main livelihood and health issues, access to health services and constraints to productivity. Responses were recorded on tablets. Anthropometric data were collected for under-fives including, weight, height and circumference of the middle arm and head. Similar data was obtained for mothers. A further survey of the same four villages using a comprehensive (open) questionnaire provided more details on economic livelihood and further data for Masters project studies. For these individual studies students developed their own questionnaires.

In addition to the systematic literature review on livelihoods, crops, livestock and health for selected cocoa-farming communities in Sulawesi, we analysed the status of the Indonesian cocoa industry, value chains, fermentation, processing, livestock enterprises as well as diet and main health indicators for the farmer population. We also reviewed the indicators of human nutrition and health as constraints to rural labour productivity in Indonesia and Australia, including associations between dietary quality (nutritional adequacy and dominance of high-mycotoxin risk foods), health and impact on livelihoods.

The introduction of mixed cocoa/goat enterprises potentially present an additional source of microbial contamination. This requires consideration in respect to the composting of manures, proximity to water sources, and contamination of cocoa or other crops (e.g. vegetables), as well as hand hygiene practices.

Data obtained from baseline and follow-up interviews on livelihoods and community health included measures for the following:

- Farm-level cocoa-farming practices
- Farm-level cocoa bean fermentation and drying
- Industry-level cocoa bean fermentation and drying and processing
- Farm-level cocoa, goat and food crop production
- Market for cocoa, goats and food crops
- Household-level labour productivity and availability, cocoa production levels and income sourced from cocoa production
- Household diets
- Household sanitary practices
- Extent of stunting and under- and over-nutrition
- Household-level sick days lost to productivity and school attendance
- Impact analysis will be applied by using econometric modelling to measure different observed variables between communities.

From the literature review, surveys and interviews we identified and evaluated a number of opportunities and interventions for cocoa-farming diversification.

Outcomes

Cocoa farm productivity, and as a consequence family farm livelihood, has been declining due to a complex set of factors. Far from becoming the largest cocoa producer globally (a goal set by the government of Indonesia), Indonesia could soon fall from its current position as the third largest cocoa producer. The majority of smallholder farmers produced 400 kg or less dry beans per year on their 1 ha farms and relied on cocoa as their sole source of farm income (Neilson et al. 2011, IPB). Thus, their income from cocoa is approximately $600 annually, and farmers need to undertake off-farm employment or plant alternative crops to support their families. Because farmers spend less time managing their cocoa, this workload is neglected, delegated to women (adding to their workloads and feminising agriculture), or left to less experienced youth.

We have identified market uncertainty, poor financial literacy, ageing farmer populations, poor rural health and nutrition as reasons for declining investment in cocoa. This project has explored approaches to improve livelihoods by integrating farming systems (reducing costs) and providing supplementary sources of income, sustainable production practices, including pest and disease management, connecting market demands and improved quality and pricing recommendations to reduce income uncertainty.

A value chain study conducted under this project at IPB indicated that price uncertainty influenced farmers and acted as a deterrent to capital and labour investments. In addition, land ownership was a key factor in access to finance, and certificates of ownership encouraged youth engagement.

We are working closely with health authorities to improve the focus and delivery of health services for smallholder cocoa farmers. The project has identified significant gaps in:

• health extension, particularly in knowledge underpinning key recommended practices
• eye and mental health
• early detection of infections, especially in children
• malnutrition
• how to address increasing incidence of non-communicable disease.

A curriculum for a village volunteer livelihood program was completed. A similar curriculum for cocoa/farm management was developed. The framework of the curriculum, which consists of different training modules, was discussed in detail with district health staff in November 2017 and 2018 during visits to Polewali Mandar by the Sydney team and staff from Hasanuddin University. The curriculum is based on key areas of farming and healthcare: preventive healthcare, infectious diseases, medication, eye health, nutrition, family planning and health promotion, and outlines practical activities at the village level to address these. The main targets of the program are village volunteers (known as kadre) who assist the government midwives based in most villages. Interviews conducted with current volunteers showed a high level of commitment, but a lack of training and knowledge regarding the causes of various health problems. The village volunteer livelihood program is being converted to a mobile phone application (mobile phone is the main form of distance communication in rural areas). Further funding from the Australia–Indonesia Centre has been obtained to pilot the Village volunteer livelihood program.

Summary of results

- Price volatility was a major deterrent to farmer investments in agricultural inputs and management practices.
- Fluctuations in international price were transmitted directly to farmer and domestic prices and, additionally, price variation was greater at the farmer level, demonstrating that investments by farmers bear higher risks than downstream players.
- Increased production requires intensification as new land for expansion of cocoa planting is restricted.
- Numerous training programs have increased farmer knowledge on Good Agriculture Practice (GAP), but the implementation of this training is limited by lack of capital for investment into planting material, fertilisers and extra labour to apply management strategies.
- Youth are not attracted to cocoa farming.
- Access to formal finance is a key constraint.

- Smallholders may use available funds to purchase new planting material but expenditure on chemical inputs and labour to intensify cocoa production is negligible.
- Technical efficiency scores are low.
- The study demonstrated access to finance is improved by financial literacy.
- Household income was higher on farms that had diversified into other crops.
- Evaluation of a mixed farm (cocoa/goat) model based demonstrated efficient use of resources and favourable cost/benefit ratios. (However, this requires capital to establish goat herd and shed, and access to capital is limited).
- The study found that premiums for fermented beans are inadequate as large trader/processors import fermented beans and source unfermented beans in Indonesia for cocoa butter and powder.

Health findings

- Health constraints to productivity were demonstrated in Polewali-Mandar, supporting the WHO-DALY estimates of substantial losses in labour productivity due to poor health and nutrition.
- Key health issues detected were:
  - high blood pressure (34.5 per cent of a subsample of adult males; 30 per cent reported by the District Health office for pregnant mothers, higher than the national average)
  - undernutrition (26.3 per cent) and malnutrition (23.7 per cent) in young children, high rates of adult obesity (31.4 per cent in females and 24.1 per cent in males)
  - joint pain (24.8 per cent in women and 30.1 per cent in men).
  - high rates of blurred vision (19.1 per cent in women and 33.1 per cent in men)
  - over 80 per cent of both genders had never had an eye examination
  - few resources are available for mental health patients
  - a high proportion of households accessed open or unprotected water sources and either lacked or had only shared access to, a latrine

- dietary diversity (especially important for young children) was low and daily consumption of vegetables was only 53.4 per cent in adult males
- gender roles are separated on cocoa farms and women generally do not attend training programs, yet they performed key roles in harvesting, drying and selling to collectors.

The results of the survey in regard to health and nutrition were similar to results from other similar surveys of cocoa farmers in Ethiopia, Cote d' Ivoire and Bougainville.

The research has also identified priority areas for further research which will be discussed with the cocoa-farming communities.

Acknowledgement

This 18-month project was funded by the Australia–Indonesia Centre (2016–18).

Case study 3: *Salmonella* Brandenburg – a One Health team approach to controlling an emerging animal and human pathogen

Stan Fenwick

Identifying the problem to be addressed

Prior to 1996, *Salmonella* outbreaks were recorded sporadically in sheep flocks in New Zealand (NZ), causing significant economic losses due to diarrhoea, abortions and deaths, with *S. Typhimurium* and *S. Hindmarsh* the principal serovars involved. Factors involved with outbreaks included periods of high stocking density, inclement weather and poor husbandry. A killed trivalent vaccine released in the 1980s (Salvexin, Schering-Plough; containing *S. Typhimurium*, *S. Hindmarsh* and *S. Bovismorbificans*) had been developed to control the disease in sheep and cattle, and this was widely used by sheep farmers in the country.

The situation changed in 1996 when a sheep farm in Mid Canterbury, in the South Island of NZ, experienced an outbreak of abortions and deaths in pregnant ewes. From that first farm, epidemics of abortions and deaths spread to other nearby farms in 1997 and by 1998 south to Otago and Southland, linked to the transport of sheep for grazing between drought-affected Canterbury and the southern provinces. Typically, around 5 per cent of ewes aborted on affected farms. *Salmonella* Brandenburg (SB), a previously uncommon isolate recovered from sporadic infections in NZ sheep, was identified as the causative organism. At the peak of the epidemic, from 1999 to 2001, over 900 farms and thousands of sheep were affected across the three regions. Economic losses were estimated at around $10,000 per farm per year. During the epidemic, sporadic cases were also seen in cattle and other animals, including cats, dogs, deer, goats, pigs, poultry, wild birds and horses. While sporadic cases were seen regularly in cattle during the epidemic peak, outbreaks in cattle gradually became more common in Southland, a primary dairy area, causing significant economic losses. Outbreaks mostly occurred in late winter to early spring, when management practices prior to the lambing period, and adverse environmental conditions, contributed to high levels of contamination and ease of transmission. Outbreak peaks appeared to be cyclical, with the highest number of affected farms in 1999–2000, and smaller peaks in 2005 and 2010. The cyclic five-year pattern was thought to be due to waning flock immunity. The disease has now become endemic in the lower South Island but interestingly has rarely been seen in other sheep farming regions of the country. Sporadic cases have been reported in the North Island, principally in veal calves, but the organism has not become established.

In addition to the effect on farm animals, SB also became an important direct zoonosis with well-defined occupational risks, which indirectly affected family members. Prior to 1996, SB was an infrequent human pathogen in NZ (around 25 cases of food poisoning per year), but a marked increase in human cases was recorded in 1998 (134 cases per year) and remained high during the epidemic years. Human cases peaked during the lambing and calving periods, from September to November, coincident with animal outbreaks. Typically, *Salmonella* infections in NZ peak in the late summer months and are largely food-borne. From 1998–2002 over 550 SB cases were notified in affected regions, approximately a fifth of the total *Salmonella* isolations from the southern South Island. Many rural workers, including veterinarians and their families, were affected. *Salmonella* Brandenburg became the predominant isolate at Southland hospital from 1997, with many isolations from extra-intestinal sites indicating invasive disease.

Getting the right team together

The evolution of a One Health team to combat the disease began gradually, with different members and stakeholders joining the outbreak response team over the first 1–2 years, adopting many different roles. Initially the disease was predominantly a sheep issue and the team thus involved farmers and large animal veterinary practitioners from affected areas, and veterinarians and laboratory scientists from the Ministry of Agriculture, Forestry and Fisheries (MAFF) regional centres in Canterbury and Otago. Once the organism responsible for the disease had been identified as *Salmonella*, scientists at the Ministry of Health (MOH) enteric reference group at the Centers for Disease Control (CDC) were involved in serotyping of the isolates. Coincidentally, staff from the microbiology laboratory at the Institute of Veterinary and Biomedical Sciences (IVABS), Massey University, became involved in molecular typing of isolates from animals at this stage and developed close links with CDC, sharing information over the next few years. Massey's involvement came about as a result of prior professional linkages with Schering-Plough, the veterinary pharmaceutical company responsible for the development and marketing of Salvexin, the original *Salmonella* vaccine sold in NZ.

Once the outbreaks had been confirmed as salmonellosis, farmers who were concerned that the vaccine they were using had somehow become ineffective initially criticised Schering-Plough. After the strain had been defined as SB, however, it was acknowledged by the scientific community that cross-immunity to the outbreak strain from the killed vaccine was lacking and that the only possible solution was to include the new strain in a multivalent vaccine. This is usually a long and formidable process involving significant R&D efforts, including small-scale efficacy and safety trials, government approval, scaling up to commercial vaccine production, product registration, marketing etc.; however, the severity of the outbreak and its effect on both humans and animals launched an unprecedented, multidisciplinary campaign to fast-track the procedures. From the outset, Schering-Plough worked closely with scientists and veterinarians from Massey University and MAFF, and also with private practitioners from affected areas, to conduct research into the efficacy of a vaccine including SB antigens. Initial experiments were performed in mice, and subsequently in sheep, and the results were encouraging enough to involve rapid commercialisation and field trials. Salvexin-B was approved and launched in 2000, 3–4 years after the initial cases had appeared.

In parallel with the multidisciplinary approach to combat the animal disease, the concomitant increase in human infections resulted in the team expanding to include members of the medical profession. Medical laboratory scientists, doctors, public health workers and epidemiologists from the hospitals, health departments and laboratories in the affected areas, and from central government, were all involved, interacting closely with their animal health and industry colleagues. This rapid and successful embracing of a One Health approach to this new disease may have been facilitated in NZ due to the prior efforts of a very farsighted epidemiologist from Massey University, Professor David Blackmore, who at least 10 years earlier had persuaded two key ministries (MOH and MAFF) to co-fund the Veterinary Human Health Advisory Group (VHHAG) to convene and share information on zoonotic diseases in the country on a regular basis. The group included representatives from many stakeholder groups involved in detection, prevention, control and research into key zoonoses in NZ, and its genesis was inspired by high levels of leptospirosis and brucellosis affecting employees in the animal industries. This body helped to smooth the way for quick and efficient collaboration and information sharing across disciplines in response to the outbreak.

Following the initial outbreak response, members of the team expanded to include scientists researching many other aspects of the disease, from microbiology to field epidemiology. Central government also became involved in research efforts due to the knock-on effect that the disease had on NZ sheep meat exports. Reports from Spain that SB had been found in NZ sheep meat resulted in several countries in Europe placing a temporary ban on imports, with severe economic ramifications for the NZ sheep industry, including farmers, abattoirs and meat exporters. A large quantitative risk analysis (QRA) was performed to examine the safety of NZ sheep meat in order to provide information to persuade overseas governments to revoke the ban. The QRA, which examined the microbiological risks from farm to carcass, involved a strong multidisciplinary effort including laboratory and field staff from MAFF and IVABS, veterinary practitioners, farmers and abattoir workers.

Other major research efforts involved identification of risk factors for spread of the disease, and environmental scientists and wildlife biologists from the Department of Conservation became important partners. Results of the research provided strong evidence for the role of wild birds in transmission between farms, principally black-backed seagulls scavenging on aborted foetuses and dead sheep, and also for contamination of waterways linking farms by birds and pasture runoff. Examination of seagull gut contents revealed very high levels of *Salmonella* carriage with no signs of illness.

Importantly, examination of isolates from all affected regions, and from multiple animal species and humans by the Massey IVABS group, in collaboration with the enteric reference laboratory at the Centers for Disease Control (CDC), showed that the *Salmonella* Brandenburg outbreak strain was clonal and very stable, i.e. all strains were identical using DNA fingerprinting technology and the fingerprint of the outbreak strain did not alter over many years. Looking retrospectively at historical SB isolates from a collection of CDC showed that the clone was markedly different from previous isolates of the serotype from food-borne infections prior to the outbreak. This encouraged intense speculation on the source of the novel strain (e.g. overseas travellers, sewage, seagulls, migratory birds) as well as providing justification for inclusion of the outbreak strain in the newly developed vaccine.

It is important to note that, throughout the outbreak years, research results continued to be shared rapidly between sectors and they were used to support the development of appropriate control measures and to provide advice to farmers and other stakeholders to limit the spread of the disease and the risk of human infections.

Engaging with communities

One Health is a movement that emphasises the importance of collaboaration by multiple disciplines to solve complex health problems, and response to this outbreak was distinguished by the strong co-operation of many sectors, including public and private sectors and local communities. Communication about the outbreak, its cause, risk factors and prevention and control measures took place at multiple levels during the first year of the outbreak. Most importantly, considerable efforts were made by multidisciplinary teams to engage directly with affected communities, especially farmers, veterinary and medical practitioners and other stakeholders. The outbreak peaked between 1998 and 1999 in the southern South Island provinces of Otago and Southland, and the scale of the problem affecting sheep farming communities led to rapid appeals for assistance from the veterinary profession, the pharmaceutical industry and the government. Schering-Plough responded quickly by providing financial support for multidisciplinary teams, including government, university and private practice veterinarians and government and private medical practitioners and microbiologists, to travel to affected areas to hold a series of town hall meetings to deliver information about the disease. Several hundred affected farmers attended the meetings and many heart-breaking stories of farms and families seriously affected by the disease were recounted. Despite limited information in the early stages of the outbreak, the different disciplines in the team provided relevant information on the origins of the disease, how the disease had progressed south from Canterbury, how it was being spread locally, how people were likely becoming infected and appropriate biosecurity, hygiene and management measures required to limit animal and zoonotic transmission. While the mood of the meetings was often tense, with particular concern about the lack of protection provided by Salvexin, local farmers and veterinarians were on the whole very pleased at the rapid response by the multiple sectors.

Following the meetings, numerous visits were also made to local veterinary practices to discuss control measures and risk factors in more detail so that the best advice could be provided to clients. At least three key veterinary practices were involved with the team and over the following months provided regular updates to agricultural communities via newsletters and farm visits. Further meetings by the OH team were held over the first couple of years to discuss new knowledge from research, to report progress on development of a new vaccine and finally to launch the new vaccine and to discuss its efficacy and usage. By engaging the community early in the piece, considerable goodwill was developed, and farmers rapidly adopted recommended control measures with some success.

In addition to communities, communication with other stakeholders, including government agencies, meat industry leaders and the veterinary and medical professions, was achieved by meetings, conferences, journal papers and media announcements. Engaging with the media early in the outbreak was an important task, as sharing relevant scientific information prevented innuendo and supposition and encouraged responsible journalism; in effect local newspaper journalists also became de facto members of the outbreak response team.

Funding the project

As this was a very complex outbreak involving multiple stakeholders, funding came from a number of different sources and for many different pieces of the puzzle. After the initial outbreak had been investigated by government agencies, Schering-Plough put a considerable amount of funding into veterinary practices to investigate the disease on individual farms and to support meetings to communicate findings with farmers and veterinarians in the affected regions. They also funded a substantial amount of research into many aspects of the disease. Although they were a commercial pharmaceutical company, the senior management in NZ felt a sense of social responsibility to the farmers and veterinary practices that had been their clients for many years, in particular as they were the only company promoting a *Salmonella* vaccine in NZ.

Once a decision had been made by the company to include SB in the Salvexin vaccine (and this involved a lot of technical meetings and discussions on feasibility and costs), Schering-Plough invested a large amount of money to fund the vital research to develop and test the vaccine. This research was performed at Massey University in the North

Island of NZ where good facilities existed for the series of experiments that needed to be conducted in mice and sheep to assess efficacy and safety and to provide data for product registration. Costs of the research were significant, in particular because the experiments had to be carried out following very strict biosecurity standards in order to avoid release of SB into the environment, with subsequent risk of spread to sheep producing regions outside the affected zones.

Recognising the importance of the disease for the economy and human health, the NZ government provided funding for research into the epidemiology of the disease, in particular the work to define the risk factors for maintenance and transmission of the organism. Once issues had arisen over the finding of SB in exports of sheep meat, the government also funded the large and complex QRA designed to provide information to importing countries on product safety.

Veterinary practices and Massey University also provided funding, through research grant allocation, and in-kind contributions. Although this was on a smaller scale and largely invisible, a number of university scientists, and veterinary practitioners in the affected regions, put a considerable amount of time and effort into working with farmers impacted by the disease, often pro bono, and with a sense of social responsibility to the communities they worked in.

Methods used

As might be imagined, over the course of the initial years of the outbreak a large number of methods were used to define and investigate the problem. At the outset, these were largely microbiological and epidemiological; however, later molecular biological methods, risk analysis, behaviour change communication, animal experimentation, pathology and environmental science methodologies were used to elucidate different aspects of the disease.

Outcomes and legacy

The outcomes of the One Health collaboration were perhaps slow to develop, but given the scale of the problem and the human, animal and environmental factors at play, this was understandable. Due to the efforts of a number of key team members, farmers put in place effective control measures that gradually resulted in the decline of the outbreak. Farmers' awareness of the issues was raised considerably by the strong emphasis that the team placed on communication, and this paid dividends as flock management strategies were changed to combat the disease and human cases dropped. Improving farm management and biosecurity had obvious flow-on benefits for the control of other endemic diseases, and this too could be considered a very good outcome.

Obviously one tangible legacy was the development of an improved, effective vaccine that could be used to control the disease, although the vaccine alone was not sufficient, and many other good management practices needed to be adopted by farmers. The combined efforts required to bring the vaccine to commercialisation showed that, in a crisis, working together is vital, and kudos must go to the many people involved in the process.

Although the disease had severe economic effects for many farmers, it also helped to strengthen community bonds in affected areas, by bringing together all the stakeholders and giving each of them a voice. This was a major outcome of the successful One Health approach that was quickly and efficiently put into effect following the outbreak and involving communities from the beginning helped to break down barriers that might have previously existed between professions and the many people affected by the disease.

In conclusion, the disease was not eradicated completely and *Salmonella* Brandenburg has become endemic, with limited numbers of cases seen each year in sheep and cattle. On the bright side, the disease has been contained to the lower South Island, and farmers have learned to live with the situation and to take effective measures to respond to cases as they arise. This was probably the largest outbreak of *Salmonella* recorded in animals worldwide and only the success of the prompt and efficient One Health response, involving multiple sectors and disciplines, prevented it from spreading to other sheep-rearing regions of New Zealand and probably globally.

Case study 4: The role of tradition in Aboriginal wellbeing

Paul Memmott

This chapter is catalysed by the continuing lack of success[2] in addressing the multifaceted disadvantage within modern Australian Aboriginal communities despite many policy shifts and goals, the most recent being the national 'Closing the Gap' policy. This disadvantage is reflected in the statistical measures and key performance indicators (KPIs) of modern neoliberal government bureaucracy such as life expectancy, incidence of life threatening diseases and risks (e.g. foetal alcohol syndrome, kidney failure, heart disease), child development vulnerability, mental health, unemployment, household crowding, substance abuse, self-injury, suicide, family violence (multiple forms), Indigenous crime rates, imprisonment, homelessness, school dropout etc. The constant framing of Aboriginal wellbeing in deficit values reflecting national standards of citizen status and conditionality, and the failure to view the circumstances from an Aboriginal leadership and cultural perspective, tends to mask, even drown, the positive attributes within Aboriginal societies and communities that can act as a community-driven platform from which to contribute strong social capital to address these issues.

Thus, this chapter attempts to model a good-practice case study on how an Aboriginal agency can establish, evolve and grow incrementally without sacrificing its independence, integrity and vision and drawing selectively on Aboriginal cultural traditions and values as drivers within the modern intercultural context of Australian society. This is despite the tendency for successive governments to impose top–down, 'we-know-best' policies that stifle grassroots, community-driven approaches. Government resources and short-term problem-solving processes are inadequate to readily solve interconnected labyrinths of health, social, economic and psychological problems; a more holistic sustainable approach that is community-value driven and community-owned is required. This quandary can be partly informed by accurate understanding of Aboriginal contact history processes for specific

---

2   According to state or federal government political time-frames since c.1893 or c.1970 depending on one's perspective.

groups and regions, and how over many decades such histories have generated longitudinal problems within Aboriginal families and societies with successive dysfunctional enculturations in descending generations that become increasingly difficult to arrest and reverse. For example, underlying the historical problems in this case study region from 1860 include disease, massacres, slave labour (30 years), decimation, taking of country, total life control (from 1898 until the mid-1970s) under the Aboriginal Acts, poor nutrition, removal to penal settlements, breakdown of social leadership cohesion and values, indentured labour for 75 years, which eventually reversed to widespread unemployment and welfare benefit dependency in the early 1970s.

Contemporary good-practice Aboriginal agencies are vexed by constantly changing governments and policies as well as inter-family and inter-group Aboriginal politics (forms of lateral violence) driven by the competition for scarce resources, rival Native Title claims and subsequent monetary distributions by developers to self-forwarding traditional owners, and inherent family nepotism mitigating against collective advancement. Thus, the way politics of tradition are operationalised may be either positive or negative towards social wellbeing and unfortunately, as witnessed by those in the Native Title industry, the latter outcome is all too common.

A recurring problem for government and Aboriginal agencies alike is where to intervene in this labyrinth. Housing, health and leadership have each been suggested as a priority. Referred to as the 'Aboriginal problem wheel' since the early 1970s, this challenge continues to vex. This case study I present has particular cultural, regional and economic contexts, but it is only one path among many simultaneously occurring in other Australian local contexts. The aim is to distil good-practice principles that can be applied and tested across the continent. Knowledge of this case study draws from action research, the author (an anthropologist and transdisciplinary researcher) having had multiple roles in the case-study agency since, and even before, its establishment.

The Indjilandji-Dhidhanu case study

This case study[3] starts with an extended family of Indjilandji-Dhidhanu people ('Indjilandji' for short) from the upper Georgina River basin, who have a commitment to Aboriginal identity and connection to tribal land and the opportunity to gain recognition for such through Native Title. They recognised that their strategic political expression of tradition could drive economic opportunity through the advantageous leverage off ILUAs (Indigenous Land Use Agreements) under the *Native Title Act*.

However, the commitment to Aboriginality was not something easily understood given the nature of colonial violence and oppression in the region since 1861. In preparing the historic-anthropological analysis for the Federal Court (Memmott 2010a), it became apparent that only one extant clan of Indjilandji-Dhidhanu people remained on country out of an estimate of 12 or so clans who were present at the time of arrival of the first colonial exploring party led by William Landsborough from the Gulf of Carpentaria (arriving December 1861). What happened to the other 11 clans? There was a complex history, initially violent during the first 60 years with the advent of the Native Mounted Police, but becoming more submissive for most of the 20th century primarily because of the *Aboriginals Protection and Restriction of Sale of Opium Act 1897*. This Act was administered by local police who instigated punitive removal of those who resisted compliance with its indentured labour requirements.

The single Indilandji clan group who managed to both survive and remain (with cultural connections) on country for 150 years, working as labourers and stock hands within the pastoral industry, became identified in the Federal Court proceedings as the *Idaya* Descent Group having descended from their ancestor *Idaya* who was alive when the first Europeans rode onto the Georgina basin at the start of the wet season in 1861 (the party of explorer William Landsborough). *Idaya's* great-great-grandson Colin Saltmere, a former Head Stockman and ATSIC Councillor, led the first self-funded Native Title claim in

---

3   This section of the paper is drawn from a number of previous publications by
     Memmott (2010b; 2012).

Australia (as opposed to government-funded through the National Native Title Tribunal). This strong sense of bush self-reliance and a life of stock-camp work ethic, combined with customary beliefs in Aboriginal Law, were basic ingredients in the development of the group's enterprise endeavour and practice style.

At the outset of their claim process (early 2000s), two significant regional economic opportunities arose in the Indjalandji country that provided income from ILUA agreements between the traditional owners and the development proponents. One was a proposed phosphate mine. The other was a state government upgrade of the Barkly Highway starting with a new bridge over the Georgina River at the border town of Camooweal. The ILUA agreement with the miner paid the professional fees to continue the Native Title claim, while the agreement with the Main Roads Department delivered a prefab donga work camp with dining room, kitchen, laundry, bore and electricity connection for an Aboriginal labour team. The mine never went ahead but the camp was named the Dugalunji Camp and became a base for successive road-building contracts. The Myuma Corporation gradually upskilled its team, recycled profits into plant purchase and a road-metal quarry and expanded its capital base. A strong partnership was established with Main Roads such that successive contracts for regional remote road maintenance are ongoing.

However, the Myuma Group (as it came to be known, with three constituent corporations soon established) understood the fickle nature of remote economies and diversified its forms of economic activity to establish a 'hybrid' economy (after Altman 2007) – see Box 7.2. One of the most successful enterprises is the establishment of a pre-vocational training scheme for young Aboriginal adults whereby industry groups, especially mining, pre-pay for up to 30 trainees at a time to undergo a 12 to 15-week course to prepare them for employment with a capacity to sustain themselves in the rigours of working life. (Many skills have to be included from basic construction tasks, to obtaining driving and plant licences, writing a CV, and workplace safety.)

While Myuma PL focused on making money, the second corporation, the Dugalunji Corporation, specialised in land management and cultural activities stemming from a strong customary ethic of caring for country. A Ranger Group was eventually formed

---

Box 7.2: The Hybrid Economy of Myuma Group (2005–18)

- Quarry products
- Road building and maintenance; road traffic control
- Road camp and mining camp village construction
- Painting and craft
- Cultural heritage clearances and inductions
- Pre-vocational training for construction and mining industries (60 to 70 trainees per year × 14 weeks). (Now 120 trainees per year × 12 weeks.)
- Prisoner workforce training
- Ranger training
- National Park management
- Fencing contracts
- Co-operative research with University of Queensland
- Remote Jobs Community Program (RJCP) – several regions in Queensland and Northern Territory
- Trade apprenticeship training
- Gas pipeline construction subcontractor.

---

and trained to provide land-care services on the Georgina basin. The Myuma Group's profits were recycled into building and expanding its Dugalunji Camp as well as allocations for regional charitable causes through its third corporation, Rainbow Gateway. Eventually, Rainbow Gateway became the vehicle for taking on the federal government regional contract of running the work-for-dole employment schemes (CDEP followed by RJCP).[4] At the time of writing, the Myuma Group had a turnover of over $15 million per annum from its various activities.

My context as researcher-author in this ethnographical essay

This summary history of the Myuma Group does not do justice to the complex evolution of this good-practice service delivery agency which

---

4   CDEP = Community Development Employment Program; RJCP = Remote Jobs and Communities Program.

is Aboriginal-owned, managed and majority staffed. The participation of white professionals to date has always been part of its commercial success story and the author is one of those persons. I commenced pure research in the region in the early 1970s, and after completing my PhD (which was a crossover from architecture into anthropology) established my own research consultancy in the early 1980s which was always dependent upon land claims and Native Title claims for income. In the early 2000s I was the expert anthropologist witness for the Indilandji-Dhidhanu claim as well as carrying out cultural heritage consultancies for the group; it brought lasting relationships with individuals covering three generations of the *Idaya* Descent Group. With the encouragement of Myuma leader Colin Saltmere we started a process of conceptual incubation which included my establishing cultural workshops in the pre-vocational courses that can number up to four courses per year. This led me into a role as the Dugalunji Camp anthropologist visiting Camooweal every month or two, enabling me to become a participant observer as applied in anthropological methodology. I became immersed into the Dugalunji Camp life seeking to understand what made it successful from the point of view of camp managers, the workers, and trainees.

Publications resulted from efforts to record and understand how Myuma's success story has unfolded (e.g. Memmott 2012). This case study analyses the three workshops regularly conducted for each group of trainees. Unpacking the curriculum which was heavily influenced by the needs of the Dugalunji Camp shows the relationship between the employment and the wellbeing of Aboriginal people in the camp. The curriculum today mirrors the camp's philosophy of integration of Aboriginal beliefs with the spiritual nature of country, psychological and social health of the workers and their connection to a sustainable workforce in the mainstream Australian economy. The potential for an empowering way out of the horrible circumstances of third or fourth generation welfare dependency that many of the incoming trainees have experienced becomes real.

The Dugalunji Camp training courses[5]

A trainee in the Dugalunji Camp may find themselves in a mixed-gender class of up to 30 individuals of whom some may come from that trainee's own home town or community, may even be related and/or with shared cultural understandings, while others come from elsewhere with diverse personalities and backgrounds. The one predictable feature is the shared sense of their Aboriginality, but how it manifests will vary. Senior training staff need to appreciate all Aboriginal/Islander cultural regions of Queensland and the types of cultural change processes they have experienced. The psychology and cultural make-up of a *Wik* trainee from Aurukun will be different from a rural town trainee from Western Queensland towns such as Dajarra or Boulia, and they in turn will be different again to a trainee from south-east Queensland towns such as Caboolture or Ipswich, or to a rainforest person from the Atherton Tableland. There remain recurring class or workshop occasions/compositions when all manner of such juxtapositions of diverse individuals occur. Because heterogeneity also reflects workplace environments, this situational context is a useful scenario in which to explore diverse worker values and behaviours and how to make sense of and develop personal operational capacity and team skills within such diverse settings.

In mid-2013, non-Aboriginal staff realised during a Myuma trainers' evaluation workshop that family violence experiences were the norm for the majority of trainees. Physical fights, strong abuse, attempted and actual suicides and sexual trauma were common experiences (true to the national statistical measures of these problems). This reflects the embeddedness of personal psychological and social dysfunction among many Aboriginal families and requires historical models of cultural change to understand the origin of this phenomenon, as well as explain it to the trainees so as to sensitise them to their personal and family problems. Creating a vision of opportunity for them to liberate themselves and their families from it to some extent is the goal; but at the very least to show them how their family

---

5 This section of the paper is based on reflexive analysis by the author from ten years of conducting these courses.

problems may undermine their employment and the need to build up their personal resilience.

The likelihood that trainees will have personal problems is high. Establishing the right environment where these issues can be identified and ameliorated requires a supportive and safe learning process within the Dugalunji Camp. The camp needs to simulate a mining or construction camp (in terms of time schedules, multi-tasking, drug and health checks, workplace safety) but one that is conducive for trainees to remain and grow psychologically. This requires an understanding of procedures for dealing with threats, with offensive behaviours, and for restoring confidence in managerial predictability. Creating an environment where people feel safe to respond to challenges will strengthen their self-confidence and identity. I refer to the complexity of the camp setting under Aboriginal leadership as an 'Aboriginal Behaviour Setting' in cross-cultural environmental psychology terms. An Indigenous Behaviour Setting involves recurring behaviour patterns in a set of culturally appropriate, designed, physical settings, such that there is a synomorphic relation or 'fit' between the human behaviour episodes that occur (with some dominance of Indigenous behaviour patterns in the various case studies) and the physical and temporal environments of the settings. They are largely controlled and managed by Indigenous people and have been designed by Indigenous leaders possibly in collaboration with an architect, to be comfortable and bring wellbeing for Indigenous clients or users. This is achieved through a combination of behavioural patterns and environmental (landscaping) features, artifactual features (built and loose structures, objects) and setting controls which are designed to be relatively comfortable, predictable, culturally secure and conducive for Indigenous people to use. There is also a sense of identity with and even ownership of such a system of settings by Indigenous people as well as of being centred in a cultural landscape. (after Memmott and Keys 2016)

Critical in this setting are clear rules and consequences and clarity about complaints and grievances from trainees or staff. At the Dugalunji Camp, complaints can be confidential and made to senior staff any time. However, structured early morning pre-start meetings provide a forum for resolving concerns. The first meeting for staff (at 7 am) is an opportunity for discussing a trainee's discordant behaviour;

the second meeting for trainees and staff (at 7:30 am) allows issues to be raised in a spirit of communal debate, notwithstanding that senior Aboriginal staff make final decisions.

The promotion of the Dugalunji Camp as a safe place is at the forefront; mutual understanding and reinforcing of rules, goals and procedures provide daily opportunities for self-achievement. The idea of a safe place is central as a trainee may have never or rarely experienced a safe residential place, or had their own private room as in the Dugalunji Camp, which they are free to personalise.

Severe behaviour breaches occur infrequently but will involve the Managing Director (Colin Saltmere) who leads the group's pre-start meeting where the potential punishment will be discussed – either expulsion from the course and/or notification of police. He deals with less serious matters in a firm, slow, reiterative, serious but at times humorous way, often drawing on his experiences as a Head Stockman and an Aboriginal survivor in a once-racist town in order to draw out behavioural principles, boundaries and lessons for the offender and others present. This can also be an exercise in learning about appropriate values and behaviours; about the clarity and consistency of the Dugalunji Camp rules. The trainees' understanding of the rule system underpins the rarity of severe breaches.

Another critical training goal is strengthening personal self-confidence and self-esteem. A range of activities are designed to strengthen these attributes. Workshops over three days contain a set of messages, knowledge and activities designed to strengthen self-identity. Beginning with personal introductions, trainees describe their own community, mob or tribe. This is followed by a three-hour session about the complexity of contact history in Queensland including its historical traumatic phases, paying particular attention to the home communities of the trainees. This provides each one with knowledge about how the collisions of history disrupted the original harmonies of their classical tribal contexts and identities. This session aims to include everyone's particular circumstances whether *Wik* from Cape York, *Jirdabal* from the rainforest, stolen generation from institutional settings, urban upbringing at Inala or stock-working families from western towns.

Trainees begin to understand how their Elders lived under the Aboriginal Acts; the hardships and injustices, including the consequences of the Stolen Generations, Stolen Wages, and Deaths in Custody. This trauma is balanced with empowering understandings of land rights, native title, and flagship Aboriginal agencies. Sharing stories and providing contexts facilitates discussion about the trainees' ancestors respectively in missions, in government penal settlements such as Palm Island, and in pastoral camps and rural towns. In many cases I knew the grandparents or other relatives of the trainees which allows me to personalise aspects of their identity even more authentically.

Trainees participate in small groups to identify their home communities and name important people, places and historical events, sacred histories, Dreaming stories, sites, customs and then present their findings to the class. For many, motivation is high in this quest for identity concepts, and they are encouraged to phone relatives to find out about their cultural background. The depth of knowledge varies between individuals, with most being minimal. The reasons for this are explained and reinforced in the historical workshop as the impacts of frontier violence, disease, removal policies, splitting up of families and separation from country and how cultural transmission was broken down or forcefully prevented are discussed. This permits a social levelling which encourages a knowledgeable trainee (e.g. the Mornington Islander with songs and sacred histories and totems) to empathise with and be respectful towards the descendant of, for example, a Stolen Generation family who might have emotional difficulty in even naming their mob.

Field excursions into different local landscapes are interspersed to better understand hunter-gatherer lifestyle, cultural landscape, appropriate behaviour at sacred sites, and Ranger-led land management activities. The workshop titled Aboriginal Religion deals with the pan-Aboriginal belief in the Dreamtime, the origin of sacred sites, how they link to humans and the nature of totemism and ceremonial functions. This lays the groundwork for exploring kinship, social organisation and land tenure and the challenges of using such knowledge to win Native Title and Land Claims. This triggers more identity expression and development among individuals and produces rapport, mutual respect and a platform to tackle challenging activities on day three about family and domestic violence, substance abuse and other social problems.

The day-three workshop starts with an overview of violence in traditional Aboriginal societies and of the institutionalised nature of punishment that was controlled and normative. An historical overview of how this governance system was broken down by the historical contact processes, and how forms of longitudinal violence spread throughout Indigenous societies as leadership, social cohesion and moral values were dismantled, is balanced by outlining a range of effective initiatives taken by Aboriginal agencies in the modern era to tackle family violence in communities.

The aim is to develop trust so that trainees can freely express themselves and share their problems. For example, when the trainees are asked about experiencing suicide in the family, usually about half the class raise their hands. When an individual is overcome with grief, Aboriginal mentors care for them until they are ready to return to the class. This session ends with the trainees, working in small groups, preparing a violence plan to combat violence in a selected home community or town based on their profiling of the types and intensities of violence in those places. They present their plans to the class. This represents a fast-track way of moving from the emotional experience of victimhood, to knowledge of causal issues, to empowerment of planning solutions. This can end the training on a positive note, having created a prospect and vision for a future role in decreasing violence.

Another outcome from the workshops is for each trainee to create a model of personal development described in Box 7.3. Trainees move from learning new work skills that recognise and overcome personal problems to becoming a proactive team member; one who helps others with both their work and personal problems; and with the potential for leadership for some. This model of self-improvement also promotes a peer group support ethic which hopefully continues once the trainees graduate and leave the Dugalunji Camp (partly or largely sustained through social media communication techniques). Social media has the potential for individuals to be supported by their own alumni group. This peer-group resilience approach is a safety net due to the

Box 7.3 A set of attributes presented to the trainees at the Dugalunji Camp as a way to encourage and discuss reflection and a vision about self-development and empowerment (source: P. Memmott, Myuma teaching materials).

Skill sets (for me)	Skill sets for helping others
1. Work skills [you start here]	Teaching others 'work skills'
2. Problem-solving skills	Teaching others 'problem-solving skills'.
3. Self-help skills	Supporting those 'helping themselves'.
4. Help-seeking skills	Giving support to those who need help.
5. Change management skills	Giving support/guiding others to change their lives.
6. Team player skills	Being a good team player by way of example; and Mentoring younger team members.

uncertainty or unavailability of mentoring schemes. It forges social capital among the trainees (as well as with staff).

In the Violence Workshop, 12 forms of violence are covered in the community violence plan including psychological violence. This segues into a discussion on workplace bullying and racism with Aboriginal mentors recalling their worst experiences, but it also leads to interpersonal relations in the Dugalunji Camp. Subtle forms of offensive behaviours may be present – such as sexist behaviours between genders – providing the opportunity to discuss appropriate and non-appropriate behaviours around both verbal and body language and personal space, and to set values around such behaviours (including unwanted touching, repeated swearing). This connects to the workshop about kinship as traditional Aboriginal values around respect, avoidance and joking relationships, which are sanctioned between particular categories of people, revealing a non-Anglo-Australian (mainstream) position. It also relates to the skill set outlined in Box 7.3 of the need to recognise when 'I' have a problem and 'I' need to seek help, or the need to help others recognise 'they' have a problem. Due to the diversity of origins of trainees and the extent of dysfunctional sociality in their communities, these problems sometimes surface and must be managed, both for the wellbeing of camp life, the personal empowerment of the trainees and their capacity to cope in the regulated workplace of their future employment.

A major challenge for the Dugalunji Camp is to prepare Aboriginal and Islander trainees (who often suffer with personal health, social and psychological vulnerabilities) for an unpredictable workplace and build a level of personal strength, resilience and peer support to cope with recurring problems that can challenge one's holding down of a job. Other parts of the success formula have not been described or analysed here, including the entry screening process, the mentoring process, the management of personal accommodation, health, recreation, diet and cuisine, psychological counselling, time out for ceremonial or sorry business, coping with climatic extremes, and challenging workplace tasks. These deal with the ultimate personal change challenge and involve life goals, strengthening self-identity and self-confidence, moral values, and understanding teamwork and responsibilities. The Camooweal publican's wife summed up this process: 'when they arrive, they hang their head in shame and talk in a whisper; when they leave, they are looking me in the eye!'

As Myuma's portfolio expanded, the people attending the pre-vocational classes diversified. The implementation of an Inland Rivers Rangers team to carry out riverine management on the Georgina, Diamantina and Thomson basins brought trainee Aboriginal rangers into the mix. In recent years, Myuma policy required all new staff employed in one of the four corporations (a Prescribed Body Corporate formed) to participate in the three-day workshop by way of orientation. Workshops are also provided to consultants in regional developments that involve cultural heritage protection of Aboriginal sites (ranging from company directors to geologists and plant operators). Another group of young Aboriginal people attending workshop classes since 2016 are those selected for Myuma's Spinifex Project, a project illustrative of the creative and transdisciplinary approach embedded in Aboriginal values.

The Myuma Spinifex Project[6]

The Spinifex Project evolved from understandings of the traditional Aboriginal uses of this prickly hummock grass, considered a pest by many, and growing over a third of the continent. The most common traditional Aboriginal use of the hummocks was for cladding domes, forming a thick insulating and rain-repellent thatch. Some 29 of the species of *Triodia* exude a sticky gum which was used as a resin for hafting stone blades to timber handles and as a medicine for a range of ailments.

Inspired by these customary uses, Myuma developed a research partnership with the University of Queensland (UQ) to study the properties of these spinifex grasses, with a view to seeking one or more modern applications that might have commercial value, and to start a cottage industry of spinifex growing and harvesting for remote Aboriginal outstation groups. Recent neoliberal governments in Australia have pressured these groups to move away from their small settlements and relocate in regional cities where services can be centralised, housing can be more cheaply maintained and where a promise of employment beckons. However, bush economies are poor and jobs are scarce in most regional towns. Myuma is vigorously developing a bush economy using a hybrid (or mixed) economic approach. Similarly, small Aboriginal outstations need to develop several strands of seasonal income so that they might remain on country. Spinifex farming could potentially be such an opportunity. The persistent desire to stay on one's tribal country is driven by the spiritual values of remaining connected to one's Dreamings, sacred histories and sites, the sources of one's totemic being and identity.

Through 2007 to 2013, the UQ research team investigated all aspects of spinifex grass: its botany, ecology, species distribution, chemistry and material properties. Traditional shelters were built by Elders and climatic performance tested. Field plots were set up to try different methods of harvesting and study capacity for regrowth. Burning experiments were conducted to better understand the role of fire in environmental sustainability. Basic building applications were

---

6   This section of the paper is drawn from Memmott et al. (2017).

explored by architects such as reinforcing earth bricks, making insulation batts, manufacturing composite materials, and making coatings from the resin to protect timber from decay and white ant attack. In the university laboratories, nano-bio engineers began to move below the micro-level to the nano-level and to the eureka moment of discovery.

If one deconstructs the fibres through descending scales of fibrils, one isolates the nano-fibres which are smaller than the eye can see. And these nano-fibres are super-strong! They can be mixed in a liquid blend with other substances to make strong biodegradable products of international commercial value. At the time of writing, industry interest was being led by the recyclable paper manufacturers who could quadruple (or more) the strength of papers with the inclusion of a small percentage of nano-fibres; and also by the latex industry which was seeking an additive of nano-fibres for stronger thinner condoms and surgical gloves. At the rear of the Dugalunji Camp, a bioprocessing plant had been constructed in preparation for commercial production of nano-fibres. Research is ongoing concerning other commercial prospects of the fibres and resin. New work teams are forming. A prospect for a new remote bush economy is growing.

Strategic planning principles

Cultural enhancement and wellbeing for Aboriginal communities can be achieved through a strategic self-led, holistic development program (enterprise–employment–wellbeing–culture) that encapsulates the following principles:

- Grow capacity and projects organically and realistically at the local level.
- Identify Aboriginal social capital, both formal (whitefeller-style agencies) and informal (traditional kinship, land owning groups, ceremony links, skins). Consider how to design both forms of such capital into the strategic approach as foundational structure.
- Plan for a balance of enterprise projects and social/health/wellbeing projects, generating some untied funds from the former to assist with projects/initiatives that are not readily funded by government or industry project funds.

- Plan for hybrid economy or mix of enterprises to protect against market fluctuations.
- Use a not-for-profit approach, with new corporations as necessary, but capacity to have capital flows between corporations to seed-fund new projects and for charitable causes.
- Build worker dignity, self-strengthening and cultural identity plans into all activities; and ways for emotionally healing people with on-country options for wellbeing.
- Aim to deliver services that can also benefit the wider region and non-Indigenous communities and economy, so as to foster a position and respect in the economic market and develop interdependent economic relationships for ongoing economic security.
- Seek strong Indigenous leadership and the community-controlled governance of service delivery.

Works cited

Case study 1

Australian High Commission (2014). *Highlights of Australia's development assistance to the Autonomous Region of Bougainville – July 2012 to June 2014.* Port Moresby, PG: Australian High Commission, Commonwealth of Australia.

Daniel, R., et al. (2011). Knowledge through participation: the triumphs and challenges of transferring Integrated Pest and Disease Management (IPDM) technology to cocoa farmers in Papua New Guinea. *Food Security* 3(1): 65–79.

Guest, D. I., R. Daniel, Y. Namaliu, J. K. Konam (2010). Technology Adoption: Classroom in the Cocoa Block. In *Knowledge and technology transfer for plant pathology. Volume 4: plant pathology in the 21st century.* N. V. Hardwick and M. L. Gullino, eds., pp.33–44. Dordrecht. NL: Springer.

Konam, J., Y. Namaliu, R. Daniel, and D. Guest (2011). *Integrated Pest and Disease Management for sustainable cocoa production: a training manual for farmers and extension workers,* 2nd edn. Monograph No. 131. Canberra: Australian Centre for International Agricultural Research.

Scales, I., and R. Craemer (2008). *Market chain development in peace building.* Canberra: AusAID.

World Bank (2008). *Papua New Guinea: Bougainville women come together to protect expecting moms and babies.* http://bit.ly/2Q0DyJY.

Case study 2

Akiyama, T., and Nishio, A. (1996). *Indonesia's Cocoa Boom: Hands-Off Policy Encourages Smallholder Dynamism.* World Bank Policy Research Working Paper No. 1580. https://bit.ly/2UL1gYt

Hafid, H., and F. McKenzie (2012). *Understanding farmer engagement in the cocoa sector in Sulawesi: a rapid assessment.* Canberra: Australian Centre for International Agricultural Research.

Neilson, J., R. Palinrungi, H. Muhammad, and K. Fauziah (2011). *ACIAR cocoa technical report: securing Indonesia's cocoa future: farmer adoption of sustainable farm practices on the island of Sulawesi.* ACIAR No. SMAR/2005/074. Canberra: Australian Centre for International Agricultural Research.

Ruf, F. (1987). Eléments pour une théorie sur l'agriculture des régions tropicales humides: de la forêt, rente différentielle au cacaoyer, capital travail. *Agronomie Tropicale,* 42(3): 218–232.

Case study 4

Altman, J.C. (2007). *Alleviating poverty in remote Indigenous Australia: the role of the hybrid economy.* Canberra: Centre for Aboriginal Economic Policy Research, Australian National University.

Memmott, P. (2010a). *Connection report for Indjalandji-Dhidhanu Native Title Claim QUD 243/2009.* Paul Memmott & Associates and the Aboriginal Environments Research Centre, University of Queensland, St. Lucia, Queensland, Australia.

Memmott, P. (2010b). *Demand responsive services and culturally sustainable enterprise in remote Aboriginal settings: a case study of the Myuma Group.* Report No. 63. Alice Springs, NT: Desert Knowledge Cooperative Research Centre. http://bit.ly/2PmcUWA.

Memmott, P. (2012). On generating culturally sustainable enterprises and demand responsive services in remote Aboriginal settings: a case study from north-west Queensland. In *Indigenous participation in Australian economies II: historical engagements and current enterprises,* N. Fijn, I. Keen, C. Lloyd, and M. Pickering, eds., 243–59. Canberra: ANU E-Press and National Museum of Australia.

Memmott, P. (2018). The re-invention of the 'behaviour setting' in the new Indigenous architecture. In *Handbook of contemporary Indigenous architecture*, E. Grant, K. Greenop, A.L. Refiti, and D.J. Glenn, eds. pp.831-868. Springer Nature Singapore Pte Ltd.

Memmott, P., and C. Keys (2016). The emergence of an architectural anthropology in Aboriginal Australia: the work of the Aboriginal Environments Research Centre. *Architectural Theory Review* 21(2): 218–36.

Memmott, P., D. Martin, and N. Amiralian (2017). Nanotechnology and the Dreamtime knowledge of spinifex grass. In *Green composites: natural and waste based composites for a sustainable future*, 2nd edn., C. Baillie and R. Jayasinghe, eds., 181–98. Dixford, UK: Elsevier.

8

One Health surveillance: monitoring health risks at the human–animal–environment interface

Siobhan M. Mor, Anke K. Wiethoelter, Peter Massey and Keith Eastwood

Effective surveillance and response relies on networks linking diverse information sources (Gresham et al. 2013). In the context of One Health, this can include gathering disease and population statistics from humans, domestic and wild animals, coupled with data on the environment and climate, and developing networks to distribute information via multiple stakeholder groups so that appropriate actions can be taken. The International Society for Disease Surveillance (ISDS) defines One Health surveillance as 'the collaborative, on-going, systematic collection and analysis of data from multiple domains (at local, national and global levels) to detect health-related events and produce information which leads to actions aimed at attaining optimal health for people, animals, and the environment' (ISDS 2017). This builds on the World Health Organization (WHO) and World Organisation for Animal Health (OIE, after the original French name Office International des Epizooties) definitions for public health and animal health surveillance, respectively.

Box 8.1 presents a case study of a disease (Rift Valley fever, RVF) that warrants a One Health approach to surveillance. Experience with RVF outbreaks has led to formulation of frameworks for collaboration and coordination across agencies for this particular disease, as will be discussed later in this chapter. In the absence of such frameworks,

Box 8.1: Surveillance and response to Rift Valley fever in Kenya
Adapted from Centers for Disease Control and Prevention (2007), Bird et al. (2008), Jost et al. (2010), and Lutomiah et al. (2014).

After a period of heavy rainfall and flooding in north-eastern Kenya and southern Somalia in late 2006, an outbreak of an unexplained febrile illness was detected in humans in Garissa district, Kenya. At the time, unexplained deaths and abortion in livestock were being reported in the same area. The first report of human death was a herdsman who presented with fever and bleeding manifestations and later died. A further 12 cases presented to the same hospital over the next week with the same clinical signs; 11 of them died. Rift Valley fever (RVF) virus was confirmed by serology and polymerase chain reaction (PCR).

Once the outbreak was confirmed, the Kenyan Ministry of Health and Ministry of Agriculture and Fisheries, supported by international agencies, established enhanced surveillance systems to monitor disease in humans and animals, respectively. Surveillance officers in all districts reported suspected or probable cases in humans, which were followed up by the rapid response team who obtained data on demographic and clinical features as well as identified risk factors for transmission. Data regarding impact on livestock and livestock production were also gathered from pastoralists using participatory epidemiology approaches. Diagnostic testing confirmed recent RVF infection in cattle, sheep, goats and camels. Wild animals, principally buffalos and giraffes, were also found to be recently infected. Entomological investigations confirmed the virus was circulating in local mosquito populations.

Village elders, chiefs, and religious leaders were consulted throughout the outbreak. Prevention messages were developed in multiple languages and distributed via radio and public meetings. A ban on livestock slaughter was implemented in affected districts and livestock markets were closed. Livestock were vaccinated in affected areas.

By the end of the epidemic (December 2006–May 2007), more than 1,000 human cases were reported (275 deaths) across Kenya, Tanzania and Somalia. Official estimates from Kenya suggest that 12.5 million cattle, 11 million goats, 8 million sheep and 850,000 camels were directly or indirectly impacted by the outbreak. Disruption to markets and the meat industry resulted in substantial economic losses to livestock producers and traders, butchers and casual labourers associated with the livestock industry. Further, food security of producers was adversely affected as a result of loss of livestock and income.

response teams managing diseases at the human–animal–environment interface are often confronted with the following questions:

- What are the potential risks to human health?
- What are the potential risks to animal health and trade?
- How is the outbreak first recognised and notified to agencies?
- What factors determine the make-up of the response team?
- Which agency assumes the role of coordination and lead?
- Who covers expenses including laboratory testing?
- Which agency is responsible for ongoing surveillance?
- Who is responsible for providing information to the media and managing public awareness?
- What are the environmental impacts and how will they be managed?

In an ideal situation, one government agency would cover all aspects of health and develop an overarching surveillance system with an integrated outbreak response unit; one that complies with a universal investigation protocol. However, there are many obstacles to overcome before this model becomes the norm. For now, it is necessary for agencies from disparate backgrounds and with different objectives to collaborate effectively when confronted with emerging threats.

In this chapter, we consider the range of surveillance options as well as challenges to monitoring disease at the human–animal–environment interface. In the first section, we compare and contrast the different sectoral approaches to disease surveillance in humans and other animals. Practitioners intending to collect, aggregate and/or synthesise data generated from such programs need to understand the methods and motivations behind surveillance in each sector as this is crucial for conceiving new approaches to monitor health risks at the interface. In the second section, we discuss challenges and opportunities to achieving One Health surveillance. We then explore how One Health surveillance is being implemented across a range of applications in the third section. We conclude by recommending ways to enhance One Health surveillance.

Sectoral approaches to surveillance

At its core – and irrespective of whether it is for human or animal populations – disease surveillance is the process of gathering, interpreting and sharing intelligence on the occurrence of disease and other health outcomes in populations. Such systems typically comprise a system for mandatory (required by law) reporting of 'notifiable' conditions to the relevant government authority(ies). The objectives of surveillance are broadly similar across sectors, namely:

- monitoring disease trends, such as estimating the magnitude or geographic distribution of a health problem
- detecting outbreaks or epidemics, including emerging diseases
- generating hypotheses regarding the aetiology and transmission pathways of disease outbreaks
- supporting decision-making regarding research priorities and healthcare/disease control programming
- directing and evaluating control strategies
- demonstrating absence of (or 'freedom from') disease.

The last objective provides assurances for trade and tourism. This is crucial in the livestock sector since animal health surveillance data are used in import risk analysis (IRA). Surveillance – specifically proof of freedom surveys[1] – permits countries or zones within a country to be declared free of disease for trade purposes. Peeler, Reese, and Thrush (2015) and the OIE handbooks on import risk analysis for animals and animal products (Bruckner et al. 2010; Murray et al. 2010) provide an overview of IRA for those wanting more information. While this last objective receives less attention in public health, monitoring of disease-free status can be useful for tourism; for example, identifying areas free of malaria.

---

1   Rather than provide an estimate of disease prevalence, proof of freedom surveys provide evidence – with a degree of statistical confidence – that a particular disease is absent in animal populations in a given country or zone. Proof of freedom surveys are an essential tool in veterinary epidemiology. They provide evidence to trading partners that certain diseases are not likely to be present in animals from the exporting country, and thus the importing country can be assured that they are not going to introduce diseases as a result of trade between the two countries.

General approaches to disease surveillance

Methods for disease surveillance are similar across human and animal health, although triggering events, disease priorities and reporting lines differ markedly between sectors (Table 8.1). It is our impression that – compared to public health surveillance – animal health surveillance encompasses a broader range of activities, such as participatory disease surveillance (see Box 8.2) and structured population-based surveys. The latter includes prevalence surveys and proof of freedom surveys which aim to make statistical inferences about the frequency (e.g. prevalence) or absence of disease, respectively, in the total animal population under surveillance. Such investigations – typically carried out in defined populations and within a discrete period of time – are commonly classified as research activity in public health sectors. The emerging use of whole genome sequencing (WGS) as a tool to monitor strains is becoming accepted practice in the public health sector and stretches traditional understanding of surveillance into the area of research (Kwong et al. 2015).

Traditional surveillance systems are designed to collect data on specific diseases (so-called indicator-based surveillance). Laboratory confirmation is usually required according to a prescribed criterion or 'case definition'. This applies to human and animal diseases, with newly emerging disease risks added to the systems as indicated. To improve timeliness, notification of serious diseases (e.g. typhoid and measles in humans; foot-and-mouth disease and highly pathogenic avian influenza in livestock and poultry, respectively) is recommended to occur on suspicion and before laboratory confirmation, based on symptoms and signs consistent with disease rather than laboratory criteria. Some surveillance systems – such as those designed to support smallpox and polio eradication or to monitor trends in gastroenteritis and influenza-like illness – rely exclusively on clinical, and not laboratory case definitions. This is sometimes called 'symptomatic surveillance' or 'syndromic surveillance'; although the latter term is also used to describe non-traditional data sources in disease surveillance (see below). Since laboratory confirmation is not required, this type of surveillance is particularly useful in resource-poor settings or as an early warning system since time to detection is more rapid (May et al. 2011)

Box 8.2: Participatory disease surveillance
'Participatory disease surveillance' refers to the use of participatory epidemiology (PE) for surveillance. These methods originated in the 1980s as part of rural development programs in low-income countries, where it was recognised that communities could identify problems and design initiatives to solve them in the absence of formal education. This challenged 'top-down' approaches to data collection and programs that positioned development professionals and researchers as the experts. In response, a suite of methods – adapted from social/medical anthropology and agroecosystem analysis – were designed to engage communities in data collection and analysis. Given their emphasis on rural populations, veterinarians and others working with livestock keepers were amongst the first to incorporate PE methods alongside conventional disease investigation methods.

PE encompasses a range of tools and approaches, including: interviews (e.g. to start an informal conversation and identify local names of diseases affecting animals in the area); ranking and scoring methods (e.g. to identify relative importance of such diseases); and visualisation methods such as proportional piling (e.g. to identify disease incidence and mortality using piles of stones to represent the herd), mapping (e.g. to identify areas where disease vectors may be present), and seasonal calendar (e.g. to identify timing of peak disease incidence or vector abundance). These methods are relatively cheap, making PE particularly suitable for resource-scarce settings. Visual tools and use of objects in place of words means that informants can participate in the discussion, whether they are literate or not. Information learned through community participation is triangulated with available data from more conventional investigation methods (e.g. post-mortem examination, laboratory tests, and meteorological records).

Participatory disease surveillance was used extensively during the rinderpest eradication campaign in Africa, and, more recently, investigation into highly pathogenic avian influenza in Asia. Increasingly, participatory methods are being adapted to investigate disease in humans. For more information on veterinary applications and methods of PE, readers are referred to Catley et al. (2012) and Allepuz et al. (2017).

Table 8.1. Properties of surveillance systems across human and animal health sectors.

	Humans	Terrestrial livestock	Aquatic animals	Wild animals	Companion animals
Intergovernmental organisation with mandate	World Health Organization (WHO)	World Organisation for Animal Health (OIE)[2]	World Organisation for Animal Health (OIE)[2]	World Organisation for Animal Health (OIE)[2] [voluntary; effective 1993]	None[3]
National agencies responsible for collating surveillance data	Ministry representing health	Ministry representing livestock/animal resources/agriculture	Ministry representing fisheries	Various. May include ministries representing livestock/animal resources/ agriculture/ fisheries, wildlife/forestry/ environment/ conservation, or tourism/finance. OIE National Focal Point for Wildlife	None[3]

	Humans	Terrestrial livestock	Aquatic animals	Wild animals	Companion animals
Disease priorities	Blood-borne diseases, gastro-intestinal diseases,[1] quarantinable diseases, sexually transmitted infections, vaccine-preventable diseases, vector-borne diseases,[1] and other zoonoses	OIE-listed diseases (trade-sensitive diseases)	OIE-listed diseases (trade-sensitive diseases)	OIE-listed diseases (trade-sensitive diseases); non-listed diseases with conservation impacts	No formal disease surveillance in most countries[3]
Triggering events	Patient visits healthcare provider	Farmer contacts veterinarian after noticing illness; livestock inspector/veterinarian detects disease at saleyard/abattoir	Observation of unusual morbidity or mortality events in fish, molluscs, crustaceans or amphibians	Observation of unusual morbidity or mortality events in wildlife	Owner takes pet to veterinary clinic

	Humans	Terrestrial livestock	Aquatic animals	Wild animals	Companion animals
Principal stakeholders in surveillance system	Patients, medical practitioners, laboratories, public health units	Farmers, livestock handlers, veterinarians, laboratories	Fishermen, veterinarians, laboratories	Wildlife biologists, ecologists, hunters, wildlife managers, rehabilitators, conservation managers	Animal owners, veterinarians, laboratories
Common methods for data collection	Passive surveillance for notifiable conditions; active surveillance; sentinel surveillance; syndromic surveillance; event-based surveillance	Passive surveillance for notifiable conditions; abattoir inspection; structured population-based surveys; sentinel surveillance	Autopsies and laboratory analysis of dead fish, molluscs, crustaceans or amphibians	Autopsies and laboratory analysis of dead animals; abattoir inspection of game meat; surveys of free-ranging wildlife or those submitted to carers/clinics	No formal disease surveillance in most countries[3]

[1] Many of these diseases have zoonotic origins.

[2] Office International des Epizooties

[3] OIE-listed diseases which occur in companion animals may be notified to the ministry representing livestock services/agriculture/fisheries.

Surveillance systems are traditionally classified as 'passive' or 'active', depending on how reporting is initiated. In passive surveillance systems, government jurisdictions receive reports from medical practitioners/ veterinarians and laboratories when a case is diagnosed. This is the most common type of surveillance for notifiable diseases in both public health and animal health sectors. Passive surveillance systems are low-input in terms of cost and labour but potentially suffer from under-reporting. It has become standard practice in some countries to provide automated electronic reporting directly from the laboratory with benefits of improved reporting completeness and reduced workload. In active surveillance systems, government agencies contact medical practitioners/ veterinarians, laboratories, pharmacists and other providers to obtain data on cases. This is particularly useful during outbreak investigations as it heightens awareness and improves case ascertainment. Active surveillance is more time-consuming and costlier than passive reporting; however, it results in more complete reporting.

In the above examples of notifiable disease surveillance data are collected on the whole population; healthcare providers and laboratories report all diagnosed cases to government authorities. In some circumstances surveillance is performed by monitoring specific sites, providers or vectors/animals (so-called sentinel surveillance). Detection of the pathogen/disease in the sentinel population(s) is then taken to reflect the risk to the wider population. A common application is the use of sentinel chicken flocks to detect arboviral activity, such as West Nile virus in the United States and Murray Valley encephalitis virus in Australia. In the animal health sector, sentinel cattle herds are used to monitor the spread of bluetongue virus in Europe and Australia. Sentinel surveillance is discussed later in the chapter.

The advent of electronic data collection, increased computing power and the internet has generated interest in non-traditional data sources for disease surveillance (also called 'syndromic surveillance') motivated principally by the desire for earlier detection of outbreaks, that is, before laboratory information is available (Figure 8.1). By monitoring clinical (e.g. emergency department admissions) or non-clinical (e.g. over-the-counter prescription sales, school absenteeism) indicators in real-time, health departments can potentially detect early signs of an adverse health event (Henning 2004). Similar approaches

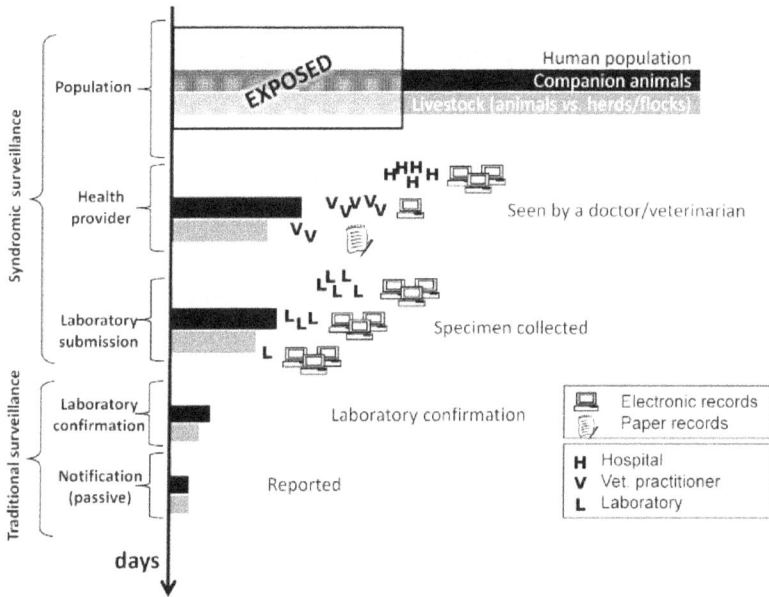

Figure 8.1 Schematic depicting the data sources used for traditional and syndromic surveillance systems. The Y axis represents the time to detection (longest = bottom). The X axis represents the (relative) number of cases detected by each approach. Adapted from Dorea, Sanchez and Revie (2011).

have been developed in animal health and are reviewed by Dorea, Sanchez, and Revie (2011). Key challenges with this approach relate to the non-specificity of the signal and defining the threshold for alert against substantial background 'noise' (Henning 2004).

Indicator-based surveillance systems can be complemented by 'event-based surveillance systems'. Under event-based surveillance, internet and media sources are scanned for information that may signal an unusual or emerging health threat. Signals may come from reports, rumours or other stories about illness in the community. Community members or news reporters may also pass on information that warrants investigation. Whereas indicator-based surveillance typically involves analysing and interpreting data collected in a standardised way and originating from within the human and animal healthcare systems, the focus of event-based surveillance is capturing, filtering and verifying non-standardised reports of potential health events from external sources. HealthMap (www.healthmap.org) is a good example of a comprehensive system combining a wide variety of indicator- and event-based data.

Disease surveillance in humans

The public health surveillance obligations of WHO member nations are described in the International Health Regulations (IHR). Early versions of these regulations focused on diseases such as smallpox, cholera, yellow fever and plague (Nuttall et al. 2014). However, with the emergence of severe acute respiratory syndrome (SARS) and its rapid spread around the world, the deficiencies of the regulations became obvious, necessitating their review. The current IHR (2005) require WHO members to develop and maintain adequate surveillance capacity to identify any event that constitutes a 'public health emergency of international concern' and to report these promptly to the WHO (WHO 2005). In 2014, the Global Health Security Agenda (www.ghsagenda.org) was launched to help countries achieve core capacities required by the IHR 2005, and is complemented on the animal health side by OIE's Performance of Veterinary Services Pathway (see below). Surveillance is also important for tracking progress towards Sustainable Development Goal (SDG) 3, which sets targets for reducing the burden of HIV, tuberculosis, malaria, and other communicable diseases (http://bit.ly/2RH2Bi0). Aggregated data showing progress towards the SDGs are publicly available via the WHO Global Health Observatory (www.who.int/gho/en/).

Disease surveillance in animals

The OIE maintains a list of notifiable conditions which is reviewed annually. The current OIE list includes 117 terrestrial and aquatic animal diseases and infections,[2] many of which occur in multiple

---

2   'Pathogen surveillance' (as opposed to 'disease surveillance') is an important
    concept in animal health surveillance, since infection with a particular

animal species, including humans and wildlife (OIE 2019). OIE member countries are obligated to report on the status of these diseases and infections (presence or absence) every six months or immediately if the disease represents an exceptional event for that country. Most countries harmonise their list of notifiable conditions with the OIE list. They are assisted by tools provided by the OIE which are used to evaluate the performance of veterinary services and strengthen national veterinary services, ensuring high quality of domestic surveillance activities and programs (OIE PVS Tool, http://bit.ly/2zKJJry). Data provided by member countries are made publicly available through OIE's World Animal Health Information System (WAHIS, http://bit.ly/2QmB49a) in an effort to improve transparency of the animal health situation in each country for trade purposes.

With trade a key driver of animal health surveillance, governments typically focus on economically important species, namely terrestrial livestock and, increasingly, aquatic animals. Passive surveillance methods and surveys to demonstrate freedom from disease comprise the bulk of surveillance activities for these species. By contrast, wild and companion animals usually fall outside of standard government structures for surveillance and different approaches are used to monitor disease in these animals.

Disease surveillance and wild animals

Compared to disease surveillance in livestock, wildlife surveillance is less regulated and responsibilities regarding wildlife health are often poorly defined. As a result, governance at the national level often falls into the jurisdiction of multiple agencies with nomination of a Focal Point for Wildlife (Table 8.1). Until recently there was no international agreement on what constituted priority diseases for surveillance in wild animals, although, as mentioned above, many of the OIE-listed diseases affect multiple species, including wildlife. The OIE Working Group

---

pathogen may not produce visible signs of disease in all species under surveillance (hence certain diseases *and* infections are notifiable). Occurrence of the pathogen is nonetheless important for understanding the potential for transmission between species, including to humans.

on Wildlife has further identified 'non-listed' diseases which countries should target for surveillance based on their importance to wildlife conservation and potential to serve as an early warning for threats to livestock and/or public health. Countries can voluntarily report these non-listed diseases affecting wild animals, through OIE's WAHIS-Wild interface (http://bit.ly/2QgBNbK). Non-listed disease data collected by OIE do not influence trade policy. Since 2016, countries reporting OIE-listed diseases occurring in wild animals do so through the regular WAHIS system.

A number of factors and issues inherent in the nature of wild animals complicate surveillance in this sector (Morner et al. 2002; Stallknecht 2007). Signs and symptoms in wildlife often differ from those in domestic animals. Many infections, being subclinical, remain undetected unless unusual events such as mass die-offs trigger investigation. Wildlife surveillance systems usually comprise opportunistic sampling to determine cause of death or disease rather than systematic sampling for specific pathogens. Because necropsy and histologic examinations are often unable to establish a cause of death or disease, laboratory diagnostic tests are required. The majority of laboratory tests, however, are only validated for humans, livestock and/or companion animals and their validity and accuracy on wildlife samples are frequently unknown. Wildlife-specific tests constitute a niche market and their development is neither cost-efficient nor industry driven, resulting in a lack of readily available diagnostic tools.

Wildlife comprises a wide range of taxa and habitats including aerial, aquatic and terrestrial animals. Many species are well camouflaged, live in areas difficult to access and sparsely populated, or undertake migration movements and frequently cross administrative boundaries. Because free-ranging wildlife is not under constant human observation, information is scarce and denominator data is lacking for calculations such as incidence or prevalence, which makes assessing the impacts of events difficult. Several techniques for estimating size and density of wildlife populations exist, including: direct (aerial surveys, drive counts) or indirect observation (tracks, nests, burrows or excretions); use of hunter harvest records; and capture–recapture methods. A collaborative project in Europe on harmonised approaches to monitoring wildlife population health and ecology and abundance

(APHAEA, http://bit.ly/2zJQwBS) has recognised the need for accurate population estimates and has compiled fact cards for key species.

Due to the specific characteristics mentioned above a co-ordinated but decentralised data collection approach supported by citizen science is well suited for wildlife surveillance to encourage and ensure observation and reporting of unusual events by as many people as possible (Lawson, Petrovan and Cunningham 2015). These approaches still have to contend with issues of reliability, standardisation and harmonisation of reports and the fear that reports of wildlife diseases may impact on livestock trade or other activities involving wildlife (hunting, tourism). In short, the management of wildlife diseases is complex. The typical livestock disease control measures (e.g. stamping out or vaccination) might not apply to wildlife, and disease detection may be counter-productive to the conservation of endangered species. Despite progress in recent years many hurdles remain including sustainable funding for the ongoing collection and analysis of wildlife data at a country level. Readers interested in learning about the approaches to wildlife surveillance are referred to OIE's training manual on surveillance and international reporting of diseases in wild animals (OIE 2015).

Surveillance in companion animals

Disease surveillance in companion animals such as dogs and cats is lacking in most countries, both high- and low-income. A number of OIE-listed diseases and infections occur in companion animals (e.g. rabies, Q fever/coxiellosis, hydatids) but, apart from rabies, few countries have surveillance systems in place to collect data and report these diseases in companion animal species (Day et al. 2012). Diseases and infections such as canine distemper virus and feline immunodeficiency virus while having a major impact on companion animals do not have implications for livestock and/or public health and so are not typically notifiable by law.

Some countries have surveillance platforms for collecting data on selected diseases (Glickman et al. 2006; Hennenfent et al. 2017; Ward and Kelman 2011). These systems rely on veterinarians entering case information using online platforms funded by the private sector or short-term government grants; at least one has been discontinued. Because these systems do not connect to any government agency responsible for companion animal health, it is unclear whether collation and analysis of information is undertaken such that a co-ordinated response to an outbreak could be mounted. Any decision to act on the information gathered through these surveillance systems sits with the end-user: the veterinary clinic inputting the data.

Challenges and opportunities in One Health surveillance

From the above discussion it is clear that, although both human and animal health sectors have similar objectives and approaches to surveillance, the motivations and reporting lines differ markedly between sectors. In addition, surveillance capacity across sectors and geographic regions differs considerably. Whereas public health and livestock surveillance is comparatively strong in high-income countries, these functions are fairly weak in low-income countries and wildlife and companion animal surveillance is virtually non-existent in most countries, both low- and high income (Institute of Medicine [IOM] and National Research Council [NRC] 2009). To improve One Health outcomes, we need to strengthen surveillance capacity within sectors as well as expand opportunities for collaboration and integration across sectors. A number of challenges exist and are discussed in this section.

Structural and organisational barriers

In most countries and states disease surveillance of humans and animals is the responsibility of multiple organisations. This governance fragmentation affects all levels of infectious disease surveillance and response: separate laboratories detecting the same pathogens; distinct units investigating and following-up cases; different agencies collating data; notifications to separate intergovernmental bodies. The divide has practical ramifications for One Health activities such as lack of harmonisation of laboratory methods, weak communication channels across sectors, and legal and technical hurdles to real-time sharing of information. Mechanisms for funding cross-sectoral initiatives are rarely in place. Gaps in information sharing between the public and private sectors are also evident (IOM and NRC 2009).

Some countries have managed these barriers by establishing multi-sectoral task forces to facilitate joint planning and budgeting, particularly during outbreak periods (Morse 2014; Stark et al. 2015). More often cross-sectoral collaboration occurs via informal networks of trusted peers (Stark et al. 2015). In trying to formalise these networks, some countries have found it helpful to conduct a network analysis to better understand the stakeholder organisations and nature of the collaboration between sectors involved in One Health activities (Kimani et al. 2016; Sorrell et al. 2015). The increasing incidence of emerging diseases has prompted a number of regional disease surveillance networks to adopt One Health approaches, such as the Mekong Basin Disease Surveillance and East African Integrated Disease Surveillance Network (EAIDSNet) (Bond et al. 2013). Networks of networks have also formed, such as the non-governmental organisation, Connecting Organizations for Regional Disease Surveillance (CORDS), with the objective of improving coordination between human, animal and environmental sectors (Gresham et al. 2013). Addressing these existing structural barriers to One Health remains an area of intense and ongoing activity.

Differing disease priorities

Related to the above structural barriers are the different mandates and priorities of agencies involved in surveillance which provide limited opportunities for direct overlap. This is true even in the context of zoonoses, which might be expected to be an area of common interest to both human and animal health sectors. To illustrate this barrier, we compared notification lists for three countries with similar surveillance capacity (Australia, the United Kingdom and the United States of America) (Table 8.2). When there was an overlapping interest it was often confined to uncommon or rare diseases which limits occasions for combining datasets to enhance epidemiological knowledge. Zoonotic diseases in animal populations such as Q fever/coxiellosis, leptospirosis and chlamydiosis/ornithosis are not necessarily notifiable by veterinarians, yet are of public health importance. This reflects the trade-emphasis of animal health surveillance and the fact that many zoonotic infections do not cause illness in animals and so are not considered a major animal health issue.

Notwithstanding differing agency priorities and data requirements there will be many occasions when collating information is mutually beneficial even if additional information is required. It may be constructive for agencies to jointly agree on those diseases deserving of enhanced, cross-sectoral surveillance and response. This can be challenging in the context of data scarcity, particularly on the animal health side. To address this challenge the US Centers for Disease Control and Prevention (CDC) has developed a decision support tool to facilitate transparent priority setting by stakeholders involved in zoonotic disease surveillance, response and research (Rist, Arriola and Rubin 2014). Importantly, the tool is suitable for use in countries where surveillance data may be lacking.

Information sharing and data linkage

Surveillance data germane to One Health is often stored in different databases and from different organisations, and there are legal and technical barriers to information sharing and data linkage. One initial obstacle to data sharing across agencies is confidentiality of information, although in our experience this is often overcome at the network level when trust has been achieved. On the other hand, while sharing of data is operationally possible, accepted and desired, barriers may still exist at the policy level that prevent sharing of data (Stark et al. 2015). Differing spatial resolutions and lack of timeliness are other barriers to real-time data linkage (Wendt, Kreienbrock and Campe 2016).

Sharing information between private and public sectors is particularly challenging in the animal health sector as disclosure of information can impact the financial standing and market access of commercial entities (Stark et al. 2015). For some pathogens, these challenges are overcome by supporting anonymous sharing of isolates by animal industries for purposes of testing and sequencing. This approach has been used for influenza virus surveillance in swine in the United States (Animal and Plant Health Inspection Service [APHIS] n.d.). This approach impedes traceability and therefore would not be suitable for all pathogens.

Disease	Australia[1]		UK		USA	
	Animal	Human	Animal	Human	Animal	Human
Australian bat lyssavirus	X	X				
Anthrax	X	X	X	X	X	X
Babesiosis	X				X	X
Brucellosis	X	X	X	X	X	X
Chlamydiosis/Ornithosis	X	X		X	X	X
Echinococcosis/Hydatids		X			X	
Hendra virus infection	X	X				
Influenza	X	X	X	X	X	X
Japanese encephalitis	X	X			X	
Leptospirosis		X		X	X	X
Nipah virus infection	X				X	
Plague (*Yersinia pestis*)		X	X			X
Q fever/Coxiellosis		X	X	X	X	X
Rabies	X	X	X	X	X	X
Rift Valley fever	X		X	X	X	
Trichinellosis	X				X	X
Tularaemia	X	X		X	X	X
West Nile virus infection	X	X	X	X	X	X

[1] Notification of diseases varies between states of Australia.

Table 8.2. A comparison of animal and human notifiable diseases for three selected countries of similar surveillance capacity. 'X' denotes those diseases that are notifiable in animals and humans.

Sharing pathogen databases also highlights the lack of harmonisation of molecular typing methods within and across sectors. Variable uptake of new diagnostic technologies and typing practices results in un-matched data collections which impede the ability to link data (Wendt, Kreienbrock and Campe 2015). The use of the WGS is advancing rapidly in public health and may replace other typing systems; however, introduction of this technology will be gradual and inevitably multiple typing systems will exist until concord is reached. WGS is yet to be incorporated into routine veterinary surveillance, leaving major gaps in our understanding of the microbial diversity of domestic and wild animals.

Human resources

Effective surveillance systems require people trained in the principles and practical aspects of monitoring diseases. Knowledge of applied epidemiology and skills in data analysis and communication help in surveillance activities (M'ikanatha et al. 2013). Field epidemiology training programs (FETPs) – modelled after the US CDC's Epidemic Intelligence Service – have been the cornerstone of applied epidemiology training globally. In recent years, a number of FETPs have specifically catered for veterinarians with the aim of strengthening field veterinary services (Iamsirithaworn et al. 2014). Some programs deliberately engage both human and animal health professionals (Becker et al. 2012; Monday et al. 2011). Combined training in One Health surveillance is an excellent foundation, bringing medical practitioners, veterinarians, and environmental health professionals from different governmental sectors together with the common purpose of disease control and prevention (Monday et al. 2011).

One Health approaches to surveillance

The different drivers and motivations underpinning surveillance in humans and other animals means that certain approaches will always be needed to meet the individual requirements of each sector. Where overlap exists, efforts to integrate information and/or undertake joint

Box 8.3: Cross-sectoral surveillance and response for Rift Valley fever (RVF). Refer to the case study presented in Box 1.
Adapted from de La Rocque and Formenty (2014).

During outbreaks of RVF, inter-ministerial taskforces are usually activated along with a principal committee to co-ordinate the technical subcommittees. Subcommittees vary country to country but typically undertake the following tasks: epidemiological investigations, surveillance and diagnostics; clinical case management; disease control at the human–animal interface; logistics and security for field operations; social and behavioural interventions; and media and communication.

Four periods are recognised in the response to RVF:

1. Forecasting and preparedness

   During this period remote sensing data are used to identify environmental conditions that might favour RVF emergence in Africa. Following confirmation of suitable conditions, public health and veterinary services in affected areas are advised to establish or enhance surveillance systems, establish clinical facilities to manage cases and prepare and disseminate educational materials targeting high-risk groups (e.g. slaughterhouse workers, veterinarians, healthcare workers). Mass vaccination of livestock may be implemented during this phase.

2. Alert phase

   During this period, a multidisciplinary response team is established to investigate rumours of suspected cases in humans and livestock. Diagnostic specimens are collected and tested.

3. Outbreak control

   Following confirmation of an outbreak, enhanced surveillance is initiated to identify cases in humans and livestock. Clinical case management of affected humans is provided by healthcare units and hospitals. Movement restrictions are imposed on livestock. Social scientists conduct active listening and dialogue with affected communities and surrounding areas. A program of tailored social and behavioural interventions is implemented to inform the public about the risks and promote effective infection control practices.

4. Post-epidemic phase

   In this period surveillance reverts to pre-epidemic levels, to ensure that sporadic cases are detected. Authorities conduct a performance evaluation.

data collection could lead to improved prediction of the risks to human and animal health, earlier detection of outbreaks and faster responses in both sectors. Such approaches have been used for some diseases, such as Rift Valley fever (see Box 8.3). Following is a discussion of areas which would benefit most from One Health surveillance.

Zoonotic diseases

Surveillance systems using a One Health approach to monitor zoonoses are generally divided into: 1) those aiming to integrate data collected through existing surveillance systems; and 2) those in which data are collected for an identified purpose using a coordinated approach. Wendt, Kreienbrock and Campe (2015) recently conducted a review of systems for integrating human and animal data on zoonoses. Of the 20 systems identified, most were established in the last decade and focused on early detection of new and emerging threats rather than endemic zoonoses. This is consistent with recent global interest and investment in the former, following major outbreaks of SARS and H5N1 influenza around 2003. These outbreaks contributed to the realisation that animals, particularly wildlife, were the sources of many recently emerged infections in humans (Jones et al. 2008) leading to proposals to redirect investment in zoonotic disease surveillance upstream, towards the wildlife source (Heymann and Dixon 2013; Karesh et al. 2012) (Figure 8.2).

At the global level, zoonotic disease surveillance systems that collate existing data include: Global Early Warning System for Major Animal Diseases, including Zoonoses (GLEWS; http://bit.ly/2zP08uZ), a joint initiative of WHO/FAO/OIE which aims to collate information on disease events gathered by each organisation; Global Public Health Intelligence Network (GPHIN), which is a web-based platform tracking disease outbreaks in humans, animals and plants reported through websites, news wires and other internet-based outlets; Global Outbreak Alert and Response Network (GOARN), which is a network of institutions and organisations providing technical support for rapid identification, confirmation and response to international outbreaks; and Program for Monitoring Emerging Diseases (ProMED-mail; www.promedmail.org) which collates information on human, animal

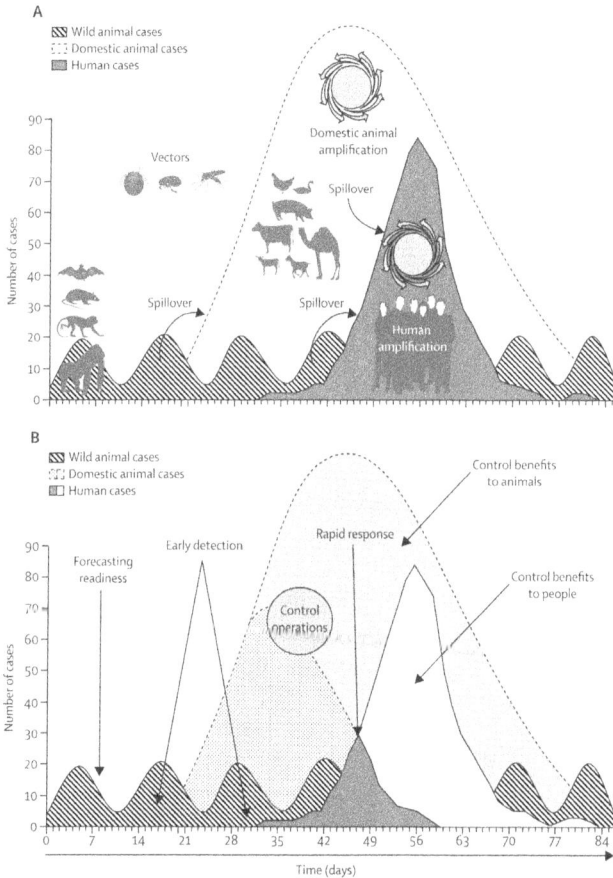

Figure 8.2 Upstream detection of zoonoses. (A) Transmission of infection and amplification in people (dark grey) occurs after a pathogen from wild animals (diagonal lines) moves into livestock to cause an outbreak (light grey) that amplifies the capacity for pathogen transmission to people. (B) Early detection and control efforts reduce disease incidence in people (white) and animals (dotted grey). Spillover arrows show cross-species transmission. Used with permission, Karesh et al. (2012).

and plant diseases retrieved from official and informal (media) reports as well as local observers.

A number of small-scale initiatives for joint data collection are reported in the literature, in particular for neglected zoonoses, such as brucellosis (reviewed by Zinsstag et al. 2015), and for disease surveillance in remote or Indigenous populations (Schurer et al. 2013; Schurer et al. 2014). Recent financial investments by international donors have resulted in the establishment of a number of large surveillance initiatives targeting high-risk populations in emerging disease 'hotspots'. For example, the Vietnam Initiative on Zoonotic Infections (VIZIONS) – funded by the Wellcome Trust – is a countrywide project that encompasses hospital surveillance of four key syndromes associated with zoonotic infections as well as active surveillance of a high-risk cohort comprising farming households and others who work with domestic and wild animals (Rabaa et al. 2015). During human disease events VIZIONS conducts sampling of animals in the household environment and subjects both human and animal samples to microbiological testing, including genomic and phylogenomic analysis, to detect known and novel viruses. Participant observation and in-depth interviews are also conducted with individuals exposed to wildlife, to assess the contextual and behavioural risk factors in these groups. Analogous projects have been initiated in Mozambique (Gudo et al. 2016) and Kenya (Thumbi et al. 2015).

Similarly, the PREDICT project – which is part of the United States Agency for International Development's (USAID) Emerging Pandemic Threats program – operates across more than 20 countries in central Africa, South and South-East Asia and parts of Latin America (Kelly et al. 2016). PREDICT works through a consortium of global and in-country partners to enhance surveillance of potential zoonotic viruses using 'risk-based approaches'. Sampling of wildlife taxa that have been found to harbour zoonotic viruses (particularly those that have spilled over into humans including non-human primates, bats and rodents; Levinson et al. 2013) is prioritised. Laboratory protocols focus on detection of known and novel viruses belonging to viral families that have previously been associated with emerging disease outbreaks in humans. Central to PREDICT's mission is development of in-country human and diagnostic capacity for wildlife disease surveillance. Training in safe and humane methods for wildlife sampling, including development of novel, non-invasive methods, is a key component of the project (Smiley Evans et al. 2015).

Whether projects such as VIZIONS and PREDICT are sustainable over the longer term is uncertain, but they illustrate the possibilities when adequate financial and political support is available. Through establishing networks of partners spanning human and animal health at national, regional and international levels, projects such as these can serve as a platform for scaling up approaches to zoonotic threats, including endemic diseases, in the future (Kelly et al. 2016).

Food-borne diseases

An important area of commonality between human and animal health is food production and a combined approach to the mitigation of food-borne disease. This includes the primary responsibility of animal feed manufacturers and farmers to ensure food safety through healthy animal production, as well as the responsibility of processors, retailers and consumers in preventing contamination further downstream. Food animals often harbour microorganisms in their normal flora that are pathogenic to humans. Poultry, for example, are often infected with *Campylobacter* and *Salmonella* resulting in frequent contamination of chicken meat and eggs. Fruit and vegetables may be contaminated with human and animal pathogens at any point during the production chain, including during the washing, packing and transportation processes. The source of outbreaks is often unknown which limits the implementation of effective whole-of-chain programs to prevent human infection (Galanis et al. 2012).

Surveillance for food-borne diseases is a core function of public health agencies and one likely to benefit from an integrated One Health approach. Use of molecular typing methods, such as pulse-field gel electrophoresis (PFGE) and multiple-locus variable number tandem repeat analysis (MLVA), enables rapid detection of clusters by identifying related isolates and establishing links between cases and potential sources. Owing to its improved discriminatory power, WGS is increasingly used in routine applications to further aid in source identification and source attribution (Vongkamjan and Wiedmann 2015). Data generated through these methods are shared via laboratory networks, such as US CDC PulseNet (http://bit.ly/2BUqNYS) and PulseNet International (http://bit.ly/2UjnotI) to better understand food-borne disease trends. To date, these techniques have primarily been used for assessing human samples and food items implicated in outbreaks. There has been limited application of these methods to food animals, feed and associated production environments.

A whole-of-chain approach to surveillance for food-borne pathogens is rare although there are some exceptions. In Canada, there have been efforts to integrate *Salmonella* data collected through several surveillance programs including data generated from (human and animal) diagnostic samples as well as active sampling of farms and feed ingredients, abattoirs, retail meats and surface water (Parmley et al. 2013). Similar approaches are being adopted in lower-income countries, such as Mexico (Zaidi et al. 2008) and Brazil (Dias et al. 2016). Enhanced molecular evaluation of potential reservoirs and vehicles – at all stages of the food chain – is contributing to improved source attribution and enabling the development of evidence-based policies. Farm-level interventions such as poultry vaccination and pre-chilling of chicken carcasses in the abattoir setting are some examples. Ongoing, integrated surveillance can be used to understand the impact of these interventions on the human burden of food-borne disease.

Antimicrobial resistance

Antimicrobial resistance (AMR) is a major threat to global health security (WHO 2014). Although often portrayed as a human health issue, AMR can be broadly framed as an ecological problem – with impacts on human, animal (domestic and wild) and plant health, as well as food hygiene and the environment (Butaye et al. 2014; Queenan, Hasler and Rushton 2016; Radhouani et al. 2014). In the context of AMR, surveillance is critical for understanding the extent of the problem, as well as evaluating the impact of interventions, such as revised infection control guidelines in (medical and veterinary) hospitals or policies regarding antimicrobial usage. Furthermore, advances in molecular characterisation of organisms have allowed a greater appreciation of the epidemiology of AMR and the movement of organisms and genes within and between environments and populations. In addition to data on the occurrence of AMR, information on antibiotic consumption is also a critical element of an AMR surveillance system, since antibiotic usage is a major cause of the problem (Queenan, Hasler and Rushton 2016).

Except for mandatory notifiable data collection (restricted to a limited range of conditions), it is difficult to obtain fully representative population-based antibiotic susceptibility data. Private laboratories in the health sector often refuse to share, citing confidentiality requirements. This results in data collections biased towards acute hospital cases; data is lacking from the general community. The limited collation of data between medical and veterinary laboratories further constrains our understanding.

The recent *WHO Global Report on Surveillance* noted major shortcomings in global capacity for AMR surveillance; specifically the lack of consensus on methodology, limited data sharing and poor co-ordination across geographic regions (WHO 2014). While a number of national and regional surveillance networks for AMR in human health have been established in recent decades, most focus on high-income countries, relate to specific pathogens, and/or data are not systematically obtained or geographically representative (Dar et al. 2016). The lack of internationally agreed standards for data collection and reporting on AMR in human health limits comparability of the data across countries and regions. In 2012 international standards on harmonisation of national AMR surveillance were adopted by OIE members (OIE 2012); however, at the time most countries lacked an official system for gathering data on antimicrobial usage in animals (Nisi et al. 2013). Lack of (medical and veterinary) microbiology diagnostic facilities remains a major constraint to AMR surveillance in low- and middle-income countries (Dar et al. 2016), and the same is true for the veterinary sector in many higher-income countries.

With these shortcomings in mind, the World Health Assembly adopted the *Global Action Plan on AMR*, in 2015 – a specific objective of which is to 'strengthen the knowledge and evidence-base through surveillance and research'. Subsequently, WHO/OIE/FAO launched a number of initiatives to support WHO member countries in developing and implementing surveillance systems for AMR and antibiotics usage in humans and animals. WHO launched the Global Antimicrobial Resistance Surveillance System (GLASS) to support standardised

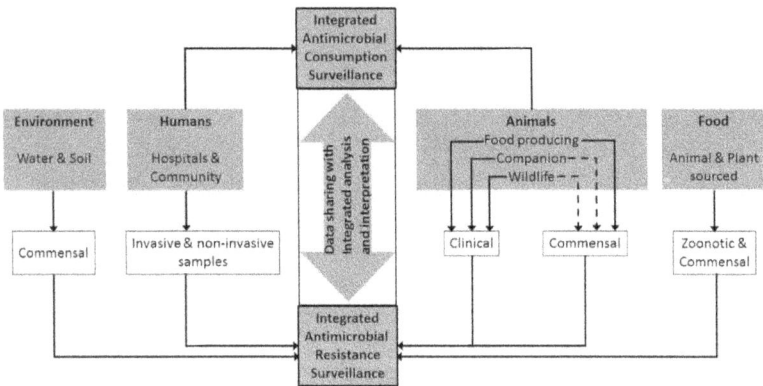

Figure 8.3 Framework for integrated surveillance on antimicrobial resistance and antimicrobial consumption. Used with permission, Queenan, Hasler and Rushton (2016).

approaches to the collection, analysis and sharing of data at the global level. Likewise, as part of the *OIE Strategy on AMR and the Prudent Use of Antimicrobials*, OIE is developing a global database on the use of antibiotics in livestock and companion animals (OIE 2016). These new initiatives – which aim to strengthen sectoral approaches to AMR surveillance – were enhanced when WHO/OIE/FAO called for improved integration of surveillance for food-borne pathogens, with coordinated sampling and testing of bacteria from livestock, foods, the environment as well as clinically ill humans (Acar and Moulin 2013) (see Figure 8.3).

A number of high-income countries have already made significant progress toward establishing integrated surveillance systems for AMR. The Danish Integrated Antimicrobial Resistance Monitoring and Research Program (DANMAP) was established in 1995 and collects and analyses data on antibiotic use and AMR in select indicator, zoonotic and pathogenic bacteria. Isolates come from a variety of sources, including: healthy animals at slaughter; sick animals subjected to diagnostic investigation; foods retrieved from wholesale and retail outlets as part of routine inspections; healthy humans; and humans subjected to diagnostic evaluation following contact with the healthcare system (Hammerum et al. 2007). Evidence generated through this integrated surveillance system was instrumental in supporting policy changes around the use of antibiotics in livestock, both in Denmark and Europe (Hammerum et al. 2007). Similar integrated surveillance systems were established in other high-income countries, and include the Canadian Integrated Program for Antimicrobial Resistance Surveillance (CIPARS) and the National Antimicrobial Resistance Monitoring System (NARMS) in the United States. Interested readers are referred to Acar and Moulin (2013) for a more comprehensive listing of such systems. More recently, lower-income countries, such as Mexico (Zaidi et al. 2008) and Colombia (Donado-Godoy et al. 2015) have established similar programs.

While integrated approaches appear to be the future of AMR surveillance, Queenan, Hasler and Rushton (2016) note that none of the current systems are fully integrated because wild and companion animals and the environment are not under surveillance. Resistant microbial populations have been detected in a variety of environmental samples, including hospital and farm effluent, sewage, and wastewater, indicating that AMR can spread through the environment (see review by Singer et al. 2016). Wild animals – rarely directly exposed to antimicrobial agents – have been found to acquire antimicrobial-resistant bacteria (Radhouani et al. 2014). Concerns about the potential for wild animals, particularly migrating birds, to disseminate resistance genes throughout the environment have been raised (see recent review by Arnold, Williams and Bennett 2016). It has been suggested that sentinel surveillance comprising sampling of high-risk environments would be an appropriate addition to enhance monitoring of AMR (Dar et al. 2016). While GLASS encourages participating countries to collect data on human bacterial pathogens, there are plans to expand data collection to the food chain and environment (WHO 2015).

Vector-borne diseases and other environmental hazards

Earlier we introduced the concept of sentinel surveillance, which involves monitoring of health events through sentinel sites, providers or vectors/ animals. With regard to the latter, sentinel surveillance has been applied to monitor circulation of various human pathogenic viruses and bacteria (see Table 8.3). These pathogens share similar features, notably a highly

Pathogen	Disease	Vector	Animal sentinel(s)
Bacillus anthracis	Anthrax	NA	Cattle and sheep
Borrelia burgdorferi	Lyme disease	Ticks	White-tailed deer
Clostridium botulinum	Botulism	NA	Waterfowl
Leishmania sp.	Leishmaniasis	Sandflies	Domestic dogs
Murray Valley encephalitis virus	Murray Valley encephalitis	Mosquitoes	Chickens
West Nile virus	West Nile fever	Mosquitoes	Crows
Yellow fever virus	Yellow fever	Mosquitoes	Non-human primates
Yersinia pestis	Plague	Fleas	Domestic cats

Table 8.3. Examples of human pathogens that are monitored through surveillance of an animal sentinel. NA, not applicable.

sensitive animal host and an environmental component to transmission. The latter may include a non-vertebrate vector or environmentally stable form such as spores. Given the sensitivity of such diseases to climate-related parameters, there has been substantial growth in methods linking meteorological data to disease data, to enhance surveillance and perform better risk analysis and prediction. For example, using data on changes in climate to predict the human health risk from Ross River virus is now an annual surveillance method deployed in Australia (Woodruff et al. 2006). Climate modelling combined with animal and human health surveillance can be used to better understand and respond to changing risk and is becoming increasingly important with global climate change. Modelling of changes to weather patterns in Zimbabwe, for example, combined with surveillance for parasitic worms in humans and snails, has shown that schistosomal risk will be reduced in some existing areas and increased in previously unaffected areas (Pedersen et al. 2014).

So far, we have only considered infectious hazards with strong links to the environment. Any discussion of environmental hazards must also consider non-infectious threats to human and animal health. According to Thacker et al. (1996), surveillance for such hazards typically encompasses three levels of investigation:

1. hazard surveillance, which establishes the presence of a particular hazard(s) in the environment (e.g. air pollution)
2. exposure surveillance, which establishes the extent of exposure to a particular toxin/chemical agent in the population (e.g. lead poisoning)
3. outcome surveillance, which monitors the frequency of adverse effects following exposure (e.g. birth defects, cancer).

In theory, all levels of investigation lend themselves to One Health approaches. In hazard surveillance, aquatic and terrestrial animals, including humans, are all potentially impacted by pollutants present in air, water and soil, and efforts to monitor and mitigate environmental release would likely benefit all species. Similarly, exposure and outcome surveillance could include monitoring chemical hazards and associated outcomes in aquatic and terrestrial animals, including humans, for the purposes of inferring dangers present to other species. Perhaps the best-known example of this is the use of canaries to detect toxic levels of carbon monoxide and methane in coalmines.

Mercury is another example where One Health surveillance may provide broad value. Mercury in the environment can have serious adverse effects across all biological systems. A striking illustration of this followed the outbreak of Minimata disease in Japan in the 1950s, when a handful of cases of a mysterious neurological illness started appearing in residents of Minimata (Harada 1995). Investigations revealed that city residents had observed strange behaviours in animals: cats were developing convulsions and dying (so-called dancing cat disease), birds were falling from the sky, and fish in Minimata Bay were floating belly-up on the surface. Many of the human patients resided on the shores of Minimata Bay and consumed fish and shellfish from the bay. Subsequent hazard surveillance confirmed high levels of organic mercury in fish, shellfish and sludge of Minimata Bay. Experimental studies in cats confirmed mercury toxicity. Regrettably, the investigation findings were not immediately accepted, allowing contamination to continue. According to official figures, around 2,252 people developed Minimata disease (1,043 died), although many thousands went undiagnosed (Harada 1995).

Lead is another case where One Health surveillance using animal sentinels has proved successful. In the town of Esperance, Western Australia, in 2006, authorities were alerted to a potential environmental disaster following a mass mortality event that affected 10,000 song birds. The deaths were attributed to lead poisoning and isotopic investigations confirmed the same signature in samples collected from birds, humans and the environment, including drinking water and soil (Gulson et al. 2009). The lead carbonate came from a nearby mine, which transported the ore through the town to the port. The sentinel event in animals triggered an investigation that showed lead dust was escaping at the port. Exposure surveillance confirmed that humans in the town had elevated blood lead levels, but very few cases of lead poisoning eventuated because of swift intervention.

Both the Minimata and Esperance incidents illustrate the potential for animals to serve as sentinels for environmental threats to human health. Readers with a particular interest in environmental health applications are referred to the Canary Database, which compiles research articles on the use of animals as sentinels of human health hazards (canarydatabase.org). It would be remiss of us not to mention that humans may also serve as sentinels for animal health events, and often do, given more comprehensive health assessment. This is how many recent emerging diseases – such as SARS – have come to be recognised.

Conclusion

This chapter has described a range of surveillance options and challenges to monitoring disease at the human–animal–environment interface. The principal objective is to design systems that meet the individual requirements of each sector, while providing a more comprehensive picture of the health risks to all populations. Without integration and an overarching appreciation of universal objectives, surveillance systems will only ever be as good as the sum of each separate component. One Health surveillance can build new understandings, give new ways of seeing issues and develop new solutions. It is the intersecting places, issues and ideas of One Health where new advances are possible.

One Health surveillance needs champions committed to harnessing the energy and building trust across sectors. Trust is more often built by deeds than words. We conclude with a challenge to readers to seek new collaborations, merge skills, share knowledge, broaden access and open up opportunities that are unattainable when we work within silos. Many One Health surveillance approaches can be developed, trialled and reported. Over time and through evaluation and sharing of learning, One Health surveillance will move from a few examples to effective and ongoing systems that benefit the whole planet.

Recommendations

These recommendations are directed at local, regional and national levels as One Health issues are not bound by borders or jurisdictions – all levels are interrelated:

- Actively develop opportunities to discuss and build One Health surveillance collaborations. In the first instance, this may occur through informal collaboration with the aim of progressing towards more formal agreements with specific terms of reference.
- Develop support at the local level for One Health surveillance through collection of data on environment, human and animal health parameters. Support may include incentives that promote inclusion and communication between diverse stakeholders.
- Develop, trial and evaluate new ways of combining surveillance data at regional and national levels to build new understandings of health risk and connectedness.
- Collaboratively and jointly report and present surveillance data in each sector.
- Advocate for political, legal and ethical frameworks for sharing surveillance data and building a One Health surveillance network.
- Engage in research collaborations using inter-agency data access and the combined skills of professionals to gather information unobtainable to individual organisations.

Works cited

Acar, J.F., and G. Moulin (2013). Integrating animal health surveillance and food safety: the issue of antimicrobial resistance. *Rev Sci Tech* 32: 383–92.

Allepuz, A., de Balogh, K., Aguanno, R., Heilmann, M., Beltran-Alcrudo, D. 2017. Review of Participatory Epidemiology Practices in Animal Health (1980-2015) and Future Practice Directions. *PLOS ONE* 12(1): e0169198. doi: 10.1371/journal.pone.0169198.

Animal and Plant Health Inspection Service. *Influenza virus surveillance in swine: program overview for veterinarians*. http://bit.ly/2AxYOft.

Arnold, K.E., N.J. Williams, and M. Bennett (2016). Disperse abroad in the land: the role of wildlife in the dissemination of antimicrobial resistance. *Biology Letters* 12(8): 2016.0137.

Becker, K.M., et al. (2012). Field epidemiology and laboratory training programs in West Africa as a model for sustainable partnerships in animal and human health. *Journal of the American Veterinary Medical Association* 241(5): 572–579.

Bird, B. H., et al. (2008). Multiple virus lineages sharing recent common ancestry were associated with a large Rift Valley fever outbreak among livestock in Kenya during 2006-2007. *Journal of Virology* 82(22): 11152–11166.

Bond, K.C., S.B. Macfarlane, C. Burke, K. Nguchusak, and S. Wibulpolprasert (2013). The evolution and expansion of regional disease surveillance networks and their role in mitigating the threat of infectious disease outbreaks. *Emerging Health Threats Journal* 6: 10.3402/ehtj.v6i0.19913.

Bruckner, G.S., et al. (2010). *Handbook on import risk analysis for animals and animal products. Volume 1: introduction and qualitative risk analysis*. Paris: World Organisation for Animal Health.

Butaye, P., E. Van Duijkeren, J.F. Prescott, and S. Schwarz (2014). Antimicrobial resistance in bacteria from animals and the environment. *Veterinary Microbiology* 171(3–4): 269–272.

Catley, A., R. G. Alders and J. L. Wood (2012). Participatory epidemiology: approaches, methods, experiences. *Veterinary Journal* 191(2): 151–160.

Centers for Disease Control and Prevention (2007). Rift Valley fever outbreak - Kenya, November 2006-January 2007. *MMWR: Morbidity and Mortality Weekly Report* 56(4): 73–76.

Dar, O.A., et al. (2016). Exploring the evidence base for national and regional policy interventions to combat resistance. *Lancet* 387: 285–95.

Day, M.J., et al. (2012). Surveillance of zoonotic infectious disease transmitted by small companion animals. *Emerging Infectious Diseases* 18(12). https://bit.ly/2HSvnvH.

Dias, M.R., et al. (2016). Molecular tracking of *Salmonella spp.* in chicken meat chain: from slaughterhouse reception to end cuts. *Journal of Food Science and Technology* 53(2): 1084–1091.

Donado-Godoy, P., et al. (2015). The establishment of the Colombian Integrated Program for Antimicrobial Resistance Surveillance (COIPARS): a pilot project on poultry farms, slaughterhouses and retail market. *Zoonoses Public Health* 62(Supplement 1): 58–69.

Dorea, F.C., J. Sanchez, and C.W. Revie (2011). Veterinary syndromic surveillance: current initiatives and potential for development. *Preventive Veterinary Medicine* 101(1–2): 1–17.

Galanis, E., J. Parmley, N. De With, and B.C. Survei (2012). Integrated surveillance of Salmonella along the food chain using existing data and resources in British Columbia, Canada. *Food Research International* 45(2): 795–801.

Glickman, L.T., et al. (2006). Purdue University–Banfield National Companion Animal Surveillance Program for emerging and zoonotic diseases. *Vector Borne Zoonotic Dis* 6: 14–23.

Gresham, L.S., M.S. Smolinski, R. Suphanchaimat, A.M. Kimball, and S. Wibulpoprasert (2013). Creating a global dialogue on infectious disease surveillance: connecting organizations for regional disease surveillance (CORDS). *Emerging Health Threats Journal* 6: 10.3402/ehtj.v6i0.19912.

Gudo, E.S., et al. (2016). Mozambique experience in implementing One Health surveillance as an innovative tool to understand the risk of spillover of emerging and zoonotic infections between wildlife and humans. *International Journal of Infectious Diseases* 45(Supplement 1): 468.

Gulson, B., et al. (2009). Windblown lead carbonate as the main source of lead in blood of children from a seaside community: an example of local birds as 'canaries in the mine'. *Environmental Health Perspectives* 117(1): 148–154.

Hammerum, A.M., et al. (2007). Danish integrated antimicrobial resistance monitoring and research program. *Emerging Infectious Diseases* 13(11): 1632–1639.

Harada, M. (1995). Minamata disease: methylmercury poisoning in Japan caused by environmental pollution. *Critical Reviews in Toxicology* 25(1): 1–24.

Hennenfent, A., V. Delvento, J. Davies-Cole, and F. Johnson-Clarke (2017). Expanding veterinary biosurveillance in Washington, DC: the creation and utilization of an electronic-based online veterinary surveillance system. *Preventive Veterinary Medicine* 138: 70–78.

Henning, K.J. (2004). What is syndromic surveillance? *MMWR: Morbidity and Mortality Weekly Report Supplement* 53: 5–11.

Heymann, D.L., and M. Dixon (2013). The value of the One Health approach: shifting from emergency response to prevention of zoonotic disease threats at their source. *Microbiology Spectrum* 1(1): 10.1128/ microbiolspec.OH-0011-2012.

Iamsirithaworn, S., K. Chanachai, and D. Castellan (2014). Field epidemiology and One Health: Thailand's experience. In *Confronting emerging zoonoses: the One Health paradigm*, A. Yamada et al., eds. Japan: Springer. doi: 10.1007/ 978-4-431-55120-1.

Institute of Medicine and National Research Council (2009). *Sustaining global surveillance and response to emerging zoonotic diseases*. Washington, DC: The National Academies Press. https://doi.org/10.17226/12625.

International Society for Disease Surveillance (2017). One Health Surveillance Workgroup. https://bit.ly/2SBiV7w.

Jones, K.E., et al. (2008). Global trends in emerging infectious diseases. *Nature* 451: 990–3.

Jost, C. C., et al. (2010). Epidemiological assessment of the Rift Valley fever outbreak in Kenya and Tanzania in 2006 and 2007. *American Journal of Tropical Medicine and Hygiene* 83(Supplement 2): 65–72.

Karesh, W.B., et al. (2012). Ecology of zoonoses: natural and unnatural histories. *Lancet* 380: 1936–45.

Kelly, T.R., et al. (2016). One Health proof of concept: bringing a transdisciplinary approach to surveillance for zoonotic viruses at the human–wild animal interface. *Preventive Veterinary Medicine* 137(Part B): 112–118. doi: 10.1016/ j.prevetmed.2016.11.023.

Kimani, T., M. Ngigi, E. Schelling, and T. Randolph (2016). One Health stakeholder and institutional analysis in Kenya. *Infection Ecology & Epidemiology* 6: 10.3402/iee.v6.31191

Kwong, J.C., N. Mccallum, V. Sintchenko, and B.P. Howden (2015). Whole genome sequencing in clinical and public health microbiology. *Pathology* 47: 199–210.

Lawson, B., S.O. Petrovan, and A. Cunningham (2015). Citizen science and wildlife disease surveillance. *EcoHealth* 12: 693–702.

Levinson, J., et al. (2013). Targeting surveillance for zoonotic virus discovery.Emerging Infectious Diseases 19(5): 743–747.

Lutomiah, J., D., et al. (2014). Blood meal analysis and virus detection in blood-fed mosquitoes collected during the 2006-2007 Rift Valley fever outbreak in Kenya. *Vector Borne and Zoonotic Diseases* 14(9): 656–664.

May, L., R.L. Katz, E. Test, and J. Baker (2011). Applications of syndromic surveillance in resource poor settings. *World Medical and Health Policy* 3(4): 1–29.

M'ikanatha, N.M., R. Lynfield, C.A. Van Beneden, and H. De Valk (2013). Infectious disease surveillance: a cornerstone for prevention and control In *Infectious disease surveillance*, 2nd edn., N.M. M'ikanatha, R. Lynfield, C.A. Van Beneden, and H. De Valk, eds. Sommerset, UK: Wiley-Blackwell.

Monday, B., et al. (2011). Paradigm shift: contribution of field epidemiology training in advancing the 'One Health' approach to strengthen disease surveillance and outbreak investigations in Africa. *Pan African Medical Journal* 10(Supplement 1): 13.

Morner, T., D.L. Obendorf, M. Artois, and M.H. Woodford (2002). Surveillance and monitoring of wildlife diseases. *Revue Scientifique et Technique* 21(1): 67–76.

Morse, S. (2014). Public health disease surveillance networks. *Microbiology Spectrum* 2(1). doi: 10.1128/microbiolspec.OH-0002-2012.

Murray, N., et al. (2010). *Handbook on import risk analysis for animals and animal products. Volume 2: quantitative risk assessment*. Paris: World Organisation for Animal Health.

Nisi, R., N. Brink, F. Diaz, and G. Moulin (2013). *Antimicrobial use in animals: analysis of the OIE survey on monitoring of the quantities of antimicrobial agents used in animals*. Paris: World Organisation for Animal Health. http://bit.ly/2EhgmAY.

Nuttall, I., K. Miyagishima, C. Roth, and S. De La Rocque (2014). The United Nations and One Health: the International Health Regulations (2005) and global health security. *Revue Scientifique et Technique* 33(2): 659–668.

Parmley, E.J., et al. (2013). A Canadian application of One Health: integration of Salmonella data from various Canadian surveillance programs (2005–2010). *Foodborne Pathogens and Disease* 10(9): 747–756.

Pedersen, U.B., et al. (2014). Modelling spatial distribution of snails transmitting parasitic worms with importance to human and animal health and analysis of distributional changes in relation to climate. *Geospatial Health* 8(2): 335–343.

Peeler, E.J., R.A. Reese, and M.A. Thrush (2015). Animal disease import risk analysis – a review of current methods and practice. *Transboundary and Emerging Diseases* 62(5): 480–490.

Queenan, K., B. Hasler, and J. Rushton (2016). A One Health approach to antimicrobial resistance surveillance: is there a business case for it? *International Journal of Antimicrobial Agents* 48(4): 422–427.

Rabaa, M.A., et al. (2015). The Vietnam Initiative on Zoonotic Infections (VIZIONS): a strategic approach to studying emerging zoonotic infectious diseases. *EcoHealth* 12: 726–35.

Radhouani, H., et al. (2014). Potential impact of antimicrobial resistance in wildlife, environment and human health. *Frontiers in Microbiology* 5: 23.

Rist, C.L., C.S. Arriola, and C. Rubin (2014). Prioritizing zoonoses: a proposed One Health tool for collaborative decision-making. *PLOS One* 9(10): e109986. doi: 10.1371/journal.pone.0109986.

Schurer, J.M., M. Ndao, H. Quewzance, S.A. Elmore, and E. Jenkins (2014). People, pets, and parasites: One Health surveillance in southeastern Saskatchewan. *American Journal of Tropical Medicine and Hygiene* 90(6): 1184–1190.

Schurer, J.M., et al. (2013). Parasitic zoonoses: One Health surveillance in northern Saskatchewan. *PLOS Negl Trop Dis* 7: e2141. doi: 10.1371/journal.pntd.0002141.

Singer, A.C., H. Shaw, V. Rhodes, and A. Hart (2016). Review of antimicrobial resistance in the environment and its relevance to environmental regulators. *Frontiers in Microbiology* 7: 1728.

Smiley Evans, T., et al. (2015). Optimization of a novel non-invasive oral sampling technique for zoonotic pathogen surveillance in nonhuman primates. *PLoS Neglected Tropical Diseases* 9(6): e0003813. doi: 10.1371/journal.pntd.0003813.

Sorrell, E.M., et al. (2015). Mapping of networks to detect priority zoonoses in Jordan. *Frontiers in Public Health* 3: 219.

Stallknecht, D. (2007). Impediments to wildlife disease surveillance, research, and diagnostics. *Current Topics in Microbiology & Immunology* 315: 445–61.

Stark, K.D., et al. (2015). One Health surveillance – more than a buzz word? *Preventive Veterinary Medicine* 120(1): 124–130.120.

Thacker, S.B., D.F. Stroup, R.G. Parrish, and H. Anderson (1996). Surveillance in environmental public health: issues, systems, and sources. *American Journal of Public Health* 86(5): 633–638.

Thumbi, S.M., et al. (2015). Linking human health and livestock health: a 'One-Health' platform for integrated analysis of human health, livestock health, and economic welfare in livestock dependent communities. *PLOS One* 10: e0120761. doi: 10.1371/journal.pone.0120761.

Vongkamjan, K., and M. Wiedmann (2015). Starting from the bench – prevention and control of foodborne and zoonotic diseases. *Preventive Veterinary Medicine* 118(2–3): 189–195.

Ward, M.P., and M. Kelman (2011). Companion animal disease surveillance: a new solution to an old problem? *Spatial & Spatiotemporal Epidemiology* 2(3): 147–157.

Wendt, A., L. Kreienbrock, and A. Campe (2015). Zoonotic disease surveillance – inventory of systems integrating human and animal disease information. *Zoonoses Public Health* 62(1): 61–74.

Wendt, A., L. Kreienbrock, and A. Campe (2016). Joint use of disparate data for the surveillance of zoonoses: a feasibility study for a One Health approach in Germany. *Zoonoses Public Health* 63(7): 503–14.

Woodruff, R.E., C.S. Guest, M.G. Garner, N. Becker, and M. Lindsay (2006). Early warning of Ross River virus epidemics: combining surveillance data on climate and mosquitoes. *Epidemiology* 17: 569–75.

World Health Organization (2005). *International Health Regulations*. Geneva: World Health Organization.

World Health Organization (2014). *Antimicrobial resistance: global report on surveillance 2014*. Geneva: World Health Organization.

World Health Organization (2015). *Global Antimicrobial Resistance Surveillance System*. Geneva: World Health Organization. http://bit.ly/2UqPF1J.

World Organisation for Animal Health (2012). *Harmonisation of national antimicrobial resistance surveillance and monitoring programmes. Terrestrial animal health code*. Paris: World Organisation for Animal Health.

World Organisation for Animal Health (2015). *Training manual on surveillance and international reporting of diseases in wild animals*. Paris: World Organisation for Animal Health.

World Organisation for Animal Health (2016). *OIE strategy on antimicrobial resistance and the prudent use of antimicrobials*. Paris: World Organisation for Animal Health. https://bit.ly/2GsR575.

World Organisation for Animal Health (2018). *OIE-listed diseases, infections and infestations in force in 2018*. Paris: World Organisation for Animal Health. http://bit.ly/2G5QmdH.

Zaidi, M.B., et al. (2008). Integrated food chain surveillance system for *Salmonella spp.* in Mexico. *Emerging Infectious Diseases* 14(3): 429–35. https://bit.ly/2t55s9O.

Zinsstag, J., et al. (2015). Brucellosis surveillance and control: a case for One Health. In *One Health: the theory and practice of integrated health approaches*, J. Zinsstag, E. Schelling, D. Waltner-Toews, M. Whittaker, and M. Tanner, eds. Wallingford, UK: CABI.

9
Health before medicine: community resilience in food landscapes

Robert G. Wallace, Robyn Alders, Richard Kock, Tammi Jonas, Rodrick Wallace and Lenny Hogerwerf

Health and disease have more than shaped civilisations past and present. They tell us how a people lived. An era's way of life confronts possible health threats with a specific array of barriers and opportunities (Dobson and Carper 1996; Engering, Hogerwerf and Slingenbergh 2013; Food and Agriculture Organization of the United Nations [FAO] 2013a; Wallace et al. 2015). Some threats are filtered out. Others are offered a fast track forward.

From our species' origins, infectious diseases, historically the greatest source of human mortality, have repeatedly emerged upon major shifts in socioeconomic and cultural practice. Early domesticated animals were sources for human diphtheria, influenza, measles, mumps, plague, pertussis, rotavirus A, tuberculosis, sleeping sickness, and visceral leishmaniasis (McNeill 1977/2010; Wolfe, Dunavan and Diamond 2007). Ecological changes that humans imposed on landscapes promoted spillovers of cholera from algae, malaria from birds, and HIV/AIDS, dengue fever, malaria, and yellow fever from wild non-human primates and monkeys. In some industrialised systems, non-communicable illnesses have replaced infectious disease as the biggest killers: heart disease, obesity, diabetes, micro-nutritional deficits, and other symptoms of a dysfunctional hypothalamic–pituitary–adrenocortical (HPA) axis, translating diet and sociopsychological stress into metabolic pathology

(Cohen et al. 2012; Lemche, Chaban and Lemche 2016; Wallace and Wallace 2013).

New juxtapositions of population health and disease regularly stimulated innovation in medicine and public health, including individual treatment and prevention, but also land and marine quarantines, compulsory burial, isolation wards, water treatment, and subsidies for the sick and unemployed (Colgrove 2002; Watts 1997). Indeed, as classic work by John McKinlay and Sonja McKinlay (1977) and Thomas McKeown (1979) showed, the declines in disease deaths that marked the first half of the 20th century in industrial countries resulted more from public health interventions than from medical advances. Social determinants can improve as well as diminish population health, with historical circumstance repeatedly resetting the clock. Each series of agricultural and industrial inventions accelerates demographic shifts and new settlement, placing susceptible host populations close to novel sources of infection and environmental exposure (Kock et al. 2012; Wallace et al. 2015).

The dynamic continues to this day. At the start of the 21st century, a large part of humanity's organising ethos orbits neoliberal capitalism (Plehwe, Walpen and Neunhöffer 2006). Neoliberalism is a program of political economy aimed at using the state to globalise laissez-faire economics for multinationals, promoting free trade and shifting state expenditures in favour of protecting private property and deregulating economic markets (Centeno and Cohen 2012; Ganti 2014; Harvey 2005). In the course of increasing the scope and pace of turning natural resources into commodity exports, the neoliberal doctrine is transforming planet Earth into planet Farm (Wallace et al. 2016). Forty per cent of the planet's ice-free land surface is dedicated to agriculture, with millions more hectares to be brought into production by 2050 (Alexandratos and Bruinsma 2012; FAO 2013a; Foley et al. 2005; Ramankutty et al. 2018). Livestock, representing over 70 per cent of vertebrate biomass, use a third of our available freshwater and a third of our cropland for feed (Herrero et al. 2013; Robinson et al. 2014; Smil 2002; Steinfeld et al. 2006; Van Boeckel 2013). Industrial animal production is a major source of greenhouse gases (Gerber et al. 2013).

Agribusiness's impact extends to the deadliest diseases. By its global expansion alone, commodity agriculture acts as a gateway through which a wide array of deadly xenospecific pathogens are migrating from the

220

deepest forests and backwater farms to the most cosmopolitan of cities (Engering, Hogerwerf and Slingenbergh 2013; FAO 2013b; Graham et al. 2008; Jones et al. 2013; Liverani et al. 2013; Wallace 2009; Wallace 2016a). Ebola, Zika, and yellow fever recently re-emerged when logging, mining, and intensive agriculture opened up neotropical forests to their escape (Dyer 2017; Wallace 2016b; Wallace and Wallace 2016: Wallace et al. 2018). Other pathogens are evolving more directly off megafarms. Nipah virus, Q fever, Middle Eastern Respiratory Syndrome (MERS), hepatitis E, salmonella, foot-and-mouth disease, antibiotic-resistant bacteria, and a veritable grocery list of novel influenza variants have emerged (Epstein et al. 2006; Graham et al. 2008; Jones et al. 2013; Khan et al. 2013; Leibler et al. 2009; McDermott and Grace 2012; Mena et al. 2016; Myers et al. 2006).

Neoliberal production appears implicated in metabolic disorders as well (Glasgow and Schrecker 2015). Schubert et al. (2011) called for disciplines such as sociology, human geography, cultural anthropology, political science, and health economics to be positioned at the centre of a new nutrition science. In one effort, Rodrick Wallace's (2016) information theoretic model finds thresholds over which an environmental/social feedback signal, acting as unresolved psychosocial stress upon the hypothalamic–pituitary adrenocortical axis (HPA), interacts with the body's regulatory systems to produce body mass pathologies. Bjorntorp (2001) and Cohen et al. (2012) show abdominal and visceral obesity (the most dangerous) originates from the chronic emotional stress that drives disorders in the HPA. Under the greatest psychosocial stresses, including an unresolved 'fight-or-flight' activation documented under globalisation's structural violence (DeVon and Saban 2012), HPA reactivity changes from relatively transient attempts to maintain homeostasis or allostasis, with temporary peaks of cortisol secretion, to a state of sensitisation and exaggerated secretion. Upon repeated challenge, homeostasis can atrophy, directing a larger than normal fraction of total body fat to visceral deposits.

The obesity pandemic (Malik, Willett and Hu 2013), extending across both global North and South, appears a metabolic correlate of a spreading (and shifting) neoliberal model of development. China, for instance, has undergone an increase in diabetes from less than 1 per cent of the population in 1980, at the start of its economic liberalisation, to 11.6 per cent in 2013 (Xu et al. 2013). The latter represents 114 million people, a third of the world's diabetes cases, with half tested showing 'prediabetic' blood glucose levels. In Africa, diabetes is spreading at an alarming rate, with prevalence predicted to increase 80 per cent in 20 years (Dalal et al. 2011).

How are we to stop or alleviate the pathogens and pathologies emerging out of such a model of food production and consumption? Biomedical approaches, from vaccines to emergency care, are necessary interventions for infectious outbreaks and metabolic disease. But in reducing health to molecular, clinical, and even ostensibly public health interactions, such approaches, consequentionalist in bias, repeatedly have proved insufficient (Muntaner and Wallace 2018; Wallace et al. 2016).

Even approaches acknowledging broader contexts can fail. The One Health approach, for instance, supplements the germ theory of disease with an ecosystemic theory: that the health of organisms in the field is relational (Zinsstag et al. 2015). Animals and their pathogens are embedded in webs of interaction across populations and species. One Health integrates investigations of wildlife, livestock, and human health in this ecological context. The approach includes medical doctors, veterinarians and wildlife biologists since many species at a locale share infectious, chronic and environmental illnesses. Who in good faith could oppose such efforts?

The One Health approach, however, repeatedly omits key sources of causality that if included can reverse preliminary conclusions (Wallace et al. 2015; Wallace and Wallace 2016). Health and disease are synonymous with no infectious agent, clinical course, or map of the ill, however conscientiously such epidemiologies are placed in the functional ecologies humans, livestock and wildlife share. Causality often extends beyond the areas where health crises are ostensibly located. The capital backing the development and production behind shifts in land use driving health crises in the global South, for instance, routinely originate in centres of capital, including New York, London and Hong Kong. Sovereign wealth funds, state-owned enterprises, government and private equity, the latter including mutual funds, banks, pension funds, hedge funds and university endowments, finance such development (Daniel 2012; Oakland Institute 2011a; Wallace 2016a; Wallace and Kock 2012).

One Health as a science can blur such contexts, even while describing multiple sources of epidemiological cause and effect (Degeling

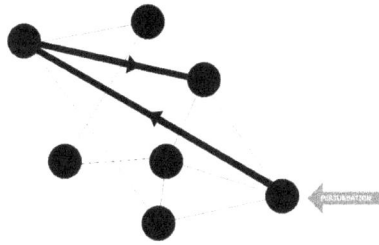

Figure 9.1a Your Schematic of resilient system defined by multiple loose ecological ties (thin lines) among participants (dots) and only a few strong ties (thick lines). Perturbation shock (indicated by the arrow) dissipates along loose ties.

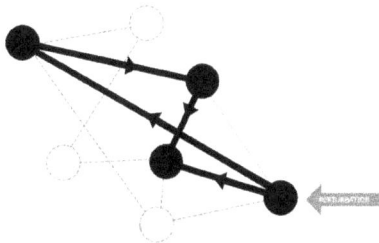

Figure 9.1b Less resilient system defined by a stronger proportion of strong ties. Such systems are often defined by less diversity and are unable to replace lost relationships (dashes) with ecological equivalents. Perturbation (indicated by the arrow) shock broadcasts through entire system, leading to a rapid shift in the very nature of the system.

et al. 2015; Kingsley and Taylor 2017; Queenan et al. 2017; Wallace et al. 2015). If the vantage is limited enough, health research treats state and market neoliberalism as a natural order that study interpretations and proposed interventions must accommodate, even should other studies show the economic system's mechanisms are central to the health crises under examination. Many studies offer rationales for the land grabs, deforestation and agricultural intensification underpinning many a health problem, including famine, in favour of the very companies and governmental agencies pursuing such efforts (and now also funding One

Health studies) (Davis 2006; Martin-Prével, Mousseau and Mittal 2016; Oakland Institute 2011b; Wallace 2016a). The kinds of community resilience at the heart of keeping infectious and chronic morbidities from emerging in the first place are foundationally interconnected with alternate models of agriculture and social organisation that reacquaint economic practice and ecological regeneration (Bennegouch and Hassane 2010; Jones, Betson and Pfeiffer 2017; Kock 2010; Scherr and McNeely 2008; Wallace and Kock 2012). In this chapter, we define resilience and explore several of the mechanisms underlying its function in food landscapes. We also present three examples from the field, from different parts of the world and in different stages of historical development.

What is community resilience?

Resilience is the capacity of a community to absorb external impacts without changing the system's fundamental properties (Chapin, Kofinas and Folke 2009; Folke 2016; Patel et al. 2017). In an agricultural context, these properties can include an area's mix of agricultural sectors, crops harvested, prevalent wildlife, typical economy, and human population densities and distribution. Localities defined by similar demographics can differ in resilience (Gunderson 2000; Holling 1973; Ives 1995; Walker et al. 2004; Wallace and Wallace 2000).

In some areas, the functional interactions among agroecosystemic players are finely structured and characterised by many 'loose' relationships of largely contingent or intermittent interaction (Figure 9.1a). Any single impact upon the community may be felt along some of the 'strong', obligatory ecological relationships, but much of the impact is dissipated along the loose ties. Strong ties lost in an impact are replaced by functional equivalents and the system retains its general character (Kéfi et al. 2016). Such systems are considered resilient.

In contrast, other areas may be defined by only a limited number of requisite strong ties (Figure 9.1b). An external shock felt by one player is more easily amplified across to other players. Such systems, often defined by lesser diversity, are less able to replace lost ecological players. In short, a system defined by only a few strong relationships more

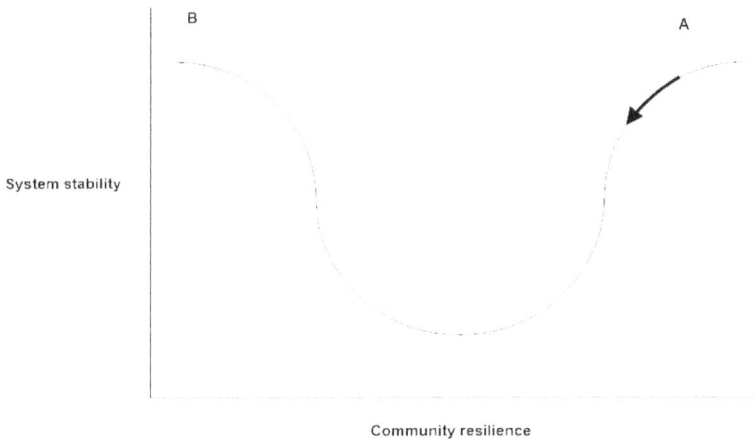

Figure 9.2 Schematic showing transition from an ecosystem defined at one quasi-equilibrium (high stability) by many loose ties and high resilience to another quasi-equilibrium defined by fewer loose ties and less resilience.

readily undergoes a sharp shift in agroecological character. Multiple impacts can degrade a system's loose ties in such a way as to transform a resilient system at one quasi-equilibrium into one less resilient at another equilibrium (Figure 9.2). The new system may stabilise but is also functionally degraded as subsequent shocks are more easily felt throughout.

The International Panel of Experts on Sustainable Food Systems (IPES-Food) (2016) attempts to socialise the resilience concept along two axes:

Environmental resilience refers to the capacity of an ecosystem to resist and recover from stresses, shocks and disturbances, be they natural events or impacts caused by human activity; livelihood resilience refers to the ability of people to secure the capabilities, assets and activities required to ensure a decent living, particularly in the face of shocks (e.g. economic crises, environmental disasters).

The IPES definition folds in a particular metaphysical model of the relationship that nature and society share, with fundamental implications for the metrics that might be used to track systemic inputs and outcomes (Bergmann 2016; Moore 2015). As farmers in any drought-prone region can testify, the two types of resilience are mutually dependent.

These relationships are also dynamic. For Folke (2006), pest and disease control efforts along the lines of 'bio-exclusion', however conscientiously implemented across agricultural sectors, often fail because of a refusal to account for the possibility that systems involve change, uncertainty and surprise, affecting even scales beyond their immediate scope:

> [The resilience perspective] is in stark contrast to equilibrium-centered, command-and-control strategies that aim at controlling the variability of a target resource (e.g. fish populations, insect outbreaks, cattle grazing), a perspective that has dominated contemporary natural resource and environmental management. These strategies tend to solve resource problems in the short term, like declining yields, but success in controlling one variable that often fluctuates, leads to changes in variables that operate at other temporal and spatial scales, like nutrients or food web dynamics. Such management creates landscapes that become spatially homogenized and vulnerable to disturbances that previously could be absorbed ...

Rotz and Fraser (2015) address such industrial landscapes explicitly. In a preliminary analysis, they show agribusiness concentration, farm-scale intensification, mechanisation, and the cost–price squeezes to which contract farmers are subjected have led to decreases in ecological and economic diversity (within and between crops, in soils, across oligopolistic markets), higher orders of spatial and organisational connectivity, and diminished decision-making power at the level of the individual farmer. Rotz and Fraser propose that, as a result, industrial food systems are becoming less resilient to external shocks, including disease and climate change.

Even in an agrosystem of expansive community resilience, complications can abound. The non-linearity, heterogeneity, dispersed interactions across space and scale, and continual adaptation displayed by resilient systems complicate recovery after impact (Folke 2006; O'Neill 1999). Such systems do not just return to a state of quasi-equilibrium. The disturbance may affect the system's ties in such a way that, when the system recovers, it appears superficially similar though not exactly the same. The system does not so much 'recover' as regenerate and reorganise. System trajectories post-impact may be unique and difficult to predict. The notion that one cannot step in the same ecosystemic river twice has inspired some researchers to abandon resilience theory for models of socioeconomic evolutionary process (Wallace 2015). Communities subject to significant perturbation experience a selection pressure that, if they survive, permanently alters their structure and the culture they pass on. The communities evolve along a path-dependent trajectory and never return to equilibrium.

Evolution and resilience need not necessarily be opposed. Communities that adapt can better buffer their core relationships (even as others may indeed evolve anew or are broken for good) (Barnes 2009; Tonts, Plummer and Argent 2014). Even in the face of an epistemic opacity by which the future cannot be predicted, in *some* cases orderly transitions (or even persistence) may be possible. Regime shifts – from one constellation of interrelationships to another – appear preceded by a variety of statistical signals, including increasing variance at multiple scales, greater autocorrelation across system variables, slower recovery after perturbation, changes in skewness, transient amplifications, and spatial indicators (Biggs, Carpenter and Brock 2009; Carpenter and Brock 2006; Dakos et al. 2008; Guttal and Jayaprakash 2008; Kleinen, Held and Petschel-Held 2003; Scheffer et al. 2015; Townley et al. 2007; van Nes and Scheffer 2007). There may be room for a field of applied resilience in food systems.

Resilience, emergent or intended, does not always produce favourable conditions. Perverse outcomes are possible. For instance, a semi-resilient community defined by great diversity but with sufficient strong ties to allow infectious disease or environmental exposure to spill over across a population (and across species) may promote disease persistence in ways that a less diverse community, assuming little geographic connectivity, cannot (Hogerwerf et al. 2010). In the latter community, the threshold of susceptibles to support a pathogen beyond an initial outbreak may not be available. When connectivity prevails, 'good' and 'bad' localities can be linked in counterintuitive large-scale relationships that render both highly sensitive to perturbation (Wallace et al. 2007). Another perversity centres about intervention. A network of weak ties that attenuates bad shocks may also retard intervention efforts (Wallace and Wallace 2000; Wallace 2004). There are, finally, the matters of *for whom* resilience is established and *at what* it is directed (Cretney 2014; Rotz and Fraser 2015). The environmental and economic costs of industrial agriculture are routinely externalised to smallholders, farmworkers, consumers, local rivers, wildlife, livestock and governments, protecting agribusiness from the shocks that its own business model promulgates across multiple biocultural domains (Wallace 2016a).

Despite, or perhaps because, of these complications, we propose the difficult, cutting-edge science of the 21st century will include studying and designing the spatiotemporal configurations across agroecological interactions best able to promote healthy outcomes before crises emerge, pre-empting acute biomedical intervention, however necessary the latter remains (Wallace et al. 2016). We next review three food-disease systems, beginning with those in Tanzania and Zambia, wherein such outcomes – producing health resilience across food landscapes – appear either in progress, switching off, in their planning stages, or combinations thereof.

Village chickens and mixed farming households in Tanzania and Zambia

Rural communities in low- to middle-income countries that rely on rain-fed crops (especially in areas with unimodal, irregular or limited rainfall) often experience severe hunger periods just prior to the major harvesting season when their stored grains have been exhausted. These significant peaks and troughs in household food availability, even in peri-urbanised landscapes, are exacerbated by low diversity in family farming activities, especially for more vulnerable households (Arnold 2008; Sibhatu, Krishna and Qaim 2015). Loss in diversity has been identified as a secular trend as far back as 10,000 years ago, from humanity's transition out of hunting and gathering to sedentary farming, decreasing dietary diversity, with, until recently, limited meat consumption and increased consumption of cereals (Kock et al. 2012; Turk 2013).

In addition to sufficient calories, the right mix of essential macro- and micronutrients is required for each stage of our lives (Alders et al. 2016; Geissler and Powers 2010; Neumann et al. 2003). If the mix is not achieved, the resulting undernutrition will affect the physical and cognitive development of children, with long-term impacts on maternal health, educational attainment, and productivity in adulthood (Black et al. 2013). Different species, and within species different populations, have converged upon various options for nutritional survival and optimal growth across the seasons (Foster and Kreitzman 2009).

Early in human history, humans moved their locations with the changing seasons. Since the advent of sedentary agriculture and large urban centres, humans have designed systems of social reproduction wherein food is moved to human settlements (Metheny and Beaudry 2015). From the late 19th century, rural households have largely switched from producing the majority of food required to survive harvest to harvest, to focusing on the production of a smaller range of food and fibre products they sell into commercial value chains (Ali 2012). Households use the money earned to purchase additional foods to meet household requirements.

The switch is as much structurally bounded as it is a household decision. In what appears a disconnect between human health agencies and their agricultural counterparts, agricultural researchers have tended to focus on developing plant varieties and animal breeds with higher yields and/or faster growth (Turk 2013; Wang et al. 2009). The 'Green Revolution' focused on producing such cheap energy-rich, nutrient-poor plant foods in low-income countries (Turk 2013). Despite increases in agricultural production over the past two decades, malnutrition rates in children have not diminished significantly in these countries. Recent reviews of agricultural interventions on childhood nutrition have shown little impact (Girard et al. 2012; Masset et al. 2012). In response to undernutrition, health-related multilateral agencies have been supporting micronutrient fortification and supplementation through national ministries of health (Alders et al. 2014). Agriculture-related multilateral agencies meanwhile had been supporting production with an emphasis on the quantity of food produced for income rather than its nutritional quality.

The long-term sustainability of these interventions is increasingly under reconsideration because many rural poor are unable to access fortified foods and increased agricultural production has tended to emphasise nutrient-poor staples such as hybrid maize (Idikut et al. 2009). Current debate has shifted focus from food security to food and nutrition security which is defined as existing 'when all people at all times have physical, social and economic access to food, which is consumed in sufficient quantity and quality to meet their dietary needs and food preferences, and is supported by an environment of adequate sanitation, health services and care, allowing for a healthy and active life' (Committee on World Food Security 2012). Other programs explicitly push for food sovereignty in which local peoples actively oppose structural inequalities and exert self-determination around their own agricultural and food policy, including around food production and consumption (Chappell 2018).

Over the past two decades, in conjunction with the new focus, increased attention has been paid to gender equity in agriculture. Empowered women who make decisions on household income and expenditure spend more money on nutritious food, healthcare and education (Quisumbing et al. 1995). Women's work can also lead to increased income, which may be spent on food, improving nutrition. According to the Food and Agriculture Organization of the United Nations, the International Fund for Agricultural Development, and the World Bank, an increase in women's income of $10 in Sub-Saharan Africa achieves the same improvements to children's nutrition and health as an increase in a man's income of $110 (Ashby et al. 2008).

These findings prompted one team to design a multi-sectoral, interdisciplinary and participatory project in Tanzania and Zambia aimed at enhancing traditional village chicken-crop systems (Alders et al. 2014; Pym and Alders 2016). The project, funded by the Australian Centre for International Agricultural Research (ACIAR), emphasised assets controlled by women as a sustainable solution to the ongoing nutritional challenges in Sub-Saharan Africa. The five-year, mixed methods, cluster-randomised controlled project staggered each study ward into the project. Project activities began in April 2014 in Sanza Ward, the semi-arid central zone of Tanzania with a mean annual rainfall of less than 600 mm.

One strategy for meeting the global international development priority of food and nutrition security is to improve village chicken health and welfare. Prior to this project, only one such intervention had been documented. Poultry meat and eggs increase household access to high quality protein, bio-available micronutrients, and income (de Bruyn et al. 2015; Wong et al. 2017). Village chickens are frequently the only livestock controlled by women in low- and middle-income countries in Africa and South-East Asia (Alders and Pym 2009).

Healthy village poultry ensures households have physical and economic access to adequate, safe and culturally appropriate nutrition (Alders et al. 2014). The project began improving chicken health with a community-led anti-Newcastle-disease vaccination campaign of four-monthly eye-drop administrations conducted on a fee-for-service basis (Alders, Bagnol and Young 2010). Manure from poultry and other livestock also improves soil fertility for producing indigenous vegetables at the household level, further diversifying the range of foods eaten.

The wet season commencing December 2014 was very poor in the project area, with rainfall totalling only 183 mm. When grain supplies are depleted, village poultry are often consumed or sold (Alders and Pym 2009; de Bruyn et al. 2015) (Figure 3). Chickens and other poultry can also scavenge feedstuffs not typically consumed by humans (de Bruyn et al. 2015). Despite the drought, data collected in two project wards demonstrated an increase in poultry from 2014 to 2015. The impact of vaccination against Newcastle disease on chicken numbers and nutrition security is under investigation. de Bruyn et al. (2016) did report that children from participating households that owned chickens had significantly improved height-for-age Z-scores than those from households without chickens (-1.76 vs. -1.90; p=0.03).

This model of cross-sectoral and interdisciplinary research collaboration incorporates producers and traders, as well as government and local and international research institutions (Pym and Alders 2016). When adapting a community-centred approach, such collaborations can target strategies with the best chance of long-term

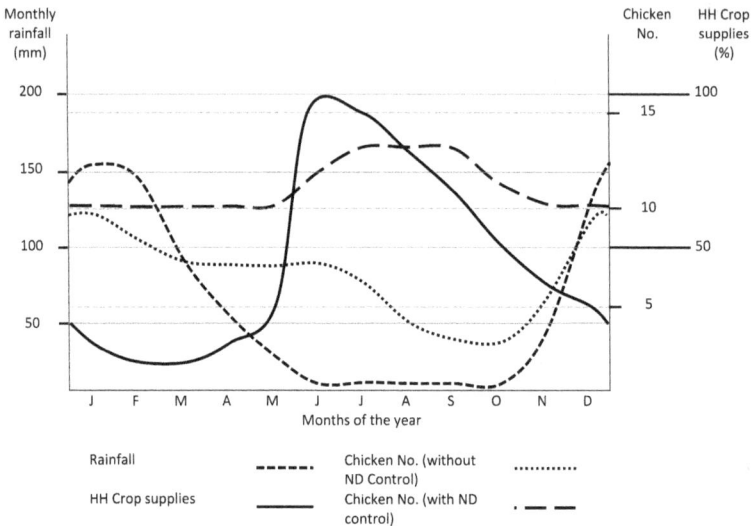

Figure 9.3 General patterns of monthly rainfall, availability of household (HH) crops, and village chickens throughout the year, with and without regular vaccination of chickens against Newcastle disease in Sanza Ward, central Tanzania.

sustainability. The research explores how an interdisciplinary and multi-sectoral team – one covering human and livestock health, food and nutrition security, and related policy-making agencies – can create a cohesive team delivering long-term solutions. The Tanzanian Country Coordinating Committee (CCC), which has oversight over the project, has already contributed to nutrition-sensitive policy interventions at district and national levels.

Linkages between the CCC and households have prompted community members to raise a broad range of nutrition-sensitive issues and interventions (Maulaga et al. 2016). Self-determination, the crux of food sovereignty, enables rural communities to direct their own course in building resilient food systems, often in the face of cheap exports, cycle migration associated with semi-proletarianisation, and other external perturbations.

Resilience shifts among the Nenets on the Yamal Peninsula

Cities and urban sprawl, driving many of the key agricultural dynamics of the ostensibly rural systems just described, are the dominant human-occupied landscape worldwide. Such systems are characterised by a separation of people from the natural land and agriculture into an artificial, serviced environment (McGranahan and Satterthwaite 2014). Retailers and service agents sell goods to consumers, including food and water, clothing, energy, transportation, medicines and other necessities. The food system is mechanised and industrialised, incorporating supply chains from sources of near-global origins (Godfray et al. 2010). Processed food products unrecognisable from their original ingredients are packaged, greatly reduced in nutrition, and carry significant health risks both for individuals and the population (Keding, Schneider and Jordan 2013; Schwingshackl et al. 2017).

These food systems have become so fast and efficient that little consideration is given to storage or preservation, apart from the time along the length of the commodity chain. There is no profit in holding or banking for the seasons, droughts and famines, the last now treated as a thing of the past or limited to villages of the global South. But can the modern family make a meal from raw food? Are the diets in this system leading to healthy bodies and minds? Are these systems resilient? Is three days' food supply adequate for supplying a modern city subjected to a collapse in transport that produces an acute shortage or even the threat of starvation? (Wallace and Wallace 2016).

Rural systems – losing land to multinational agribusiness, men to the cycle migration associated with urban industrialisation, and lifestyles to peri-urban integration – are also being pulled apart in these socioeconomic transitions (M. Davis 2006; D.K. Davis, 2006). Communities remaining on the land and whose food cultures are embedded in local production systems and livelihoods, with livestock and crop diversity consciously cultivated, can survive external impacts putatively more sophisticated societies might struggle with under the worst conditions. Many such communities that survive still access cyclical resources along ancient terraces or routes of transhumance and nomadism, often based on livestock systems (Catley, Lind and Scoones 2013; Tessema, Ingenbleek and van Trijp 2014). They remain cash-poor but largely healthy societies in the relative absence of external inputs and limited healthcare. The seasons are respected. Physical activity is the norm and the need to replenish the ecosystems from which they draw their wealth is a daily duty. Some of these cultures and their diets, such as the Mediterranean, are recognised as world heritage.

The indigenous communities on the Yamal Peninsula, an autonomous region of the Russian Federation, offer one example. The Nenets people were early migrants from southern Asia between 500–1100 AD, moving there during the upheaval of the emerging Mongols (Fedorova 1998). A frozen remote landscape perhaps offered better prospects than life on the steppe with pillaging armies. The Nenets live on a flat peninsula of land the size of England, devoid of forest, bar a few riverine pines (Figure 9.4a–c). Their socioecological system survived the traumatic histories of the Soviet era better than other regions, as has been described by Forbes and colleagues (2009; 2013). Jutting into the Arctic seas of the far north, temperatures during the long dark winter nights are as low as -60 degrees Celsius and hot summer days are marked by exceptional mosquito populations dependent on the blood they find. The vegetated tundra includes a few herbs, grasses, and lichens clinging to impoverished soils, interspersed with myriad lakes and the snaking Orb River and its fish supply.

The Nenets have survived on fish and reindeer, supplemented by berries and a few plant-based foods. They migrate with their herds up to 1,200 km annually (Stammler 2005), retreating from the northern Arctic chill in winter and returning north before from the insect storms from the South in summer. The Nenets remain a rare example of the pastoral or nomadic lifestyle. The reindeer are semi-domesticated, with available food resources determining migration patterns. The herds provide most essentials, including transport and when slaughtered food, warm clothing, skins for constructing household tents, and binding for sleighs. Fish, mostly caught in summer with occasional catches through winter ice-holes, supply valuable protein supplements and essential oils. Trade in these products also provides a small income for purchasing imported goods. Satellite dishes and mobile phones are now in evidence but purchased for their usefulness in the context of communication across their dispersed community and, when necessary, the rest of the world, rather than primarily as a platform for entertainment (Stammler 2009).

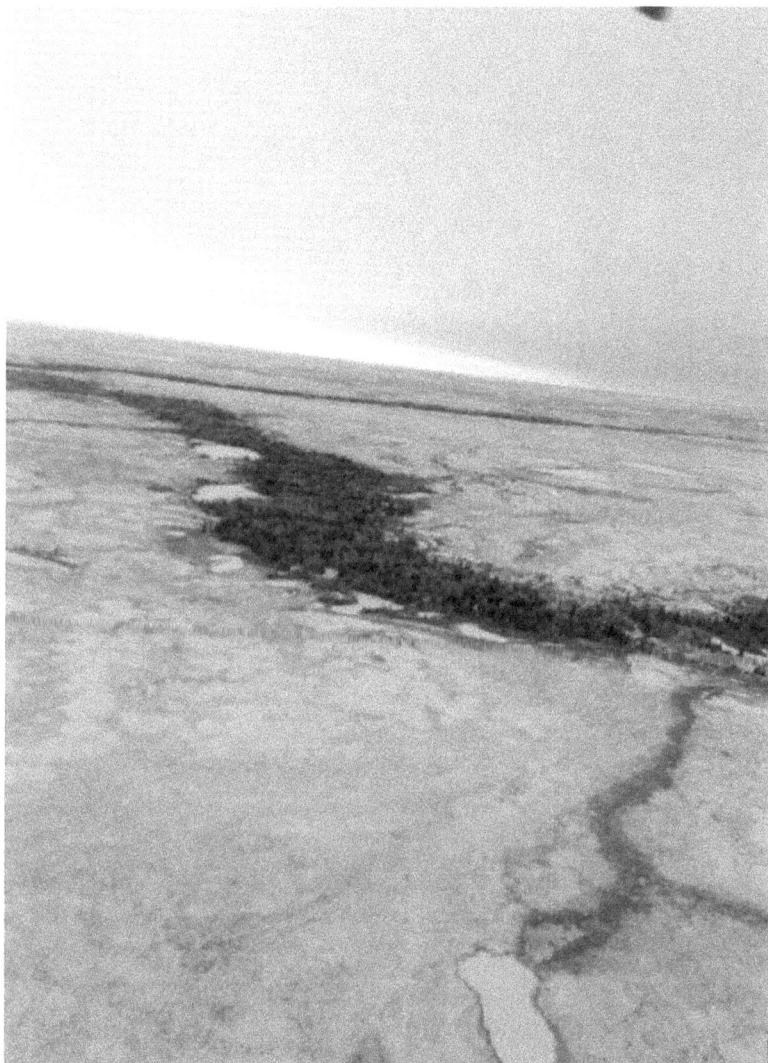

Figure 9.4a Aerial photograph of the frozen Yamul Peninsula within the Arctic Circle with meandering rivers, scant riverine forest, and interfluvial tundra.

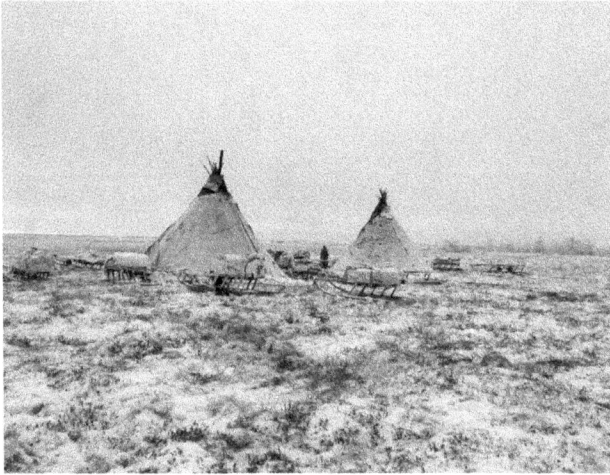

Figure 9.4b Traditional shelters of the migratory Nenets, along the Yamul Peninsula, who are dependent on reindeer and fish for food.

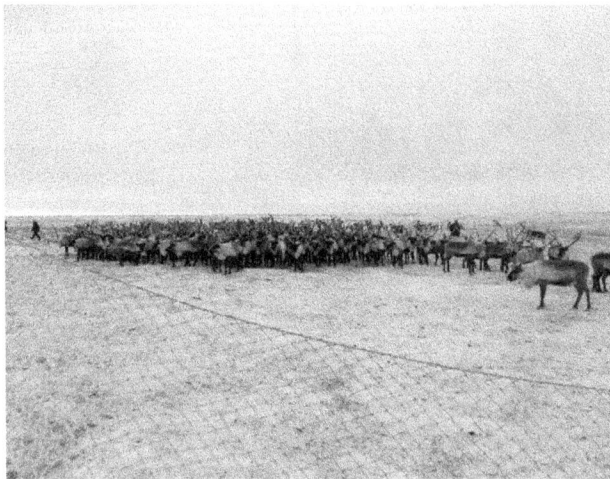

Figure 9.4c Semi-domesticated reindeer herded by dogs and Nenets on sleighs along the Yamul Peninsula.

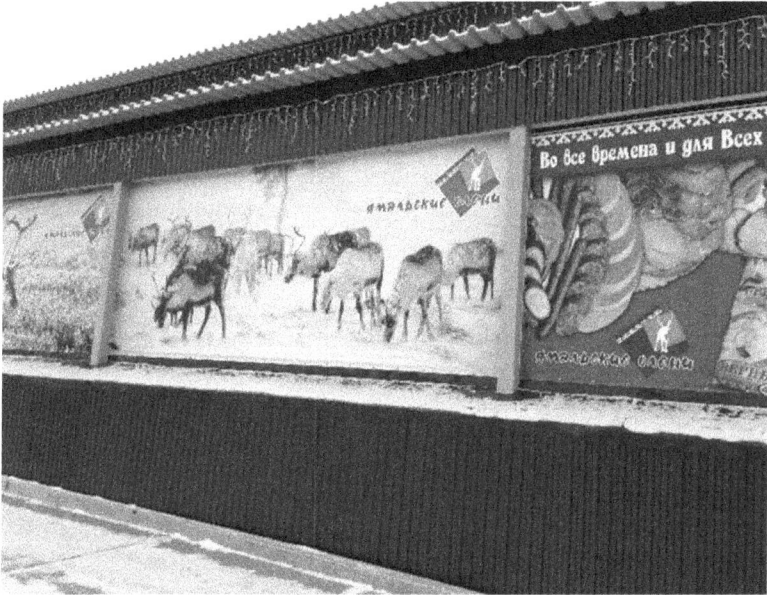

Figure 9.4d An abattoir and marketing company set up for the Nenets to improve their income and enable a more modern lifestyle with schooling, access to communications, and other consumables.

The Nenets population survived for centuries in modest numbers of a few tens of thousands, and about 350,000 reindeer, with limited, if any, support from outside the ecosystem. The ecosystem still functions in the face of ongoing change, including the suppression of carnivores mostly by non-natives and impacts on vegetation from burgeoning numbers of herbivores (Forbes 1999; Kyrazhimsky et al. 2012). At times these impacts are associated with dramatic infectious outbreaks. Over the last century, anthrax, associated with soil exposures, periodically surfaced, with its most recent appearance in 2016 when climatic warming likely led to exposure of previously frozen reindeer carcasses carrying the bacterium (Simonova et al. 2017).

Even as authorities tread cautiously around the Nenets culture, centres of trade and growing administrative hubs have been established, mostly engaged in seeking, exploiting and supporting natural resources extraction in the region, primarily oil and gas (Degteva and Nelleman 2013). These small cities are visible by their columns of smoke from coal-fired boilers, heating large buildings, and vehicles and helicopters moving to-and-fro. The centres offer some benefits to the Nenets, including abattoirs for the reindeer and a small industry in processing reindeer meat for export. These facilities enable some cash liquidity and readier access to modern consumables, medicine and education.

On the other hand, gas-field construction, commercial fishing in the Kara Sea, and increasing environmental damage to lake systems together with construction and industrial activity associated with vast storage and processing facilities, roads, and industrial housing for large workforces have disturbed reindeer and fish migration and reduced fish stocks, resulting in a lower fish intake among Nenets (Degteva and Nelleman 2013; Forbes 2013).

Fishers and traders meanwhile seek the higher prices paid by the new industrial and urban communities, which, when combined with highly processed food and an increasing percentage of Nenets becoming sedentary, is shifting the nutrient composition of their diet. With alcohol and cigarettes added, the prevalence of cardiovascular disease (CVD) is now comparable to urban counterparts in Russia where there are exceptional levels of obesity, CVD, diabetes and ill health especially among women (Petrenya 2014). Kozlov et al. (2014) demonstrate a decline in vitamin D status in these populations as they shift from a traditional diet to a Westernised one. The health shift may exemplify the sociospatial connectivity across systems that, as pointed out above, can drive even a resilient order under (Wallace et al. 2007).

Will Nenets children, now placed in state boarding schools and offered a pathway to modernity, continue to follow the traditional lifestyle? Is health resilience shifting as presented in Figure 9.2? Will sedentary urban life become prevalent, with reindeer herding at best a tourism venture? Will an industrialised diet and associated habits pushed by the prevalent political economy – increasing consumerism, dependence on fossil fuels, access to material goods, inactivity, and alternate transportation and housing – end the community as we know it? Will this unique human culture disappear in the local wake of global circuits of capital?

The lesson underpinning the current scientific debate is less about what is possible and what is 'productive', but rather the value, sustainability and beauty that remains of environmentally integrated communities. Should metrics of Nenets health and wellbeing extend to cultural mode? This is not to suggest that the population return to an arbitrary point in the past. Growing evidence implies, however, that development narratives are often connected to ill-supported and expedient assumptions about progress (Wallace et al. 2015). The health and wellbeing of integrated human–animal communities extend to self-determination. Respecting cultures may be as utilitarian as it is 'just'. Regime shifts may unexpectedly reverse as humanity crosses environmental tipping points, infusing life in the frozen north, even buffeted by climate change, with a greater appeal than the system failures of capital-led globalisation.

Regionalising a 'probiotic' food landscape in Victoria, Australia

Other alternatives are growing from the centres of modern food production. The shires of Hepburn, Macedon Ranges and Mount Alexander in the central highlands of Victoria, Australia, northwest of Melbourne, are well-beaten trails for food connoisseurs (Municipal Association of Victoria 2009). Their restaurants and cafes are bustling while other country towns decline. Where the town of Daylesford is arguably the heart of regional tourism, Castlemaine is affectionately known as 'north Northcote', marking its growing population of urban refugees from Melbourne's northern suburbs. Kyneton and Woodend are corridor towns for those commuters still split between the livelihood of the city and the lifestyle of the country. Hepburn Springs, just north of Daylesford, is home to Australia's largest concentration of mineral springs (Department of Transport, Planning and Local Infrastructure 2014). 'Spa Country' was the first draw for tourism in the 19th century, coupled with the architectural heritage of the region's early Swiss and Italian settlers who prospected for gold in the 1850s.

The rich red volcanic soils make for high quality cropping country, long supporting a major potato-growing sector. But over the past decade, global food giant McCain Foods, the country's main buyer, gutted the crop system, marginalising local farmers in favour of cheap imports. The decline in contract potato was concurrent with growth in small-scale agroecological farming – free-range pigs and poultry, organic and heirloom vegetables – and an emerging niche wine sector. The pairing has increased farms for the first time in decades. In a major break from the model of industrialised commodity farming, most of the new producers sell directly to consumers.

The significant market advantage of its locality – just over an hour from a major international city with a reputation as the food capital of Australia (House 2014) – gives the central highlands the impetus to test strategies in agroecology and resilience across larger regional food production. Can a system of ecosystemically integrated production be developed in the face of a variety of challenges, including a highly centralised food system, climate change and an historically prevalent ethos of rugged individualism that can undermine collective action?

Benedict Anderson (1991) famously coined the phrase 'imagined communities' in his seminal work on the roots of nationalism, applicable to such an agricultural community already rethinking its identity and landscape. A group of disparate people, neighbours and strangers, have over the past two decades begun to view themselves as part of a community of growers, makers and eaters of artisanal, ecological and ethical food. For thousands of years, the area was defined by another imaginarium – of the dreamtime of the Dja Dja Wurrung people, with traditional inhabitants, the Munal gundidj clan, living closest to present-day Daylesford (Clark 1995). The region is still scored by scar trees, rock wells, seed grinding grooves, oven mounds, shell middens and Aboriginal place names (Stewart 2009). Squatters grazing sheep and cattle undertook the earliest of settler expropriation, largely between the late 1830s – when the Blood Hole and Campaspe Plains massacres were perpetrated – and 1850s when gold fever produced a population boom.

A hundred years later, what started with the food-focused cultures of the Swiss and Italians transitioned into fine dining for tourists travelling to Hepburn for the mineral waters. As the restaurant culture grew, so did the population of producers who supply the hospitality market. Good soils, enviable rainfall in a very dry state, proximity to

Melbourne, and a thriving tourism industry rationalised a new model of farming across the central highlands. The population of new farmers includes former chefs, academics and professionals.

The new farmers grow an impressive variety of heritage breeds of animals, fruits and vegetables, and until recently did so with camaraderie but without co-ordination or collectivisation. While most confirm the importance of biodiversity and incorporate it on their farms, the farmers are only now thinking about planning biodiversity for agroecological resilience at the regional level. The new vision includes operationalising the benefits of shared value-chain infrastructure and collaborative distribution.

Regional pig farmers appear ahead of their poultry counterparts in growing heritage and rare-breed pigs and moving away from industrial breeds. The Wessex Saddleback is a local success story championed first by Fiona Chambers of Fernleigh Free Range who worked through the 1990s and 2000s to restore the breed from near extinction in Australia (Chambers 2004). Today there are over a hundred breeding sows of Wessex Saddleback across the country. Tamworth, Berkshire and large black pigs have also risen in popularity. Conscious narratives around the ethics and quality of meat from paddock-raised animals, as opposed to conventional agricultural yield set by corporate buyers at the farm gate, have enabled farmers to price their meat accordingly.

Whereas the slower growth rates of heritage breeds were once considered commercially unviable in an industry that over the past century was totally reliant on purpose-grown grain for animal feed, the new farmers look to predecessors for inspiration and solutions. The farmers are innovating access to and processing so-called waste-stream produce to create nutritious feed. They are weaning themselves off industrial grain, with financial and ecological benefits. Localising supply chains and utilising one farm's surplus yield as another's primary feed source reduces reliance on petrochemicals and strengthens local relationships.

Poultry farmers have also started diversifying breeds of chickens and ducks. One of Australia's best-known pastured chicken farmers raises a new breed bred from old genetics, the Sommerlad bird, in a diverse silviculture that provides shade, protection from aerial predation, and seasonal fodder for these excellent foragers (Sommerlad

Poultry 2016). However, most meat chicken farmers still rely on the industrial Ross and Cobb birds, bought as day-olds and flown in from Queensland. Regional farmers have long been attuned to the welfare of industrial birds grown too fast, a mode of production inducing stress morbidities, including pecking wounds and tibial dyschohdroplasia. The community is now developing understanding of the role biodiversity across farms plays in protecting each farm's husbandry from major ecological and public health threats should a virulent strain of influenza or other pathogen emerge out of the industrial sheds to the north and south of the region (Deng et al. 2012; Regional Development Victoria 2016; Wallace 2018).

In tandem with the Australia-wide movement of new regenerative farmers collaborating and learning by way of social media and at Deep Winter Agrarians, an annual off-season convergence, local farmers have founded a new collective, the Central Highlands Deep Roots Farmers and Allies. The collective is moving towards building a regional abattoir on the old Daylesford abattoir site to regain control of the last part of the supply chain that currently eludes them. The site already hosts an emerging food hub, with farmers and makers processing, packing, storing and distributing a variety of food goods, including wild fermented vegetables, kombucha and pastured eggs.

While the early focus has been on improving local farmers' access to value chain infrastructure in the region, the community is also sharing agroecological methods for continual improvement. Regional farmer-to-farmer sharing of knowledge, itself a pillar of agroecological practice (FAO 2017), includes notes on potential supplies of waste-stream feed; watering systems that are designed to support the growth of new trees for shade, protection and fodder as well as for watering animals in mobile systems; and the ecological and cultural benefits of biodiversity of animals and seeds. Another complication still requires address in the central highlands: connecting the ecological to the economic. How are farmers to overcome the commercial difficulties of working with slow-growing animals with limited genetic pools from which to draw?

From production to processing to distributing the fruits of their labour, these central highlands farmers of Victoria are re-localising the food system, reducing reliance on external inputs, cycling nutrients on their farms, and increasing biodiversity on-site and across the region. They are building greater resilience to epizootic and economic perturbations into their ecological and social structures. Could such a program in agroecological resilience successfully juxtapose regional economic and ecological demands and services?

Conclusion

A recent editorial in *Monthly Review*, a political journal, denounced the concept of socioecological resilience because neoliberals and neocons had appropriated it as the next generation in eugenics (Editors 2017). Affluent societies, the argument goes, are better able to survive disasters. But are they inherently better? A 'survival of the most resilient' philosophy that places claims upon our global future and naturalises the market economy is one that destroys the poorest societies (Cox and Cox 2016). Detailed study, however, indicates that 'advanced' countries are turning increasingly fragile under the very neoliberal programs they celebrate (Rotz and Fraser 2015; Wallace et al. 2007; Wallace and Wallace 2016). So the starting premise holds little support. In addition, it seems terrible strategy abandoning key scientific concepts because proponents of policies to which we object aim to appropriate the ideas for their own uses.

Resilience is indubitably a political object (Armitage and Johnson 2006; Cretney 2014; Hornborg 2009; Robertson 2007). Indeed, new political practices must be instituted from the local village to the global economy. If a community's wealth is found in part in its landscape, a notion upon which our three examples here converge, rather than solely in wages from externally sourced capital or a small plot's seasonal output, then taking care of the land and local wildlife, and cultivating probiotic ecologies able to self-modulate biological control against pathogens and metabolic disorders, turns into a prime directive even in a global marketplace (Wallace 2016; Wallace and Kock 2012). Wealth – in a shared commons of human, wildlife and livestock population health – turns back into the kind of value neoclassical economics has long abandoned. Lauderdale's paradox, by which the market rewards efforts to destroy earth's remaining resources, may be better resolved in favour of populations that conserve the environments they consume (Foster, Clark and York 2010; Wallace and Kock 2012).

Resilience, putting health before medicine, arises in part from communal ownership of resolving the problem of the metabolic rift between ecology and economy, including recycling physical and social resources for the next season, the next year, and the next generation. Such communities in common are unlikely – even unable – to engage in the 'spatial fixes' routinely undertaken by agribusiness as operational practice, skirting from plot to plot when surplus capital is locked up or resources depleted, species by species, mineral by mineral, and region by region (Harvey 1982/2006; Wallace and Kock 2012).

Because political economies are embedded in relational geographies spanning the world, the political project of resilience extends beyond immediate landscapes to unpacking the machinery of global expropriation, the assumptions and practices of which have been stitched into the fabric of capitalist metaphysics as early as 1419 (Moore 2015; Patel and Moore 2017). The International Panel of Experts on Sustainable Food Systems (IPES-Food) (2016) offers one such program, noting, 'The way food systems are currently structured allows value to accrue to a limited number of actors, reinforcing their economic and political power, and thus their ability to influence the governance of food systems'. Qualman (2017) reports that over the past three decades, transnational agribusiness has captured 98 per cent of Canadian farmers' revenues by extracting almost all value from the value chain with sales for inputs and services, leaving farmers with little, in some years placing a nation of farmers collectively in debt. The remaining contract farmers have survived on off-farm employment, federal subsidies, and loans. The concentration of political power rationalises measures of success synonymised with company margins, unbreakable path dependency, export-led production, productivist narratives of 'feeding the world' at the world's expense, and expectations of cheap food that short-changes farmers across the globe (Chappell 2018; Clapp and Fuchs 2009).

IPES-Food summarises a variety of interventions that are turning these lock-ins into entry points for change (Figure 9.5). As the villages of Tanzania and Zambia show, food systems can develop new indicators of sustainability. Outside Melbourne, as elsewhere, shorter supply chains and alternate retail structures are emerging. Agroecology can

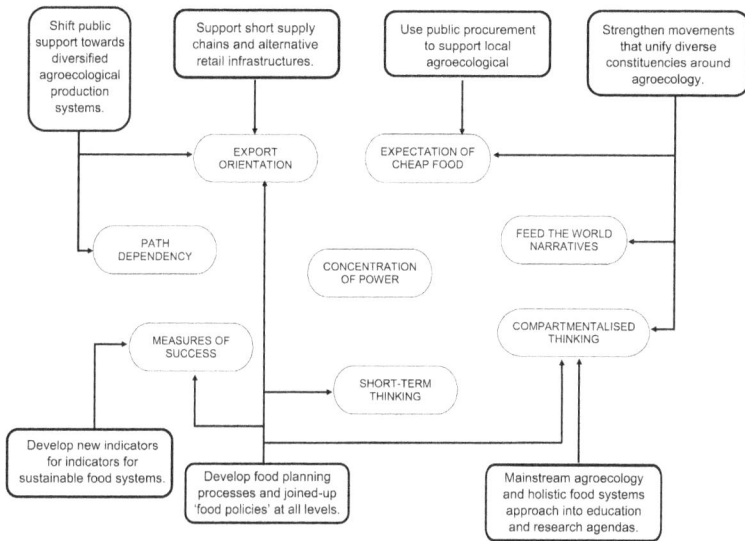

Figure 9.5 Schematic showing interventions that turn sociopolitical lock-ins in industrial food production into entry points for change compatible with agroecological resilience. Adapted from International Panel of Experts on Sustainable Food Systems (2016).

also be strengthened both in research and as a political platform behind which the public can rally in support. As to community resilience directly, Rotz and Fraser (2015), connecting ownership structure to ecosystemic outcomes, recommend:

- Policy should be directed toward creating incentives for more diversified farming systems.
- While acknowledging the utility of agricultural trade, resilience will be enhanced if there is a greater degree of regional autonomy within food systems.
- Increases need to be made to the degree to which farmers are able to act autonomously and choose management practices suitable for their farms. This requires that farmers not only gain political

and economic power (see the next point) but also the skills and knowledge required to farm using more agroecological practices.

- To achieve these ends, there is a need to correct power imbalances in the food system.
- Industrialisation, corporate concentration, and standardisation in the food system have facilitated shifts in both power and practice. In the end, the policy goal ought to embody transformative shifts in system connectivity, diversity and decision-making autonomy that improve ecological resilience on the farm, within the processing and distribution process, and throughout the food system as a whole.

Chappell (2018) warns food system reformers that even shovel-ready programs, however necessary, are insufficient. Success is dependent upon whether the problem, policy and politics streams of society align enough to take advantage of suddenly open policy windows. As agribusiness loses its credibility and authority, alienating a growing roster of constituencies upon which it externalises costs of production – governments, indigenous peoples, farmers, food labour, consumers, taxpayers and environmentalists – such alignments become more likely (Montenegro de Wit and Iles 2016; Wallace 2016). The future of agroecologically resilient food landscapes may be already here. The transitions appear to be arising out of a combination of conscious design and historically emergent practice across nature and society.

Acknowledgements

Funding provided by the Australian government, especially the Australian Centre for International Agricultural Research (FSC/2012/ 023), the Food and Agriculture Organization of the United Nations, and the Crawford Fund in support of research on disease prevention and improved food and nutrition security is gratefully acknowledged.

Works cited

Alders, R.G., et al. (2014). Using a One Health approach to promote food and nutrition security in Tanzania and Zambia. *Planet@Risk* 2(3): 187–90.

Alders, R.G., B. Bagnol, and M.P. Young (2010). Technically sound and sustainable Newcastle disease control in village chickens: lessons learnt over fifteen years. *World's Poultry Science Journal* 66(3): 433–40.

Alders, R.G., et al. (2016). Approaches to fixing broken food systems. In *Good nutrition: perspectives for the 21st century*. M. Eggersdorfer et al., eds., 132–44. Basel, CH: Karger. https://bit.ly/2QTAJGe.

Alders, R.G., and R.A.E. Pym (2009). Village poultry: still important to millions, eight thousand years after domestication. *World's Poultry Science Journal* 65(2): 181–90.

Alexandratos, N., and J. Bruinsma (2012). *World agriculture towards 2030/2050: the 2012 revision*. ESA Working Paper 12-03. Rome: Food & Agriculture Organization of the United Nations. https://bit.ly/1lIkiWx.

Ali, T.O. (2012). The envelope of global trade: the political economy and intellectual history of jute in the Bengal Delta, 1850s to 1950s. Doctoral dissertation, Harvard University.

Anderson, B. (1991). *Imagined communities: reflections on the origin and spread of nationalism*, London: Verso.

Armitage, D.R., and D. Johnson (2006). Can resilience be reconciled with globalization and the increasingly complex conditions of resource degradation in Asian coastal regions? *Ecology & Society* 11(1): 2. https://bit.ly/2CneC5F.

Arnold, J.E.M. (2008). Managing ecosystems to enhance the food security of the rural poor. A situation analysis prepared for the International Union for the Conservation of Nature. https://bit.ly/2DbrjCq.

Ashby, J., et al. (2008). Investing in women as drivers of agricultural growth. Gender in agriculture. World Bank, Food and Agriculture Organization of the United Nations, and International Fund for Agricultural Development. https://bit.ly/2N2H0Po

Barnes, G. (2009). The evolution and resilience of community-based land tenure in rural Mexico. *Land Use Policy* 26(2): 393–400.

Bennegouch, N., and M. Hassane (2010). MOORIBEN: the experience of a system of integrated services for Nigerian farmers. *Farming Dynamics. SOS Faim Newsletter*, September 2010. https://bit.ly/2tgklpR

Bergmann, L. (2016). Towards economic geographies beyond the nature–society divide. *Geoforum* 85: 324–35.

Biggs, R., S.R. Carpenter, and W.A. Brock (2009). Turning back from the brink: detecting an impending regime shift in time to avert it. *Proceedings of the National Academy of Sciences of the United States of America* 106(3): 826–31.

Bjorntorp, P. (2001). Do stress reactions cause abdominal obesity and comorbidities? *Obesity Reviews* 2(2): 73–86.

Black, R.E., et al. (2013). Maternal and child undernutrition and overweight in low-income and middle-income countries. *Lancet* 382(9890): 427–51.

Brock, W.A., and S.R. Carpenter (2006). Variance as a leading indicator of regime shift in ecosystem services. *Ecology & Society* 11(2): 9. https://bit.ly/2FuRDcW.

Catley, A., J. Lind, and I. Scoones, eds. (2013). *Pastoralism and development in Africa: dynamic change at the margins.* London: Routledge and Earthscan.

Centeno, M.A., and J.N. Cohen (2012). The arc of neoliberalism. *Annual Review of Sociology* 38: 317–40.

Chambers, F. (2004). Status of pig breeds in Australia.

Chapin, F.S., G.P. Kofinas, and C. Folke, eds. (2009). *Principles of ecosystem stewardship: resilience-based natural resource management in a changing world.* New York: Springer Verlag.

Chappell, M.J. (2018). *Beginning to end hunger: food and the environment in Belo Horizonte, Brazil, and beyond.* Berkley: University of California Press.

Clapp, J., and D. Fuchs (2009). *Corporate power in global agrifood governance.* Cambridge, MA: MIT Press.

Clark, I.D. (1995). *Scars in the landscape. A register of massacre sites in western Victoria 1803–1859.* Canberra: Aboriginal Studies Press.

Cohen, S., et al. (2012). Chronic stress, glucocorticoid receptor resistance, inflammation, and disease risk. *Proceedings of the National Academy of Sciences of the United States of America* 109: 5995–9.

Colgrove, J. (2002). The McKeown Thesis: a historical controversy and its enduring influence. *American Journal of Public Health* 92: 725–9.

Committee on World Food Security (2012). *Comprehensive framework for action.* CFS 2012/39/4. Rome: United Nations Committee on World Food Security. https://bit.ly/2Hofece.

Cox, S., and P. Cox (2016). *How the world breaks: life in catastrophe's path, from the Caribbean to Siberia.* New York: The New Press.

Cretney, R. (2014). Resilience for whom? Emerging critical geographies of socio-ecological resilience. *Geography Compass* 8(9): 627–40.

Dakos, V., et al. (2008). Slowing down as an early warning signal for abrupt climate change. *Proceedings of the National Academy of Sciences of the United States of America* 105(28): 14308–12.

Dalal, S., et al. (2011). Non-communicable diseases in sub-Saharan Africa: what we know now. *International Journal of Epidemiology* 40: 885–901.

Daniel, S. (2012). Situating private equity capital in the land grab debate. *Journal of Peasant Studies* 39(3–4): 703–29.

Davis, D.K. (2006). Neoliberalism, environmentalism, and agricultural restructuring in Morocco. *The Geographical Journal* 172: 88–105.

Davis, M. (2006). *Planet of slums*. London: Verso.

de Bruyn, J., et al. (2016). *Village chicken ownership, irrespective of location of overnight housing, has a positive impact on height-for-age Z-scores of infants and young children in central Tanzania.* One Health EcoHealth Conference, Melbourne, Australia, 5–7 December 2016, Abstract Booklet No. 583.

de Bruyn, J., J. Wong, B. Bagnol, B. Pengelly, and R. Alders (2015). Family poultry and food and nutrition security. *CAB Reviews* 10(013): 1–9.

Degeling, C., et al. (2015). Implementing a One Health approach to emerging infectious disease: reflections on the socio-political, ethical and legal dimensions. *BMC Public Health* 15: 1307. doi.org/10.1186/s12889-015-2617-1

Degteva, A., and C. Nelleman (2013). Nenets migration in the landscape: impacts of industrial development in Yamal peninsula, Russia. *Pastoralism: Research, Policy & Practice* 3: 15. doi.org/10.1186/2041-7136-3-15

Deng, Y.M., et al. (2012). Transmission of influenza A(H1N1) 2009 pandemic viruses in Australian swine. *Influenza & Other Respiratory Viruses* 6(3): e42–e47.

Department of Transport, Planning and Local Infrastructure (2014). Central Highlands Regional Growth Plan. https://www2.delwp.vic.gov.au/

DeVon, H.A., and K.L. Saban (2012). Psychosocial and biological stressors and the pathogenesis of cardiovascular disease. In *Handbook of stress, coping, and health: implications for nursing research, theory, and practice*, 381–408. V.H. Rice, ed. Thousand Oaks, CA: SAGE Publications.

Dobson, A.P., and E.R. Carper (1996). Infectious diseases and human population history. *BioScience* 46(2): 115–26.

Dyer, O. (2017). Yellow fever stalks Brazil in Zika's wake. *BMJ* 356: j707.

Editors (2015). Interdisciplinary science must break down barriers between fields to build common ground. *Nature* 525: 289–90.

Editors (2017). Notes from the editors. *Monthly Review* 68(9): 2.

Elgert, L. (2016). 'More soy on fewer farms' in Paraguay: challenging neoliberal agriculture's claims to sustainability. *Journal of Peasant Studies* 43(2): 537–61.

Engering, A., L. Hogerwerf, and J. Slingenbergh (2013). Pathogen host environment interplay and disease emergence. *Emerging Microbes and Infections* 2(1):1–7.

Epstein, J.H., H.E. Field, S. Luby, J.R. Pulliam, and P. Daszak (2006). Nipah virus: impact, origins, and causes of emergence. *Current Infectious Disease Reports* 8(1): 59–65.

Fedorova, N. (1998). *Gone to the hills.* Yekaterinburg: Institute of History and Archaeology, Russian Academy of Sciences.

Foley, J., et al. (2005). Global consequences of land use. *Science* 309(5734): 570–4.

Folke, C. (2006). Resilience: the emergence of a perspective for social-ecological systems analyses. *Global Environmental Change* 16(13): 253–67.

Folke, C. (2016). Resilience. In *Oxford research encyclopedia of environmental science.* Oxford: Oxford University Press. https://bit.ly/2QOcPMp.

Food and Agriculture Organization of the United Nations (2013a). *FAO statistical yearbook 2013.* Rome: Food & Agriculture Organization of the United Nations.

Food and Agriculture Organization of the United Nations (2013b). *World livestock 2013: changing disease landscapes.* Rome: Food & Agriculture Organization of the United Nations.

Food and Agriculture Organization of the United Nations (2017). Sustainable pathways: smallholders' ecology. https://bit.ly/2HhJxpQ.

Forbes, B.C. (1999). Reindeer herding and petroleum development on Poluostrov Yamal: sustainable or mutually incompatible uses? *Polar Record* 35(195): 317–22.

Forbes, B.C. (2013). Cultural resilience of social-ecological systems in the Nenets and Yamal-Nenets Autonomous Okrugs, Russia: a focus on reindeer nomads of the tundra. *Ecology & Society* 18(4): 36. https://bit.ly/2T4wdq4.

Forbes, B.C., et al. (2009). High resilience in the Yamal-Nenets social-ecological system, West Siberian Arctic, Russia. *Proceedings of the National Academy of Sciences of the United States of America* 106(52): 22041–8.

Foster, J.B., B. Clark, and R. York (2010). *The ecological rift: capitalism's war on the earth.* New York: Monthly Review Press.

Foster, R.G., and L. Kreitzman (2009). *Seasons of life: the biological rhythms that enable living things to thrive and survive.* London: Profile Books.

Ganti, T. (2014). Neoliberalism. *Annual Review of Anthropology* 43: 89–104.

Geissler, C., and H. Powers (2010). *Human nutrition,* 12th edn. London: Churchill-Livingston Elsevier.

Gerber, P.J., et al. (2013). *Tackling climate change through livestock – a global assessment of emissions and mitigation opportunities.* Rome: Food & Agriculture Organization of the United Nations. https://bit.ly/1cTMGEx.

Girard, A., J. Self, C. McAuliffe, and O. Oludea (2012). The effects of household food production strategies on the health and nutrition outcomes of women and young children: a systematic review. *Paediatric & Perinatal Epidemiology* 26(Supplement 1): 205–22.

Glasgow, S., and T. Schrecker (2015). The double burden of neoliberalism? Noncommunicable disease policies and the global political economy of risk. *Health & Place* 34: 279–86.

Godfray, H.C.J., et al. (2010). The future of the global food system. *Philosophical Transactions of the Royal Society B: Biological Sciences* 365: 2769–77.

Graham, J.P., et al. (2008). The animal–human interface and infectious disease in industrial food animal production: rethinking biosecurity and biocontainment. *Public Health Reports* 123(3): 282–99.

Gunderson, L.H. (2000). Ecological resilience – in theory and application. *Annual Review of Ecology & Systematics* 31: 425–39.

Guttal, V., and C. Jayaprakash (2008). Changing skewness: an early warning signal of regime shifts in ecosystems. *Ecology Letters* 11(3): 450–60.

Harvey, D. (1982/2006). *The limits to capital*. 2nd edn. New York: Verso.

Harvey, D. (2005). *A brief history of neoliberalism*. Oxford: Oxford University Press.

Herrero, M., et al. (2013). Biomass use, production, feed efficiencies, and greenhouse gas emissions from global livestock systems. *Proceedings of the National Academy of Sciences of the United States of America* 110(52): 20888–93. doi: 10.1073/pnas.1308149110.

Hogerwerf, L., et al. (2010). *Agroecological resilience and protopandemic influenza. Project final report, Animal and Health Production*. Rome: Food & Agriculture Organization of the United Nations.

Holling, C. (1973). Resilience and stability of ecological systems. *Annual Review of Ecology & Systematics* 4: 1–23.

Hornborg, A. (2009). Zero-sum world: challenges in conceptualizing environmental load displacement and ecologically unequal exchange in the world-system. *International Journal of Comparative Sociology* 50(3–4): 237–62.

House, A. (2014). Melbourne named among world's top 18 foodie cities. *Escape*, 18 October. https://bit.ly/2TPT4G3.

Idikut, L., A.I. Atalay, S.N. Kara, and A. Kamalak (2009). Effect of hybrid on starch, protein and yields of maize grain. *Journal of Animal & Veterinary Advances* 8(10): 1945–7.

International Panel of Experts on Sustainable Food Systems (2016). From uniformity to diversity: a paradigm shift from industrial agriculture to diversified agroecological systems. https://bit.ly/2SFAljI.

Ives, A.R. (1995). Measuring resilience in stochastic systems. *Ecological Monographs* 65(2): 217–33.

Jones, B.A., M. Betson, and D.U. Pfeiffer (2017). Eco-social processes influencing infectious disease emergence and spread. *Parasitology* 144(1): 26–36.

Jones, B.A., et al. (2013). Zoonosis emergence linked to agricultural intensification and environmental change. *Proceedings of the National Academy of Sciences of the United States of America* 110(21): 8399–404.

Keding, G.B., K. Schneider, and I. Jordan (2013). Production and processing of foods as core aspects of nutrition-sensitive agriculture and sustainable diets. *Food Security* 5(6): 825–46.

Kéfi, S., V. Miele, E.A. Wieters, S.A. Navarrete, and E.L. Berlow (2016). How structured is the entangled bank? The surprisingly simple organization of multiplex ecological networks leads to increased persistence and resilience. *PLOS Biology* 14(8): e1002527. doi.org/10.1371/journal.pbio.1002527

Khan, S.U., K.R. Atanasova, W.S. Krueger, A. Ramirez, and G.C. Gray (2013). Epidemiology, geographical distribution, and economic consequences of swine zoonoses: a narrative review. *Emerging Microbes & Infections* 2: e92. doi: 10.1038/emi.2013.87.

Kingsley, P., and E.M. Taylor (2017). One Health: competing perspectives in an emerging field. *Parasitology* 144(1): 7–14.

Kleinen, T., H. Held, and G. Petschel-Held (2003). The potential role of spectral properties in detecting thresholds in the Earth system: application to the thermohaline circulation. *Ocean Dynamics* 53(2): 53–63.

Kock, R., R. Alders, R. Wallace, W. Karesh, and C. Machalaba (2012). Wildlife, wild food, food security and human society. In *Animal health and biodiversity: preparing for the future. Compendium of the OIE Global Conference on Wildlife, Paris, France, 23-25 February 2011*, W. Karesh, ed., 71–9. Paris: World Organisation for Animal Health.

Kock, R., M. Kock, S. Cleaveland, and G. Thomson (2010). Health and disease in wild rangelands. In *Wild rangelands: conserving wildlife while maintaining livestock in semi-arid ecosystems*, J. du Toit, R. Kock, and J. Deutsch, eds., 98–128. Oxford: Wiley-Blackwell.

Kozlov, A., Y. Khabarova, G. Vershubsky, Y. Ateeva, and V. Ryzhaenkov (2014). Vitamin D status of northern indigenous people of Russia leading traditional and 'modernized' way of life. *International Journal of Circumpolar Health* 73(1): 26038.

Kryazhimskiy, F.V., K.V. Maklakov, L.M. Morozova, and S.N. Ektova. (2012). Simulation modelling of the system "Vegetation Cover – Domestic Reindeer" in the Yamal Peninsula: Could global warming help to save the traditional way of land use? *Procedia Environmental Sciences* 13: 598–605.

Leibler, J.H., et al. (2009). Industrial food animal production and global health risks: exploring the ecosystems and economics of avian influenza. *EcoHealth* 6(1): 58–70.

Lemche, E., O.S. Chaban, and A.V. Lemche (2016). Neuroendorine and epigentic mechanisms subserving autonomic imbalance and HPA dysfunction in the metabolic syndrome. *Frontiers in Neuroscience* 10: 142. doi: 10.3389/fnins.2016.00142.

Liverani, M., et al. (2013). Understanding and managing zoonotic risk in the new livestock industries. *Environmental Health Perspectives* 121(8): 873–7.

Malik, V.S., W.C. Willett, and F.B. Hu (2013). Global obesity: trends, risk factors and policy implications. *Nature Reviews Endocrinology* 9(1): 13–27.

Martin-Prével, A., F. Mousseau, and A. Mittal (2016). *The unholy alliance: five western donors shape a pro-corporate agenda for African agriculture*. Oakland, CA: The Oakland Institute. https://bit.ly/1XNVKSH.

Masset, E., L. Lawrence Haddad, A. Cornelius and J. Isaza-Castro (2012). Effectiveness of agricultural interventions that aim to improve nutritional status of children: systematic review. *BMJ* 344: d8222.

Maulaga, W., et al. (2016). *Supporting policy implementation through collaboration: sustainable solutions to the food and nutrition security challenge in Tanzania*. International One Health EcoHealth Conference, Melbourne, Australia, 3–7 December 2016, Abstract Booklet No. 959.

Mcdermott, J., and D. Grace (2012). Agriculture-associated diseases: adapting agriculture to improve human health. In *Reshaping agriculture for nutrition and health*, S. Fan and R. Pandya-Lorch, eds. 103–11 Washington, DC: International Food Policy Research Institute.

McGranahan, G., and D. Satterthwaite (2014). *Urbanisation concepts and trends*. IIED Working Paper. London: International Institute for Environment and Development. https://bit.ly/2HcSuAU.

McKeown, T. (1979). *The role of medicine: dream, mirage or nemesis?* Oxford: Basil Blackwell.

McKinlay, J.B., and S.M. McKinlay (1977). The questionable contribution of medical measures to the decline of mortality in the United States in the twentieth century. *Milbank Memorial Fund Quarterly* 55(3): 405–28.

McNeill, W.H. (1977/2010). *Plagues and peoples*. New York: Anchor Books.

Mena, I., et al. (2016). Origins of the 2009 H1N1 influenza pandemic in swine in Mexico. *Elife* 5.pii:e16777.

Metheny, K.B., and M.C. Beaudry (2015). *Archaeology of food: an encyclopedia*. Lanham, MD: Rowman & Littlefield.

Montenegro de Wit, M., and A. Iles (2016). Toward thick legitimacy: creating a web of legitimacy for agroecology. *Elementa Science of the Anthropocene* 4:p.000115. http://doi.org/10.12952/journal.elementa.000115.

Moore, J. (2015). *Capitalism in the web of life: ecology and the accumulation of capital*. New York: Verso.

Municipal Association of Victoria (2009). Submission – inquiry into the impact of the Global Financial Crisis on regional Australia. https://bit.ly/2SHd1ll

Muntaner, C., and R.G. Wallace (2018). Confronting the social and environmental determinants of health. In *Under the knife: beyond capital in health*, H. Waitzkin, ed. 224–38. New York: Monthly Review Press.

Myers, K., et al. (2006). Are swine workers in the United States at increased risk of infection with zoonotic influenza virus? *Clinical Infection & Disease* 42(1): 14–20.

Neumann, C.G., et al. (2003). Animal source foods improve dietary quality, micronutrient status, growth and cognitive function in Kenyan school children: background, study design and baseline findings. *Journal of Nutrition* 133(11, Supplement 2): 3941S–3949S.

Oakland Institute (2011a). Special investigation phase one: understanding land investment deals in Africa. https://bit.ly/2AJc41V.

Oakland Institute (2011b). Special investigation phase two: understanding how land deals contribute to famine and conflict in Africa. https://bit.ly/2TRE5eL.

O'Neill, R.V. (1999). Recovery in complex ecosystems. *Journal of Aquatic Ecosystem Stress & Recovery* 6(3): 181–7.

Patel, R., and J.W. Moore (2017). *A history of the world in seven cheap things: a guide to capitalism, nature, and the future of the planet*. Berkeley: University of California Press.

Patel, S.S., M.B. Rogers, R. Amlôt, and G.J. Rubin (2017). What do we mean by 'community resilience'? A systematic literature review of how it is defined in the literature. *PLOS Currents Disasters* Feb 1 (Edition 1). https://bit.ly/2AL6zzx.

Petrenya, N. (2012). A study of fish consumption and cardiometabolic risk factors among the Circumpolar population of the rural Nenets Autonomous Area in comparison with the urban population of Arkhangelsk County. Doctoral thesis, Faculty of Health Sciences, Department of Community Medicine, University of Tromsø Norway. https://bit.ly/2GozRsc

Plehwe, D., B. Walpen, and G. Neunhöffer, eds. (2006). *Neoliberal hegemony: a global critique*. New York: Routledge.

Pym, R., and R. Alders (2016). Helping smallholders to improve poultry production. In *Achieving sustainable production of poultry meat*, S.C. Ricke, ed. 441–71. Cambridge, UK: Burleigh Dodds Science Publishing.

Qualman, D. (2017). Agribusiness takes all: 90 years of Canadian net farm income. https://bit.ly/2Cp5Jc4.

Queenan, K., et al. (2017). Roadmap to a One Health agenda 2030. *CAB Reviews* 12(014): 1–17.

Quisumbing, A.R., L.R. Brown, H.S. Feldstein, L. Haddad, and C. Pena (1995). *Women: the key to food security*. Food Policy Statement No. 21. Washington, DC: International Food Policy Research Institute.

Ramankutty, N., et al. (2018). Trends in global agricultural land use: implications for environmental health and food security. *Annual Review of Plant Biology* 69: 789–815.

Regional Development Victoria (2016). Victoria's broiler industry. https://bit.ly/2WXxX6V

Robertson, M.M. (2007). The neoliberalization of ecosystem services: wetland mitigation banking and the problem of measurement. In *Neoliberal environments: false promises and unnatural consequences*, N. Heynen, J. McCarthy, S. Prudham, and P. Robbins, eds. 114–25. New York: Routledge.

Robinson, T., et al. (2014). Mapping the global distribution of livestock. *PLOS One* 9(5): e96084. doi: 10.1371/journal.pone.0096084.

Rotz, S., and E.D.G. Frase (2015). Resilience and the industrial food system: analyzing the impacts of agricultural industrialization on food system vulnerability. *Journal of Environmental Studies and Sciences* 5(3): 459–73.

Scheffer, M., S.R. Carpenter, V. Dakos, and E.H. van Nes (2015). Generic indicators of ecological resilience: inferring the chance of a critical transition. *Annual Review of Ecology, Evolution & Systematics* 46: 145–67.

Scherr, S.J., and J.A. McNeely (2008). Biodiversity conservation and agricultural sustainability: towards a new paradigm of 'ecoagriculture' landscapes. *Philosophical Transactions of The Royal Society B Biological Sciences* 363(1491): 477–94.

Schubert, L., D. Gallegos, W. Foley, and C. Harrison (2011). Re-imagining the 'social' in the nutrition sciences. *Public Health Nutrition* 15(2): 352–9.

Schwingshackl, L., et al. (2017). Food groups and risk of type 2 diabetes mellitus: a systematic review and meta-analysis of prospective studies. *European Journal of Epidemiology* 32(5): 363–75.

Sibhatu, K.T., V.V. Krishna, and M. Qaim (2015). Production diversity and dietary diversity in smallholder farm households. *Proceedings of the National Academy of Sciences of the United States of America* 112(34): 10657–62.

Simonova, E.G., et al. (2017). Anthrax in the territory of Yamal: assessment of epizootiological and epidemiological risks. *Infektsii* 1: 89–93.

Smil, V. (2002). Eating meat: evolution, patterns, and consequences. *Population & Development Review* 28: 599–639.

Sommerlad Poultry (2016). https://bit.ly/2HgKPBu.

Stammler, F. (2005). *Reindeer nomads meet the market: culture, property and globalisation at 'the end of the land'*. Berlin: Lit Verlag.

Stammler, F. (2009). Mobile phone revolution in the tundra? Technological change among Russian reindeer nomads. *Folklore: Electronic Journal of Folklore* 41: 47–78. https://bit.ly/2He1jKr.

Steinfeld, H., et al. (2006). *Livestock's long shadow: environmental issues and options*. Rome: Food & Agriculture Organization of the United Nations.

Stewart, A. (2009). Windows onto other worlds: the role of imagination in outdoor education. Paper presented at *Outdoor education research and theory: critical reflections, new directions*, the Fourth International Outdoor Education Research Conference, La Trobe University, Beechworth, Victoria, Australia, 15–18 April 2009. https://bit.ly/2RwbVsV.

Tessema, W.K., P.T.M. Ingenbleek, and H.C.M. van Trijp (2014). Pastoralism, sustainability, and marketing: a review. *Agronomy for Sustainable Development* 34(1): 75–92.

Tonts, M., P. Plummer, and N. Argent (2014). Path dependence, resilience and the evolution of new rural economies: perspectives from rural Western Australia. *Journal of Rural Studies* 36: 362–75.

Townley, S., D. Carslake, O. Kellie-Smith, D. McCarthy, and D. Hodgson (2007). Predicting transient amplification in perturbed ecological systems. *Journal of Applied Ecology* 44(6): 1243–51.

Turk, J.M. (2013). Poverty, livestock and food security in developing countries. *CAB Reviews* 8(033): 1–8.

Van Boeckel, T. P. (2013). Intensive poultry production and highly pathogenic avian influenza H5N1 in Thailand: statistical and process-based models. Doctoral thesis, Université Libre de Bruxelles.

van Nes, E.H., and M. Scheffer (2007). Slow recovery from perturbations as a generic indicator of a nearby catastrophic shift. *American Naturalist* 169(6): 738–47.

Walker, B., C.S. Holling, S.R. Carpenter, and A. Kinzig (2004). Resilience, adaptability and transformability in social-ecological systems. *Ecology & Society* 9(2): 5. http://www.ecologyandsociety.org/vol9/iss2/art5/

Wallace, D., and R. Wallace (2000). Life and death in Upper Manhattan and the Bronx: toward an evolutionary perspective on catastrophic social change. *Environment & Planning A* 32(7): 1245–66.

Wallace, R. (2015). *An ecosystem approach to economic stabilization: escaping the neoliberal wilderness*. New York: Routledge.

Wallace, R. (2016). Visceral obesity and psychosocial stress: a generalized control theory model. *Connection Science* 28(3): 217–25.

Wallace, R., and D. Wallace (2013). *A mathematical approach to multilevel, multiscale health interventions: pharmaceutical industry decline and policy response*. London: Imperial College Press.

Wallace, R., D. Wallace, J. Ahern, and S. Galea (2007). A failure of resilience: estimating response of New York City's public health ecosystem to sudden disaster. *Health & Place* 13(2): 545–50.

Wallace, R., and R.G. Wallace (2016). The social amplification of pandemics and other disasters. In *Neoliberal Ebola: modeling disease emergence from finance to forest and farm*. R.G. Wallace and R. Wallace, eds., 81–93. Basel, CH: Springer.

Wallace, R., L.F. Chaves, L.R. Bergmann, C. Ayres, L. Hogerwerf, R. Kock, and R.G. Wallace (2018). *Clear-cutting disease control: capital-led deforestation, public health austerity, and vector-borne infection*. Switzerland: Springer.

Wallace, R.G. (2003). AIDS in the HAART era: New York's heterogeneous geography. *Social Science & Medicine* 56(6): 1155–71.

Wallace, R.G. (2004). Projecting the impact of HAART on the evolution of HIV's life history. *Ecological Modelling* 176(3-4): 227-253.

Wallace, R.G. (2009). Breeding influenza: the political virology of offshore farming. *Antipode* 41(5): 916–51.

Wallace R.G. (2016a). *Big farms make big flu: dispatches on infectious disease, agribusiness, and the nature of science*. New York: Monthly Review Press.

Wallace, R.G. (2016b). Losing the forest for the trees. https://bit.ly/1XQBWfw.

Wallace, R.G. (2018). *Duck and cover: epidemiological and economic implications of ill-founded assertions that pasture poultry are an inherent disease risk*. The Australian Food Sovereignty Alliance. https://bit.ly/2Tpo8wM.

Wallace, R.G, et al. (2015). The dawn of structural One Health: a new science tracking disease emergence along circuits of capital. *Social Science & Medicine* 129: 68–77.

Wallace, R.G., and R.A. Kock (2012). Whose food footprint? Capitalism, agriculture and the environment. *Human Geography* 5(1): 63–83.

Wallace, R.G., et al. (2016). Did neoliberalizing West African forests produce a new niche for Ebola? *International Journal of Health Services* 46(1): 149–65

Wallace, R.G., and R. Wallace, eds. (2016). *Neoliberal Ebola: modeling disease emergence from finance to forest and farm*. Basel, CH: Springer.

Wang, Y., C. Lehane, K. Ghebremeskel, and M.A. Crawford (2009). Modern organic and broiler chickens sold for human consumption provide more energy from fat than protein. *Public Health Nutrition* 13(3): 400–8.

Wolfe, N.D., C.P. Dunavan, and J. Diamond (2007). Origins of major human infectious diseases. *Nature* 447(7142): 279–83.

Wong, J.T., et al. (2017). Small-scale poultry and food security in resource-poor settings: a review. *Global Food Security* 15: 43–52. doi: 10.1016/j.gfs.2017.04.003.

World Bank (2006). Why invest in nutrition? In *Repositioning nutrition as central to development: a strategy for large-scale action*, 21–41. Washington, DC: World Bank.

Xu, Y., et al. (2010). China Noncommunicable Disease Surveillance Group, 2013. Prevalence and control of diabetes in Chinese adults. *Journal of the American Medical Association* 310(9): 948–59.

Zinsstag, J., E. Schelling, D. Waltner-Toews, M. Whittaker, and M. Tanner, eds. (2015). *One Health: the theory and practice of integrated health approaches.* Wallingford, UK: CABI.

10
A clash of appetites: food-related dimensions of human–animal conflict and disease emergence

Sean C.P. Coogan, Robyn Alders, Richard Kock, David Raubenheimer and Siobhan M. Mor

In 2011 the human population crossed the 7 billion threshold, more than doubling the global population just 50 years earlier, leading to radical changes in human food production systems (Food and Agriculture Organization Corporate Statistical Database [FAOSTAT] 2014; United Nations Population Fund 2011). While 66 per cent of people lived rurally in 1961, more than half now live in cities (FAOSTAT 2014). Land clearing for human food production – including growing crops for human consumption or production of livestock/fish feed, as well as grazing livestock – has converted around 40 per cent of the earth's surface to cropland and pasture (Foley et al. 2005) (Figure 10.1a). Demand is largely met with increases in production per land area, as a result of technological advances (e.g. fertiliser and irrigation), improvements in plant and livestock genetics, and intensification of livestock industries. Taken together, humans and livestock now make up approximately 96 per cent of global mammal biomass (Bar-On et al. 2018). Simultaneous with increasing population and food production, rising per capita incomes in recent decades have changed human diets. The average human now consumes 2,870 kilocalories (kcal) per person per day, up from 2,196 kcal per person per day in 1961, with a larger proportion of the diet comprising food of domestic animal origin (FAOSTAT 2014; Kearney 2010).

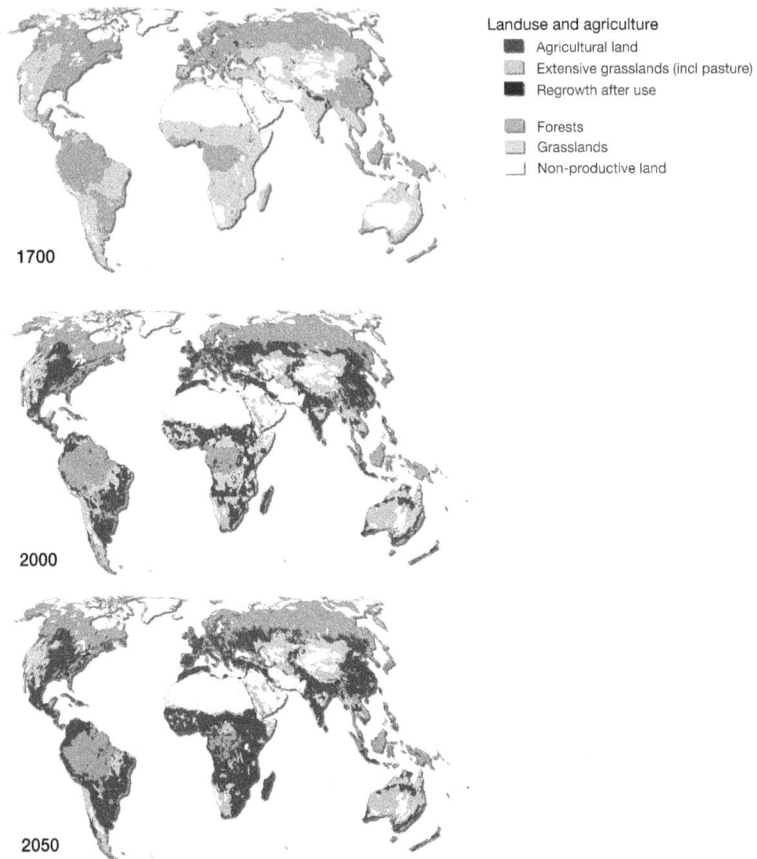

Figure 10.1a Land use and agriculture and biodiversity loss.

These rapid changes are problematic for the health of humans, other species and the environment. Industrialisation of the food chain has contributed to a global incidence of overweight and obesity of approximately 1.5 billion, despite some 1–2 billion people suffering from inadequate calorie or macro/micronutrient intake (Bhutta and Salam 2012; Nordin et al. 2013). Concurrently, the anthropogenically dominated landscape is profoundly impacting non-human species.

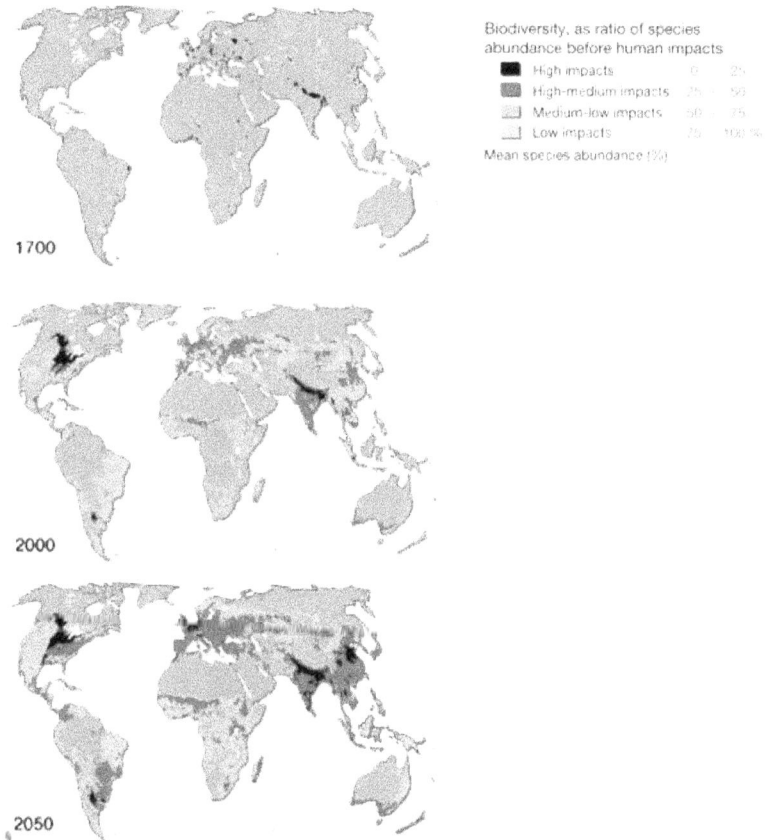

Figure 10.1b Land use and agriculture 1700 to 2050. Source: Hugo Ahlenius, United Nations Environment Programme/Global Resource Information Database-Arendal.

Habitat loss and fragmentation is a primary threat to many endangered wild species, with agricultural expansion a major contributor (Baillie et al. 2004; Can et al. 2014). Between 1970 and 2014, animal species populations are estimated to have declined by 60 percent, with freshwater species declining by 83% according to the living planet index (WWF/ZSL 2018). The speed of decline indicates that a sixth mass-extinction is underway (Ceballos et al. 2005). Other human-influenced biotic and abiotic factors are also fundamentally changing the planetary geophysical and chemical systems. For example, global agriculture and human food production is estimated to contribute 25 per cent of all greenhouse gases, which are driving rapid warming of the planet's climate (Edenhofer et al. 2014). Climate change is predicted to have far-ranging impacts across the biosphere, with a recent meta-analysis estimating that around one in six (16 per cent) species could become extinct under current policies (Urban 2015). Conservation efforts have had limited success, but they have not reversed the current rate of biodiversity loss (Hoffman et al. 2010) (Figure 10.1b).

Competition between humans and non-human animals over resources such as food and space damages both populations. Human–wildlife conflict arising through depredation of livestock by large predators (Boitani et al. 2015) or agricultural crops by herbivores such as elephants (Mamo et al. 2015) negatively impacts on farmer livelihoods and often results in retaliatory attacks on wildlife. Further, encroachment of humans and livestock on wildlife habitat has created new opportunities for emergence and exchange of infectious agents. Scientists have identified an increase in new and emerging infectious diseases in humans, a majority of which had their origins in non-domesticated animals (Jones et al. 2008; Morse et al. 2012). Many such pathogens are now independently maintained in humans (e.g. human immunodeficiency virus, HIV) and their domestic animals (e.g. highly pathogenic avian influenza, HPAI). Changing human food production systems as a key driver for disease emergence is relatively well understood (Jones et al. 2013; Keesing et al. 2010; McFarlane, Sleigh and McMichael 2013), but rarely have the resource-related needs of non-human animals been discussed in this context.

In this chapter, we investigate the biological dimensions of conflict between humans and non-human animals. Human–wildlife conflict is any interaction between humans and wildlife where the needs and behaviour of wildlife negatively impact the goals, needs and behaviours of humans, and vice versa (Cline, Sexton and Stewart 2007; Madden 2004). Infectious diseases are an example of a negative impact as a result of interaction between species. Competition over resources – and food in particular – is a key driver of human–wildlife conflict and disease emergence. Using four case studies ranging from sociobehavioural and habitat-related issues to the nutritional preferences of animals, we show how diverse synthesis can improve understanding of the complex nature of this topic and influence the development of strategies that facilitate the cohabitation of human and non-human animals.

The carnivores

Our first case study explores the African wild dog (*Lycaon pictus;* AWD) in carnivore–human conflict, noting its relevance to other species. When carnivores come into conflict with humans – worldwide – they are more vulnerable to extinction (Ripple et al. 2014). Strict carnivores such as large cats (Felidae) and wolves (*Canis lupus*) cause livestock depredation which is a major cause of human–wildlife conflict (Chapron et al. 2014; Inskip and Zimmermann 2009; Ripple et al. 2014; Treves and Karanth 2003). The impact of livestock depredation and fear of carnivores can lead to negative public perception and persecution (Zedrosser et al. 2011). In Nepal, endangered snow leopards (*Panthera uncia*) attacked livestock raised by resident agro-pastoralists, resulting in an estimated loss of more than US$44,000 in less than two years, culminating in retaliatory killings of snow leopards and other predators (Aryal et al. 2014). Situations such as these are a global problem involving several carnivore species, ranging from wolverine (*Gulo gulo*) in Scandinavia (Boitani et al. 2015) to dingoes (*C. l. dingo*) and domestic crosses in Australia (Fleming et al. 2001).

Case study 1: African wild dogs (AWD)

AWDs belong to a unique genus (i.e. distinct from *Canis*) within the dog family (Canidae) and are proficient predators, hunting in packs, never scavenging. They were once a successful species, ranging across the savannahs of Africa where they thrived on abundant antelope prey for over a million years (Savage 1978). With the evolution and expansion of humans and associated livestock and the decline of wild herbivore populations, this wide-ranging species is now extinct in all but a few locations; today it is classified as endangered on the

International Union for Conservation of Nature (IUCN) 2015 Red List (Woodroffe and Sillero-Zubiri 2012). Research on causes of mortality in free-ranging populations of AWD across Africa showed that 73 per cent of adults and 16 per cent of pups died from human-caused road/ train accidents, shooting, poisoning and snaring (Woodroffe, McNutt and Mills 2004). While deaths occur inside and outside of protected areas the majority of the conflict is in the community or privately owned lands. The wild dog is particularly susceptible to this, as their home range usually exceeds that of the available protected areas. A further 5 per cent die from diseases, such as rabies and canine distemper contracted from the domestic dog reservoir (Woodroffe, McNutt and Mills 2004). Insufficient protected land for this species and subsequently competition over resources is at the root of the conservation challenge. The recent history of the WDA provides an excellent illustration of depredation and human food–wildlife conflict.

In wildlife protected, private or community wildlife areas AWD are mostly welcomed, and considered important for eco tourism (Lindsey et al. 2005). In game ranches where hunting, game consumption and livestock farming occur, a perception exists that the AWD compete with other species for trophy animals or food (Lindsey et al. 2005). Research shows that AWDs tend to select weak and poor trophy animals suggesting that, far from being a competitor, they provide an ecosystem service by ensuring selection pressure for better quality animals (Pole et al. 2004). Studies also show that AWDs are less relevant in this conflict than the lion, hyena and leopard (Ogada et al. 2003; Woodroffe et al. 2005), and that livestock are more likely to die due to disease or theft than depredation (Frank 1998; Rasmussen 1999). Nevertheless, there are documented examples of livestock losses due to AWD affecting both extensive community systems and more intensive livestock systems and ranches (Davies and du Toit 2004; Kock et al. 1999; Rasmussen 1999; Woodroffe et al. 2005).

A survey of attitudes among Southern African livestock and game farm owners (mostly ranchers from ethnically European, English and Afrikaans speaking communities) provides insight into the problem (Lindsey et al. 2005). Notably, depredation by AWD appears to be worse with small and fenced properties, or where offtake for commercial purposes was high, requiring artificially high densities of livestock. In open systems, such as conservancies (i.e. multiple properties cooperating and removing fencing) with less restrictions on animal movement, the presence of AWDs was better tolerated. In more traditional African communities, such as pastoral systems in Eastern Africa, nomadic livestock keepers tolerate the AWD even though the level of cattle husbandry is high. Protection is via the use of fortified enclosures ('bomas'), guarded by humans and dogs, and more recently with the use of 'lion lights' for night protection (Ogada et al. 2003; Pimm 2012). But there are communities in Eastern Africa – mainly agro-pastoralists with settled livestock – that are more likely to persecute AWDs when they pass through their land. They fear the animal and suffer from raids in the absence of protective measures (Kock et al. 1999).

The usual behaviour of AWD in areas of abundant herbivorous wildlife is to select natural prey species and avoid contact with humans and livestock. The loss of natural prey in human settled environments is associated with increased depredation – previously reported in southern Africa (Woodroffe et al. 2005). Sometimes AWDs occupy community lands despite adjacent protected areas having abundant prey, perhaps reflecting competition pressures with other larger carnivores. Lions seek out and kill AWD (Kock et al. 1999) and, in protected areas like the Serengeti National Park (SNP), lions survive in high densities where they are effectively over-protected by the absence of humans. In contrast, AWD was extirpated from the SNP in the late 1980s, and only small populations were rarely observed to survive on the periphery.[1] Further, learned behaviour around livestock (i.e. modified based on experience) occurs given the inability of some domestic animals to respond appropriately to predator attacks (Rasmussen unpublished. Data in: Woodroffe, McNutt and Mills 2004). One account describes a small pack of young AWDs – a breakaway group from larger packs present on the lowlands – that learned to

---

1   Recently AWD have been reintroduced into SNP and are now more commonly observed with at least two packs establishing. Ranging behaviour takes these animals in and out of the SNP and as far as the central Rift in Kenya. Losses continue when migrating these vast distances.

attack flocks of merino sheep on the slopes of Mount Kenya (Kock personal observation 1996; Kock et al. 1999). The sheep tended to form a compact unit rather than flee when under attack, resulting in a frenzy of killing or maiming, with no attempt to feed on or remove the carcasses. This behaviour was rarely if ever reported in the pastoral lands, where sheep and goats are more feral. As with other carnivores, learned behaviours around predation of livestock (or humans) are usually fatal to the pack or individual and therefore self-limiting. Evidence suggests that learning is also affected by the individual needs of the animal, such as lack of prey or from degradation of the habitat making hunting difficult. The intensification of agricultural systems, crop agriculture alongside rangelands, artificially high prey densities in game ranches, fencing systems and human settlements all influence AWDs ranging and hunting behaviours. These landscape changes degrade the ecosystem and create sinks – areas where losses produce a vacuum for expansion of adjacent populations – sometimes leading to overall decline in a species population (Delibes, Gaona and Ferreras 2001).

Sharing the land

Because humans inhabit the same area as domesticated and non-domesticated animals, strategies are required to better manage wildlife that forage in anthropogenic environments. There have been some successes. In Europe, large carnivore populations are on the increase despite close proximity to humans, due to management practices and positive public perception (Chapron et al. 2014). However, in addition to increased human–wildlife conflict, close proximity brings risk of disease to all involved. Coyotes (*Canis latrans*) which forage in urban areas around North America, for example, tend to have higher incidences of sarcoptic (*Sarcoptes scabiei*) mange (Murray et al. 2015).

Case study 2: Bat to basics

Sharing habitat with wildlife is particularly germane to highly mobile, aerial species such as birds and flying mammals. As a keystone species, fruit bats – such as those belonging to the genus *Pteropus* ('flying foxes') – provide essential ecosystem services including seed dispersal and pollination (McConkey et al. 2006). Flying foxes respond to food supply by migrating throughout the landscape and occupying specific sites based on proximity to preferable food sources (Schmelitschek, French and Parry-Jones 2009). They roost in camps during the day and feed at night. Fruit bats are considered 'sequential specialists', meaning they feed on items in a hierarchy of preference until they are depleted or seasonally unavailable (Parry-Jones and Augee 2001). The grey-headed flying-fox (*P. poliocephalus*), on the east coast of Australia, displays a preference for nectar and pollen from eucalypts, melaleucas and banksias (Department of Environment, Climate Change and Water [DECCW] 2009; Parry-Jones and Augee 2001). When these are unavailable, dietary intake of forest fruits increases, with native figs (*Ficus* spp.) becoming a major component of the seasonal diet (Parry-Jones and Augee 2001; Schmelitschek, French and Parry-Jones 2009).

Along with numerous other *Pteropus* species, *P. poliocephalus* is listed as vulnerable on the IUCN 2015 Red List owing to continuing population declines (Lunney, Richards and Dickman 2015). In contrast to the AWD, where habitat fragmentation and conflict with humans is the primary threat (Woodroffe and Sillero-Zubiri 2012), loss of foraging and roosting habitat is the primary threat to *P. poliocephalus* (Duncan et al. 1999). One study which examined the full geographic extent of *P. poliocephalus* found 50 per cent loss of native vegetation (Eby and Law 2008). Although stone fruit are relatively low in the feeding hierarchy (Parry-Jones and Augee 2001), flying foxes feed on commercial fruit crops when native food sources are scarce which brings them into conflict with orchardists (DECCW 2009).

Loss of native habitat and urban expansion (Markus and Hall 2004), as well as anthropogenic effects on local climate (Parris and Hazell 2005), may be influencing this historically temperate/tropical forest-dwelling species to utilise southern, urban environments. The number and size of urban flying-fox camps has increased (Tait et al. 2014), with some urban camps occupied year round (Parry-Jones and Augee 2001; van der Ree et al. 2006). Urbanisation may be a behavioural response to the advantages offered by this landscape (Tait et al. 2014); since European settlement there has been a dramatic increase in availability of food in urban centres (Williams et al. 2006), with figs in particular providing a year round source at some sites (Parry-Jones and Augee 2001). Street trees in suburban areas appear to have had nutritional benefit for flying foxes (McDonald-Madden et al. 2005), but it comes at a cost of increased interaction with humans and domesticated animals.

Flying foxes have been implicated as the host to several newly discovered viruses of public health concern (Table 10.1). While bats may be unique for their ability to tolerate some of the most deadly viral zoonoses known (Wang, Walker and Poon 2011), the sudden spillover to humans and other intermediate hosts – and thus discovery of these viruses – appears to be driven by factors other than the presence of these viruses in fruit bats. For example, efforts to understand why Hendra virus (HeV) recently emerged in Australia have centred around the changing behaviour and feeding ecology of flying foxes. HeV is spread from flying foxes to horses, and from horses to humans. Since horse and human population density are related (McFarlane, Becker and Field 2011), urban aggregation of flying foxes increases opportunities for contact with horses (Plowright et al. 2011). Indeed, spatial analysis reveals clustering of equine HeV cases at around 40 km – consistent with nocturnal foraging range of flying foxes (Smith et al. 2014). Risk of HeV transmission to horses is also known to increase during periods of flying-fox reproduction and nutritional stress. In one study, bats sampled during a blossom and nectar shortage had a 14–42 times higher odds of seropositivity, compared to bats studied in other seasons (Plowright et al. 2008). The high seroprevalence in this context may be due to increased viral susceptibility or an adaptive behavioural response to nutritional stress, such as crowding around restricted food sources or sharing food with other bat species that are more competent at transmitting HeV. Further research indicates that decreased migratory behaviour also affects infection dynamics; with a lower probability of HeV reinfection of camps, the proportion of immunologically naive (i.e. never before exposed) offspring accumulates. When HeV is subsequently reintroduced, high-intensity outbreaks follow, resulting in spillover to horses and potentially humans (Plowright et al. 2011).

Virus	Drivers
Severe acute respiratory syndrome-coronavirus (SARS-CoV)	Economic growth Desire for game meat Live wild animal trading in wet markets International travel
Ebola virus	Desire for game meat Live wild animal trading Burial practices
Marburg virus	Infected monkeys used for research Mining Tourism
Hendra virus	Population growth/urbanisation/human encroachment/synanthrophy Climate change Starvation Reproductive stress
Nipah virus (Bangladesh)	Date palm juice (food source) Cultural tradition
Nipah virus (Malaysia)	Agricultural intensification (dual land use) Encroachment into forested areas Movement of pigs to grower piggeries within Malaysia Food processing in Singapore Trade Habitat destruction Stress
Lyssaviruses, e.g. rabies, Australian bat lyssavirus (ABLV)	Urbanisation Deforestation Synanthrophy

Table 10.1. Drivers for selected emerging bat zoonotic viruses. Adapted from Smith and Wang 2013.

Similar links between bat foraging behaviour, land use changes, and disease spillover have been established for Nipah virus (NiV). In this instance, emergence in Malaysia was facilitated by the practice of growing fruit trees (particularly mango) alongside pigsties (an example of 'dual-use agriculture'), thus creating opportunities for contact between the two species. Further, repeated introductions of NiV into the index farm – a high-turnover, commercial pig farm (i.e. with continuous supply of naive hosts) – allowed the virus to persist, leading to increased transmission among pigs, and from pigs to humans (Pulliam et al. 2012). Thus, anthropogenic events and actions that alter food availability to flying foxes – such as habitat loss, urbanisation and specific agricultural practices – are key reasons why emerging diseases like HeV and NiV have suddenly appeared in the human population (Plowright et al. 2008).

Case study 3: Water wars: wild birds, poultry and people

Pigs and poultry are particularly adaptable to industrial farming systems, since they can tolerate high-grain diets and more efficiently convert this feed into edible products such as meat and eggs compared to ruminants (Food and Agriculture Organization of the United Nations [FAO] 2009; O'Mara 2012). These markets have undergone rapid expansion in recent decades, consistent with the shift away from pasture-based farming systems and rising demand for affordable meat (FAO 2009; Steinfeld et al. 2010) (Figure 10.2). Although industrial farming systems were developed in the West, much of the growth in livestock production is now occurring in low- and middle-income countries (the so-called livestock Revolution [Delgado et al. 1991]) many of which ship products to the high-income countries.

An efficient commercial poultry industry requires feed and water to be delivered to birds with precision throughout the year (FAO 2009). This contrasts with migratory wild birds which move vast distances to access climatic and feed resources to support their life cycles (Chu 2007). Migratory bird flyways link areas where birds can find fresh water and feed, including lake, pond and riverine habitats. The dramatic increase in commercial poultry production has resulted in more fresh water resources being used to supply commercial poultry

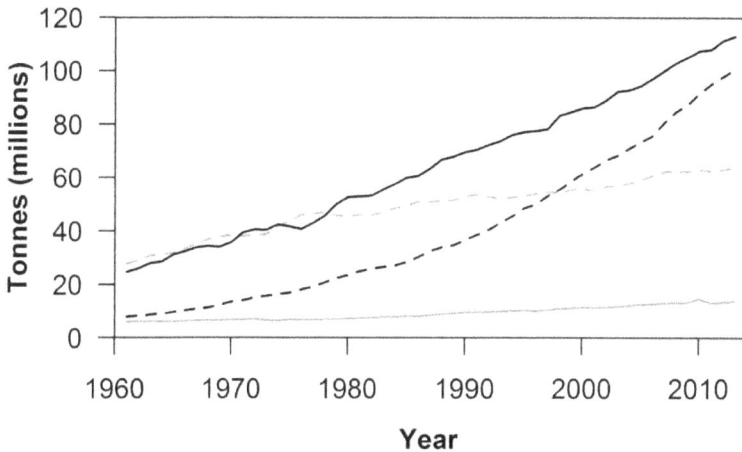

Figure 10.2 Global production of meat, by type, 1961–2013. The plot depicts total global production of meat from cattle (grey-stippled line), sheep and goats (grey-solid line), pigs (black-solid line) and poultry, including chickens and ducks (black-stippled line). Data from FAOSTAT 2014.

units (FAO 2009), contributing to the 87 per cent of fresh water reserves now consumed globally for agriculture (Postel, Daily and Ehrlich 1996). Commercial poultry farms in Australia have used treated water for their birds for years (Department of Agriculture, Fisheries and Forestry 2009) but this treatment is not applied uniformly throughout the world, notably where human water supplies are untreated. Free-range production of poultry (i.e. ducks in Asia and layer chickens in many parts of the world) has provided new opportunities for sedentary and migratory birds to source their feed and water from the same supplies (FAO 2008).

This resource conflict between commercial birds and wild birds has facilitated the emergence of novel strains of the influenza virus. Low pathogenic avian influenza (LPAI) virus occurs naturally in populations of wild and domesticated birds without signs of clinical disease (Alexander 2007; Capua and Alexander 2009). Outbreaks of HPAI in commercial chickens have occurred in Australia (Bulach et al. 2010) and elsewhere (Alexander 2007) when untreated fresh water became contaminated with LPAI from wild bird faeces. The genetic homogeneity and high-density production of the commercial chicken industry favours genetic drift or reassortment of low pathogenic strains of avian influenza into high pathogenic strains (Alders et al. 2014). The HPAI subtype H5N1 – which causes fatal infections in humans – emerged in conjunction with the massive increases in both human and commercial chicken and duck populations in Asia. The commercial duck population increased five-fold during the two decades prior to the H5N1 outbreak in China (Li et al. 2015). These commercial operations (poultry production and rice cultivation) utilised natural and semi-natural waterbodies that were occupied permanently or seasonally by wild birds. The practice of applying untreated animal waste on land (as fertiliser) and in ponds (as fish feed in aquaculture) compounded the problem because undigested grains are an attractant to wild birds (Graham et al. 2008).

The nutritional dimension

Many animals, including bats and wild birds, migrate or move between habitats to obtain food. While the focus on foods is informative, recent research shows that understanding and predicting the behaviour of animals (including humans) based on the combinations of nutrients in foods and diets is valuable (Simpson and Raubenheimer 2012). The relative balance of macronutrients (fats [F], carbohydrates [C], and proteins [P]) in foods has been shown to exert a dominant influence in this regard. The macronutrient preferences of strict carnivores are relatively high in protein, followed by lipids, while carbohydrate preferences are relatively low (Kohl, Coogan and Raubenheimer 2015). One study showed the diet of feral cats (*Felis catus*) was composed of 52P:46F:2C (per cent of energy) from wild prey (Plantinga, Bosch and Hendriks 2011) while wild wolves had a diet of 54P:45F:1C (Bosch, Hagen-Plantinga and Hendriks 2015). The macronutrient ratios selected by domestic cats (*F. catus*) in controlled experimental studies involving manufactured feeds (Hewson-Hughes et al. 2013) were similar to the ratios selected by feral cats in the wild, demonstrating that these ratios are specifically targeted rather than due to constraints on available foods in the wild. Many species of omnivores and herbivores likewise regulate their macronutrient intake, typically to lower ratios of protein than carnivores (Simpson and Raubenheimer 2012). Micronutrients (e.g. essential minerals) also play a role in animal foraging and migratory behaviour, as observed in the giant panda (*Ailuropoda melanoleuca*; Nie et al. 2015). Such nutrient-specific foraging may be useful in predicting and understanding why animals target certain foods.

Case study 4: Anthropogenic food-related human–bear conflict

Both black (*Ursus americanus*) and grizzly (*U. arctos*) bears come into conflict with humans in North America, often through livestock depredation (Gunther et al. 2004; Witmer and Whittaker 2001). In contrast to strict carnivores, both black and grizzly bears are omnivorous carnivores and consume a wide range of anthropogenic foods and garbage (Baruch-Mordo et al. 2008; Can et al. 2014; Follmann and Hechtel 1990; Gunther et al. 2004). Yellowstone National Park (YNP), has a relatively long anthropogenic food-related history with bears (Craighead, Sumner and Mitchell 1995; National Park Service [NPS] 2008). From the turn of the 20th century to the 1940s, visitors to YNP were entertained by 'bear shows' – spectators would gather around garbage dumps to watch bears forage on human discards (Craighead, Sumner and Mitchell 1995; NPS 2008). By the 1970s, the population density of bears in the park was high, with bears attaining relatively large body sizes. When a bear management strategy that included closing garbage dumps in and around the park was introduced in the 1970s, the grizzly bear population decreased substantially and incidences of human–bear conflict greatly increased, resulting in over 140 human-caused grizzly bear mortalities (Craighead et al. 1988; Craighead, Sumner and Mitchell 1995; NPS 2008). Access to large amounts of garbage in other regions has also resulted in high-density populations of relatively large bears including with shorter foraging and denning periods (Baldwin and Bender 2010; Beckmann and Berger 2003). The bear population in YNP has again increased (NPS 2008), and while grizzly bears are currently a threatened species in the USA

(FWS 1975) the Yellowstone population was recently, and controversially, considered for delisting (Doak and Cutler 2014; Morello 2014); a decision to delist had not been made at the time of writing. The controversy centres in large part on a key food of grizzly bears – the seeds of white bark pine (WBP) (*Pinus albicaulis*). White bark pine is in decline due to climate-induced changes in the occurrence of a pest which kills the tree, leading to concerns that its loss will negatively impact the bear population.

In North America, human–bear conflict incidents increase from spring through the early and late autumn "hyperphagic" season (Gunther et al. 2004) when bears attempt to eat enough to gain sufficient fat and lean mass to support hibernation, and, for females, reproduction (Lopez-Alfaro et al. 2013). In the Greater Yellowstone Ecosystem (GYE) incidents of bears obtaining anthropogenic foods, raiding gardens/orchards for fruits and vegetables, and obtaining honey from domestic beehives and apiaries peak during late hyperphagia (September to den entrance), while livestock depredation peaks in early hyperphagia (mid-July to end August) (Gunther et al. 2004). Human–bear conflict also increases when natural foods are scarce, especially during the hyperphagic season (Gunther et al. 2004; Mattson, Blanchard and Knight 1992; Peine 2001). When the autumn availability of high-fat WBP seeds and army cutworm moths (*Euxoa auxiliaris*) in the Yellowstone ecosystem was poor, conflicts due to grizzly bears obtaining anthropogenic foods increased significantly (Gunther et al. 2004). Likewise, black bear–human conflicts in Tennessee rose dramatically in autumn following a late frost and summer drought which resulted in a autumn mast-crop failure (Peine 2001). These food-related conflicts often end tragically for bears. Incidences of human-caused grizzly bear mortality in the GYE increased when WBP seed production was low (Mattson, Blanchard and Knight 1992). Anthropogenic food-conditioned bears are more likely to damage property in search of food, and are now a problem for human communities close to wild bear populations (Peine 2001).

Bears are especially susceptible to anthropogenic food attractants which often leads to conflict with humans because being omnivorous, they have a preference for a higher dietary proportion of non-protein macronutrients relative to protein 17P:83non-P, (per cent of metabolisable energy) (Erlenbach et al. 2014). This means they feed on a wider range of carbohydrate- and fat-rich anthropogenic foods that are not attractive to strict carnivores (Coogan and Raubenheimer 2016) (Figure 10.3). Diets balanced in this way maximise mass gain in grizzly bears, which is an indicator of fitness. For example, bears need to gain enough fat and lean mass to endure long periods of hibernation without eating, and larger body size offers an advantage in dominance interactions for resources (e.g. mates and food). In the wild, bears forage on a range of naturally occurring foods which may allow them to mix their diet in optimal proportions (Coogan et al. 2014). Sources of carbohydrates and lipids are often limiting to wild bears relative to protein, and natural foods rich in non-protein macronutrients are generally only abundant during the late summer and autumn periods, such as fruit and hard mast (e.g. seeds and nuts of trees and shrubs). In the absence of suitable natural foods (such as during a berry crop failure in the autumn) anthropogenic food sources can offer bears a rich source of carbohydrates and lipids which may optimise their diet prior to hibernation and likely exacerbates bear–human conflict during this time (Coogan and Raubenheimer 2016). The nutritional preferences of animals, and the ability for anthropogenically altered environments to provide those preferences, requires serious consideration as the human environment continues to encroach on wild habitats.

The future

These examples show how unintended consequences arise when the human appetite for resources impinges on the requirements of other species. With human population projected to grow to 9.7 billion by 2050, modelling has suggested that a 70 per cent increase in food production will be required to meet human food requirements (FAO 2009). This is seemingly inevitable, unless food waste can be reduced significantly, which currently amounts to about 40 per cent of production. This would also more or less cancel out the over-consumption, and under-consumption, of food in different parts of the world thereby improving the health of all. Importantly, reducing food waste will reduce the need to expand agriculture, and thus contribute to

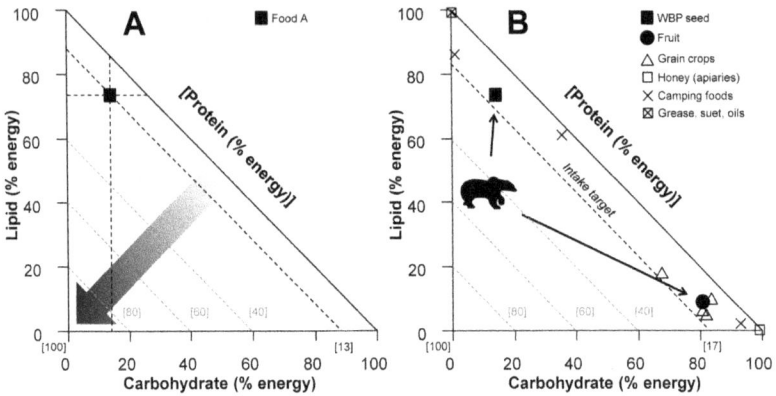

Figure 10.3 **Panel A**: right-angled mixture triangle illustrating the macronutrient (carbohydrate, lipid, and protein) composition of a hypothetical food (Food A) as a percentage of energy derived from the sum of these components. Food A contains approximately 73 per cent lipid and 14 per cent carbohydrate. The remaining 13 per cent of energy from protein is read on the implicit axis (negatively sloped black dashed line). Any mixture of macronutrients that falls along this line contains 13 per cent protein energy with non-protein energy varying accordingly. The value of the implicit axis is inversely related to the plot origin, as illustrated by the arrow with a gradient showing values of protein from low (white) to high (black). Dashed-grey lines at 40, 60 and 80 per cent protein energy have been added for reference. **Panel B**: we demonstrate how the macronutrient composition of foods can be used to understand patterns of human–wildlife conflict using data for the grizzly bear (*Ursus arctos*). The ratio of protein to non-protein energy (intake target) that was self-selected by grizzly bears in a captive trial is plotted (17 per cent protein:83 per cent non-protein energy). Grizzly bears generally consume a diet high in protein relative to their preferences (as demonstrated by the bear icon) until late summer and fall when highly sought after high-fat or high-carbohydrate foods such as white bark pine (WBP) seed and fruit are available. By consuming these foods (black arrows) bears are able to reach their intake target thereby optimising their mass gain before hibernation. When such foods are scarce or unavailable, grizzly bears may consume anthropogenic foods high in non-protein energy which may lead to increased incidences of conflict with humans. To illustrate, the nutrient composition of a selection of anthropogenic foods which grizzly bears have been documented to feed upon is shown. Figure adapted from Coogan and Raubenheimer 2016.

reducing or reversing the decline in biodiversity. The changing global climate, increasing economic growth, and resulting ecological impact are compounding challenges. A business-as-usual approach that fails to consider the resource needs of other species will extend human–wildlife conflict, accelerate species extinction and the spillover of infectious diseases from non-human animals to humans. These examples show that conflicting appetites are best managed using an integrated ecological approach, one that moves beyond the simplistic dichotomy of 'anthropogenic vs natural' and considers all species, including humans, domesticated and un-domesticated animals, as participants in an increasingly globalised ecology.

One of the most challenging and instructive scenarios involves predators. In terrestrial environments, large predators are not typically being threatened because they are harvested for food, but rather because of their large habitat requirements, depleted food base, and the threat they pose to humans and associated domesticated species (i.e. persecution). Because predators play an important role in ecosystems (Schmitz and Suttle 2001) it is imperative that conflict situations are better managed. In the case of the AWD, where protected areas are insufficient, the most effective strategies have included more open landscape management (conservancies), with multiple land use and ownership, including wildlife economy and livestock-based agriculture (Lindsey et al. 2005). By conserving a broad range of resources from pastures to bushland or forests, food sources are available for the prey species and habitat for the carnivores. This strategy combined with community conservation actions will have benefits such as losses from depredation compensated by alternative income sources. An integrated approach that looks after the interests of animals, humans and the environment provides the best hope of a future for the AWD and other carnivores in Africa. In this way, conservationists can improve the population status of wildlife species, as well as the livelihoods and diets of malnourished communities that share the landscape with African wildlife.

The bat and bird examples illustrate how the high mobility of some species ensures contact with humans and domesticated species. In both cases, the potential conflict is not competition for food (although this is a dimension in the human interaction with fruit bats), but rather complex multi-species interactions in a shared environment, involving humans, domesticated and non-domesticated animal hosts and their microbes. For bats, transmission of infectious agents is facilitated by depletion of their natural habitat and/or establishment of attractive alternatives within urban and agricultural environments. For migratory birds, the mode of contact is principally indirect, involving the shared use of riparian and aquatic habitats by non-domesticated bird species and high-intensity poultry production for human consumption. Whereas rich biodiverse communities tend to have a sterilising effect (so-called dilution effect), the placement of high-density, homogenous (farmed) animal communities adjacent to complex systems breaches biological norms and creates opportunities for species jumps and microbial evolution in new hosts (Civitello et al. 2015; Keesing et al. 2010). In the case of HeV, NiV, H5N1 influenza, and other pathogens, the results can be devastating to domesticated animals and pose a serious threat to humans. To be successful in the long term, intensive livestock production will require improved biosecurity and biocontainment practices as well as waste management strategies. These are essential for preventing zoonotic transfer of pathogens from animals in high-density settings (Graham et al. 2008). The role and significance of wildlife–livestock interface in disease ecology has been neglected; more research and surveillance on specific interfaces is warranted to mitigate the risk of disease emergence in humans (Alders and Kock 2017; Kock 2018; Wiethoelter et al. 2015). This is a challenge for low- and middle-income countries where veterinary and wildlife infrastructure is often weak and unable to predict or contain emerging disease events due to inadequate capacity and funding. These are the very same areas where pig and poultry production is on the increase, especially in tropical and subtropical environments, where microbial diversity is rich and potential for species jumping is high.

A recurring theme is conflict over shared resources, particularly foods. The case of the grizzly bear shows they are not in competition with humans for food *per se* but for specific combinations of nutrients on which they rely. When particular nutrients are scarce because of human impacts or ecological stochasticity, we can predict that anthropogenic sources of those specific nutrients, rather than foods *per se*, will provide a flashpoint for bear–human conflict. This conflict can be reduced by minimising the availability of, or reducing access to, the targeted nutrients in bear habitat (e.g. fruit orchards). Omnivores like bears use a wide range of foods as interchangeable sources of nutrients. The same reasoning might apply to crop raiding by herbivores such as elephants (Koirala et al. 2016), and carnivores more generally (Kohl, Coogan and Raubenheimer 2015). Understanding specific needs of the species with which we interact is an essential starting point for finding solutions to the conflicts that arise over competition for resources.

The main drivers of wildlife conservation issues are likely to be locally case-specific, involving different environmental, cultural, economic and geopolitical circumstances and requiring multidisciplinary effort to resolve. What is clear is that the old conservation paradigm of protected areas is now totally insufficient to maintain biodiversity and society needs to revisit integrated systems, where humans share landscapes with wildlife. This effort is required if we are to coexist with non-human species in this human dominanted landscape. As urban consumers become increasingly remote from their food sources (Satterthwaite, McGranahan and Tacoli 2010), we have to advocate for food value chains and extractive industry practices that ensure access to nutritionally balanced, ecologically sustainable diets for all species.

Works cited

Alders, R., J.A. Awuni, B. Bagnol, P. Farrell, and N. de Haan (2014). Impact of avian influenza on village poultry production globally. *EcoHealth* 11: 63–72. doi: 10.1007/s10393-013-0867-x.

Alders, R., and R. Kock (2017). What's food and nutrition security got to do with wildlife conservation?. Australian Zoologist 39: 120-126. doi: 10.7882/AZ.2016.040

Alexander, D.J. (2007). Summary of avian influenza activity in Europe, Asia, Africa, and Australasia, 2002–2006. *Avian Diseases* 51: 161–6. doi: 10.1637/7602-041306r.1.

Aryal, A., D. Brunton, W.H. Ji, R.K. Barraclough, and D. Raubenheimer (2014). Human–carnivore conflict: ecological and economical sustainability of predation on livestock by snow leopard and other carnivores in the Himalaya. *Sustainability Science* 9: 321–9. doi: 10.1007/s11625-014-0246-8.

Baillie, J.E.M., et al. (2004). *2004 IUCN Red List of Threatened Species. A global species assessment.* Cambridge, UK: The World Conservation Union. http://bit.ly/2BW4IJq.

Baldwin, R.A., and L.C. Bender (2010). Denning chronology of black bears in Eastern Rocky Mountain National Park, Colorado. *Western North American Naturalist* 70: 48–54. doi: 10.3398/064.070.0106.

Bar-On, Y.M., R. Phillips, and R. Milo (2018). The biomass distribution on Earth. Proceedings of the National Academy of Sciences USA 115: 6506-6511. doi: 10.1073/pnas.1711842115.

Baruch-Mordo, S., S.W. Breck, K.R. Wilson, and D.M. Theobald (2008). Spatiotemporal distribution of black bear–human conflicts in Colorado, USA. *Journal of Wildlife Management* 72: 1853–62. doi: 10.2193/2007-442.

Beckmann, J.P., and J. Berger (2003). Rapid ecological and behavioural changes in carnivores: the responses of black bears (*Ursus americanus*) to altered food. *Journal of Zoology* 261: 207–12. doi: 10.1017/S0952836903004126.

Bhutta, Z.A., and R.A. Salam (2012). Global nutrition epidemiology and trends. *Annals of Nutrition & Metabolism* 61: 19–27. doi: 10.1159/000345167.

Boitani, L., et al. (2015). *Key actions for large carnivore populations in Europe.* Rome: Institute of Applied Ecology. http://bit.ly/2E5tFUb.

Bosch, G., E.A. Hagen-Plantinga, and W.H. Hendriks (2015). Dietary nutrient profiles of wild wolves: insights for optimal dog nutrition? *British Journal of Nutrition* 113: S40-S54. doi: 10.1017/S0007114514002311.

Bulach, D., et al. (2010). Molecular analysis of H7 avian influenza viruses from Australia and New Zealand: genetic diversity and relationships from 1976 to 2007. *Journal of Virology* 84: 9957–66. doi: 10.1128/Jvi.00930-10.

Can, O.E., N. D'Cruze, D.L. Garshelis, J. Beecham, and D.W. Macdonald (2014). Resolving human–bear conflict: a global survey of countries, experts, and key factors. *Conservation Letters* 7: 501–13. doi: 10.1111/Conl.12117.

Capua, I., and D.J. Alexander (2009). Avian influenza infection in birds: a challenge and opportunity for the poultry veterinarian. *Poultry Science* 88: 842–6. doi: 10.3382/ps.2008-00289.

Ceballos, G., et al. (2015). Accelerated modern human-induced species losses: entering the sixth mass extinction. *Science Advances* 1: e1400253. doi: 10.1126/sciadv.1400253.

Chapron, G., et al. (2014). Recovery of large carnivores in Europe's modern human-dominated landscapes. *Science* 346: 1517–9. doi: 10.1126/science.1257553.

Chu, M. (2007). *Songbird journeys: four seasons in the lives of migratory birds.* New York: Walker & Company.

Civitello, D.J., et al. (2015). Biodiversity inhibits parasites: broad evidence for the dilution effect. *Proceedings of the National Academy of Sciences of the United States of America* 112: 8667–71. doi: 10.1073/pnas.1506279112.

Cline, R., N. Sexton and S.C. Stewart (2007). *A human-dimensions review of human–wildlife disturbance: a literature review of impacts, frameworks, and management solutions.* US Geological Survey, Open-File Report 2007–1111. https://doi.org/10.3133/ofr20071111

Coogan, S.C.P., and D. Raubenheimer (2016). Might macronutrient requirements influence grizzly bear–human conflict? Insights from nutritional geometry. *Ecosphere* 7: e01204. doi: 10.1002/ecs2.1204.

Coogan, S.C.P., D. Raubenheimer, G.B. Stenhouse, and S.E. Nielsen (2014). Macronutrient optimization and seasonal diet mixing in a large omnivore, the grizzly bear: a geometric analysis. *PLOS One* 9: e97968. doi: 10.1371/journal.pone.0097968.

Craighead, J.J., K.R. Greer, R.R. Knight, and H.I. Pac (1988). *Grizzly bear mortalities in the Yellowstone ecosystem 1959–1987.* Bozeman: Montana Department of Fish Wildlife & Parks.

Craighead, J.J., J.S. Sumner, and J.A. Mitchell (1995). *The grizzly bears of Yellowstone: their ecology in the Yellowstone ecosystem, 1959–1992.* Washington, DC: Island Press.

Davies, H.T., and J.T. du Toit (2004). Anthropogenic factors affecting wild dog *Lycaon pictus* reintroductions: a case study in Zimbabwe. *Oryx* 38: 32–9. doi: 10.1017/S0030605304000067.

Delgado, C., M. Rosegrant, H. Steinfeld, and S. Ehui (1991). *Livestock to 2020: the next food revolution.* Food, Agriculture, and the Environment Discussion Paper 28. Washington, DC: International Food Policy Research Institute. http://bit.ly/2Sx80bC

Delibes, M., P. Gaona, and P. Ferreras (2001). Effects of an attractive sink leading into maladaptive habitat selection. *American Naturalist* 158: 277–85. doi: 10.1086/321319.

Department of Agriculture, Fisheries and Forestry (2009). *National farm biosecurity manual – poultry production.* Canberra: Australian Commonwealth Department of Agriculture, Fisheries & Forestry. https://bit.ly/2BLiuhA

Department of Environment, Climate Change and Water (2009). *Draft national recovery plan for the grey-headed flying-fox* Pteropus poliocephalus. Canberra: NSW Department of Environment Climate Change and Water. http://bit.ly/2zMuBK1.

Doak, D.F., and K. Cutler (2014). Re-evaluating evidence for past population trends and predicted dynamics of Yellowstone grizzly bears. *Conservation Letters* 7: 312–22. doi: 10.1111/Conl.12048.

Duncan, A., et al. (1999). *The action plan for Australian bats.* Canberra: Environment Australia. https://bit.ly/2SZdK1H

Eby, P., and B. Law (2008). Ranking the feeding habitats of grey-headed flying foxes for conservation management. http://bit.ly/2Ge6yJA.

Edenhofer, O., et al., eds. (2014). *Climate Change 2014: mitigation of climate change. Working Group III contribution to the Fifth Assessment Report of the Intergovernmental Panel on Climate Change.* New York: Cambridge University Press.

Erlenbach, J.A., K.D. Rode, D. Raubenheimer, and C.T. Robbins (2014). Macronutrient optimization and energy maximization determine diets of brown bears. *Journal of Mammalogy* 95: 160–8. doi: 10.1644/13-Mamm-a-161.

Fleming, P., L. Corbet, R. Harden, and P. Thomson (2001). *Managing the impacts of dingos and other wild dogs.* Canberra: Bureau of Rural Sciences. http://bit.ly/2PnkPDd.

Foley, J.A., et al. (2005). Global consequences of land use. *Science* 309: 570–4. doi: 10.1126/science.1111772.

Follmann, E.H., and J.L. Hechtel (1990). Bears and pipeline construction in Alaska. *Arctic* 43: 103–9.

Food and Agriculture Organization Corporate Statistical Database (2014). FAOSTAT (online database). http://faostat3.fao.org/.

Food and Agriculture Organization of the United Nations (2008). *Biosecurity for highly pathogenic avian influenza: issues and options.* Rome: Food & Agriculture Organization of the United Nations. http://bit.ly/2BWrLnk.

Food and Agriculture Organization of the United Nations (2009). *How to feed the world in 2050.* Rome: Food & Agriculture Organization of the United Nations. http://bit.ly/2KZPVAp.

Food and Agriculture Organization of the United Nations (2009). *The state of food and agriculture: livestock in the balance.* Rome: Food & Agriculture Organization of the United Nations. http://bit.ly/2UjZQVL.

Frank, L.G. (1998). *Living with lions: carnivore conservation and livestock in Laikipia District, Kenya.* Bethesda, MD: Development Alternatives Inc. http://bit.ly/2Eixk1I.

Fish and Wildlife Service (1975). Endangered and threatened wildlife – grizzly bear. *Federal Register* 40: 31733–6.

Graham, J.P., et al. (2008). The animal–human interface and infectious disease in industrial food animal production: rethinking biosecurity and biocontainment. *Public Health Reports* 123: 282–99.

Gunther, K.A., et al. (2004). Grizzly bear–human conflicts in the Greater Yellowstone ecosystem, 1992–2000. *Ursus* 15: 10–22.

Hewson-Hughes, A.K., et al. (2013). Consistent proportional macronutrient intake selected by adult domestic cats (*Felis catus*) despite variations in macronutrient and moisture content of foods offered. *Journal of Comparative Physiology B: Biochemical, Systems, & Environmental Physiology* 183: 525–36. doi: 10.1007/s00360-012-0727-y.

Hoffmann, M., et al. (2010). The impact of conservation on the status of the world's vertebrates. *Science* 330: 1503–9. doi: 10.1126/science.1194442.

Inskip, C., and A. Zimmermann (2009). Human–felid conflict: a review of patterns and priorities worldwide. *Oryx* 43: 18–34. doi: 10.1017/S003060530899030x.

Jones, B.A., et al. (2013). Zoonosis emergence linked to agricultural intensification and environmental change. *Proceedings of the National Academy of Sciences of the United States of America* 110: 8399–404. doi: 10.1073/pnas.1208059110.

Jones, K.E., et al. (2008). Global trends in emerging infectious diseases. *Nature* 451: 990-4. doi: 10.1038/Nature06536.

Kearney, J. (2010). Food consumption trends and drivers. *Philosophical Transactions of the Royal Society B: Biological Sciences* 365: 2793–807. doi: 10.1098/rstb.2010.0149.

Keesing, F., et al. (2010). Impacts of biodiversity on the emergence and transmission of infectious diseases. *Nature* 468: 647–52. doi: 10.1038/Nature09575.

Kock, R.A. (2019) Is it time to reflect, not on the "what" but the "why" in emerging wildlife disease research?. Journal of Wildlife Diseases 55: 1-2. doi: 10.7589/2019-01-000.

Kock, R., J. Mwanzia, T. Fitzjohn, T. Manyibe, S. Kambe, and D. Lergoi (1999). *African hunting dog translocation from Mount Kenya (Timau) to Tsavo West National Park Kenya 1996–1998*. Nairobi: World Wildlife Fund.

Kohl, K.D., S.C.P. Coogan, and D. Raubenheimer (2015). Do wild carnivores forage for prey or nutrients? *BioEssays* 37: 701–9. doi: 10.1002/bies.201400171.

Koirala, R.K., W. Ji, A. Aryal, J. Rothman, and D. Raubenheimer (2016). Dispersal and ranging patterns of the Asian elephant (*Elephas maximus*) in relation to their interactions with humans in Nepal. *Ethology, Ecology & Evolution* 28: 221–31. doi: 10.1080/03949370.2015.1066472.

Li, X.L., et al. (2015). Highly pathogenic avian influenza H5N1 in mainland China. *International Journal of Environmental Research & Public Health* 12: 5026–45. doi: 10.3390/ijerph120505026.

Lindsey, P.A., R.R. Alexander, J.T. du Toit, and M.G.L. Mills (2005). The potential contribution of ecotourism to African wild dog *Lycaon pictus* conservation in South Africa. *Biological Conservation* 123: 339–48. doi: 10.1016/j.biocon.2004.12.002.

Lindsey, P.A., J.Y. du Toit and M.G.L. Mills (2005). Attitudes of ranchers towards African wild dogs *Lycaon pictus*: Conservation implications on private land. *Biological Conservation* 125: 113–121. doi: 10.1016/j.biocon.2005.03.015.

Lopez-Alfaro, C., C.T. Robbins, A. Zedrosser, and S.E. Nielsen (2013). Energetics of hibernation and reproductive trade-offs in brown bears. *Ecological Modelling* 270: 1–10. doi: 10.1016/j.ecolmodel.2013.09.002.

Lunney, D., G. Richards, and C. Dickman (2015). *Pteropus poliocephalus*. The IUCN Red List of Threatened Species, version 2015.1. www.iucnredlist.org/.

Madden, F. (2004). Creating coexistence between humans and wildlife: global perspectives on local efforts to address human–wildlife conflict. *Human Dimensions of Wildlife* 9: 247–57.

Mamo, D., H. Bouer, and Y. Tesfay (2014). Crop damage by African elephants assessment in Kaftasheraro National Park, Ethiopia. *African Journal of Ecology* 52: 138–43. doi: 10.1111/Aje.12094.

Markus, N., and L. Hall (2004). Foraging behaviour of the black flying-fox (*Pteropus alecto*) in the urban landscape of Brisbane, Queensland. *Wildlife Research* 31: 345–55. doi: 10.1071/Wr01117.

Mattson, D.J., B.M. Blanchard, and R.R. Knight (1992). Yellowstone grizzly bear mortality, human habituation, and whitebark-pine seed crops. *Journal of Wildlife Management* 56: 432–42. doi: 10.2307/3808855.

McConkey, K.R., and D.R. Drake (2006). Flying foxes cease to function as seed dispersers long before they become rare. *Ecology* 87: 271–6. doi: 10.1890/05-0386.

McDonald-Madden, E., E.S.G. Schreiber, D.M. Forsyth, D. Choquenot, and T.F. Clancy (2005). Factors affecting grey-headed flying-fox (*Pteropus poliocephalus*: Pteropodidae) foraging in the Melbourne metropolitan area, Australia. *Austral Ecology* 30: 600–8. doi: 10.1111/j.1442-9993.2005.01492.x.

McFarlane, R., N. Becker, and H. Field (2011). Investigation of the climatic and environmental context of Hendra virus spillover events 1994–2010. *PLOS One* 6(12): e28374. doi: 10.1371/journal.pone.0028374.

McFarlane, R.A., A.C. Sleigh, and A.J. McMichael (2013). Land-use change and emerging infectious disease on an island continent. *International Journal of*

Environmental Research & Public Health 10: 2699–719. doi: 10.3390/
ijerph10072699.

Morello, L. (2014). Yellowstone grizzlies face losing protected status. *Nature* 505:
465–6. doi: 10.1038/505465a.

Morse, S.S., et al. (2012). Prediction and prevention of the next pandemic
zoonosis. *Lancet* 380: 1956–65. doi: 0.1016/S0140-6736(12)61684-5.

Murray, M., M.A. Edwards, B. Abercrombie, and C.C. St Clair (2015). Poor health
is associated with use of anthropogenic resources in an urban carnivore.
Proceedings of the Royal Society B: Biological Sciences 282: 20150009. doi:
10.1098/Rspb.2015.0009.

National Park Service (2008). Yellowstone grizzly bears. *Yellowstone Science* 16:
1–48.

Nie, Y.G., et al. (2015). Obligate herbivory in an ancestrally carnivorous lineage:
the giant panda and bamboo from the perspective of nutritional geometry.
Functional Ecology 29: 26–34. doi: 10.1111/1365-2435.12302.

Nordin, S.M., M. Boyle, T.M. Kemmer, and Academy of Nutrition and Dietetics
(2013). Position of the Academy of Nutrition and Dietetics: nutrition security
in developing nations: sustainable food, water, and health. *Journal of the
Academy of Nutrition & Dietetics* 113: 581–95. doi: 10.1016/
j.jand.2013.01.025.

Ogada, M.O., R. Woodroffe, N.O. Oguge, and L.G. Frank (2003). Limiting
depredation by African carnivores: the role of livestock husbandry.
Conservation Biology 17: 1521–30. doi: 10.1111/j.1523-1739.2003.00061.x.

O'Mara, F.P. (2012). The role of grasslands in food security and climate change.
Annals of Botany 110: 1263–70. doi: 10.1093/Aob/Mcs209.

Parris, K.M., and D.L. Hazell (2005). Biotic effects of climate change in urban
environments: the case of the grey-headed flying-fox (*Pteropus poliocephalus*)
in Melbourne, Australia. *Biological Conservation* 124: 267–76. doi: 10.1016/
j.biocon.2005.01.035.

Parry-Jones, K.A., and M.L. Augee (2001). Factors affecting the occupation of a
colony site in Sydney, New South Wales, by the grey-headed flying-fox
Pteropus poliocephalus (Pteropodidae). *Austral Ecology* 26: 47–55. doi:
10.1111/j.1442-9993.2001.01072.pp.x.

Peine, J.D. (2001). Nuisance bears in communities: strategies to reduce conflict.
Human Dimensions of Wildlife 6: 223–37. doi: 10.1080/108712001753461301.

Pimm, S. (2012). Lion lights – a home grown solution to saving lions and
livestock. http://bit.ly/2G6ekFq.

Plantinga, E.A., G. Bosch, and W.H. Hendriks (2011). Estimation of the dietary
nutrient profile of free-roaming feral cats: possible implications for nutrition

of domestic cats. *British Journal of Nutrition* 106: S35-S48. doi: 10.1017/ S0007114511002285.

Plowright, R.K., et al. (2008). Reproduction and nutritional stress are risk factors for Hendra virus infection in little red flying foxes (*Pteropus scapulatus*). *Proceedings of the Royal Society B: Biological Sciences* 275: 861-9. doi: 10.1098/rspb.2007.1260.

Plowright, R.K., et al. (2011). Urban habituation, ecological connectivity and epidemic dampening: the emergence of Hendra virus from flying foxes (*Pteropus spp.*). *Proceedings of the Royal Society B: Biological Sciences* 278: 3703-12. doi: 10.1098/rspb.2011.0522.

Pole, A., I.J. Gordon, M.L. Gorman, and M. MacAskill (2004). Prey selection by African wild dogs (*Lycaon pictus*) in southern Zimbabwe. *Journal of Zoology* 262: 207-15. doi: 10.1017/S0952836903004576.

Postel, S.L., G.C. Daily, and P.R. Ehrlich (1996). Human appropriation of renewable fresh water. *Science* 271: 785-8. doi: 10.1126/science.271.5250.785.

Pulliam, J.R.C., et al. (2012). Agricultural intensification, priming for persistence and the emergence of Nipah virus: a lethal bat-borne zoonosis. *Journal of the Royal Society Interface* 9: 89-101. doi: 10.1098/rsif.2011.0223.

Rasmussen, G.S.A. (1999). Livestock predation by the painted hunting dog *Lycaon pictus* in a cattle ranching region of Zimbabwe: a case study. *Biological Conservation* 88: 133-9. doi: 10.1016/S0006-3207(98)00006-8.

Raubenheimer, D. (2011). Toward a quantitative nutritional ecology: the right-angled mixture triangle. *Ecological Monographs* 81: 407-27. doi: 10.1890/10-1707.1.

Ripple, W.J., et al. (2014). Status and ecological effects of the world's largest carnivores. *Science* 343: 1241484. doi: 10.1126/Science.1241484.

Satterthwaite, D., G. McGranahan, and C. Tacoli (2010). Urbanization and its implications for food and farming. *Philosophical Transactions of the Royal Society B: Biological Sciences* 365: 2809-20. doi: 10.1098/rstb.2010.0136.

Savage, R.J.G. (1978). Carnivores. In *Evolution of African mammals*, V.J. Maglio and H.B.S. Cooke, eds., 249-67. Cambridge, MA: Harvard University Press.

Schmelitschek, E., K. French, and K. Parry-Jones (2009). Fruit availability and utilisation by grey-headed flying foxes (Pteropodidae: *Pteropus poliocephalus*) in a human-modified environment on the south coast of New South Wales, Australia. *Wildlife Research* 36: 592-600. doi: 10.1071/Wr08169.

Schmitz, O.J., and K.B. Suttle (2001). Effects of top predator species on direct and indirect interactions in a food web. *Ecology* 82: 2072-81. doi: 10.1890/0012-9658(2001)082[2072:Eotpso]2.0.Co;2.

Simpson, S.J., and D. Raubenheimer (2012). *The nature of nutrition: a unifying framework from animal adaptation to obesity.* Princeton, NJ: Princeton University Press.

Smith, C., C. Skelly, N. Kung, B. Roberts, and H. Field (2014). Flying-fox species density – a spatial risk factor for Hendra virus infection in horses in eastern Australia. *PLOS One* 9: e99965. doi: 10.1371/journal.pone.0099965.

Smith, I., and L.F. Wang (2013). Bats and their virome: an important source of emerging viruses capable of infecting humans. *Current Opinion in Virology* 3: 84–91. doi: 10.1016/j.coviro.2012.11.006.

Steinfeld, H., H.A. Mooney, F. Schneider, and L.E. Neville, eds. (2010). *Livestock in a changing landscape: drivers, consequences, and responses.* Washington, DC: Island Press.

Tait, J., H.L. Perotto-Baldivieso, A. McKeown, and D.A. Westcott (2014). Are flying-foxes coming to town? Urbanisation of the spectacled flying-fox (*Pteropus conspicillatus*) in Australia. *PLOS One* 9: e109810. doi: 10.1371/journal.pone.0109810.

Treves, A., and K.U. Karanth (2003). Human–carnivore conflict and perspectives on carnivore management worldwide. *Conservation Biology* 17: 1491–9. doi: 10.1111/j.1523-1739.2003.00059.x.

United Nations Population Fund (2011). *The state of world population 2011.* New York: United Nations Population Fund. http://bit.ly/2BUbnDU.

Urban, M.C. (2015). Accelerating extinction risk from climate change. *Science* 348: 571–3. doi: 10.1126/science.aaa4984.

van der Ree, R., M.J. McDonnell, I. Temby, J. Nelson, and E. Whittingham (2006). The establishment and dynamics of a recently established urban camp of flying foxes (*Pteropus poliocephalus*) outside their geographic range. *Journal of Zoology* 268: 177–85. doi: 10.1111/j.1469-7998.2005.00005.x.

Wang, L.F., P.J. Walker, and L.L. Poon (2011). Mass extinctions, biodiversity and mitochondrial function: are bats 'special' as reservoirs for emerging viruses? *Current Opinion in Virology* 1: 649–57. doi: 10.1016/j.coviro.2011.10.013.

Wiethoelter, A.K., D. Beltrán-Alcrudo, R. Kock, and S.M. Mor (2015). Global trends in infectious diseases at the wildlife–livestock interface. *Proceedings of the National Academy of Sciences of the United States of America* 112: 9662–7. doi: 10.1073/pnas.1422741112.

Williams, N.S.G., M.J. McDonnell, G.K. Phelan, L.D. Keim, and R. Van der Ree (2006). Range expansion due to urbanization: increased food resources attract grey-headed flying-foxes (*Pteropus poliocephalus*) to Melbourne. *Austral Ecology* 31: 190–8. doi: 10.1111/j.1442-9993.2006.01590.x.

Witmer, W.G., and D.G. Whittaker (2001). *Dealing with nuisance and depredating black bears.* Staff Publications 581. National Wildlife Research Center, United States Department of Agriculture. http://bit.ly/2rruwa1.

Woodroffe, R., P. Lindsey, S. Romanach, A. Stein, and S.M.K. ole Ranah (2005). Livestock predation by endangered African wild dogs (*Lycaon pictus*) in northern Kenya. *Biological Conservation* 124: 225–34. doi: 10.1016/j.biocon.2005.01.028.

Woodroffe, R., and C. Sillero-Zubiri (2012). *Lycaon pictus.* The IUCN Red List of Threatened Species, version 2015.1. www.iucnredlist.org/.

Woodroffe, R.B., J.W. McNutt, and M.G.L. Mills (2004). African wild dog. In *Foxes, wolves, jackals and dogs: status survey and Conservation Action Plan,* C. Sillero-Zubiri, M. Hoffmann, and D.W. Macdonald, eds., 174–83. Gland, CH: International Union for Conservation of Nature.

World Wildlife Fund (2018). *Living planet report 2018.* Gland, CH: World Wildlife Fund. http://bit.ly/2L0JkFQ.

Zedrosser, A., S.M.J. Steyaert, H. Gossow, and J.E. Swenson (2011). Brown bear conservation and the ghost of persecution past. *Biological Conservation* 144: 2163–70. doi: 10.1016/j.biocon.2011.05.005.

11
Visualising One Health

Conor Ashleigh

I am a documentarian and storyteller and over the past decade my work has taken me to more than 50 countries. My photographs explore themes of individual identity and document stories of sentient beings. The canvas for my photography is the landscape itself – how it is used; how it is nourished, protected or neglected. This includes communicating the impact of development on communities and their response to development and research.

Preparing the photographs for One Health was an opportunity to visually respond to the breadth of topics and themes in this book. One photograph can convey many stories. Similarly, One Health research involves many disciplines with multiple stories but with one goal – to make the planet a better place for humans, animals and the environment. These photographs document some of their stories.

We must reframe our engagement with the planet and the lived environment. A One Health approach offers those working in the community, such as community development workers, communicators and researchers as well as institutions, government agencies and non-governmental organisations, the potential to try something different in partnership with the many communities seeking ways to improve their livelihoods and protect the environment.

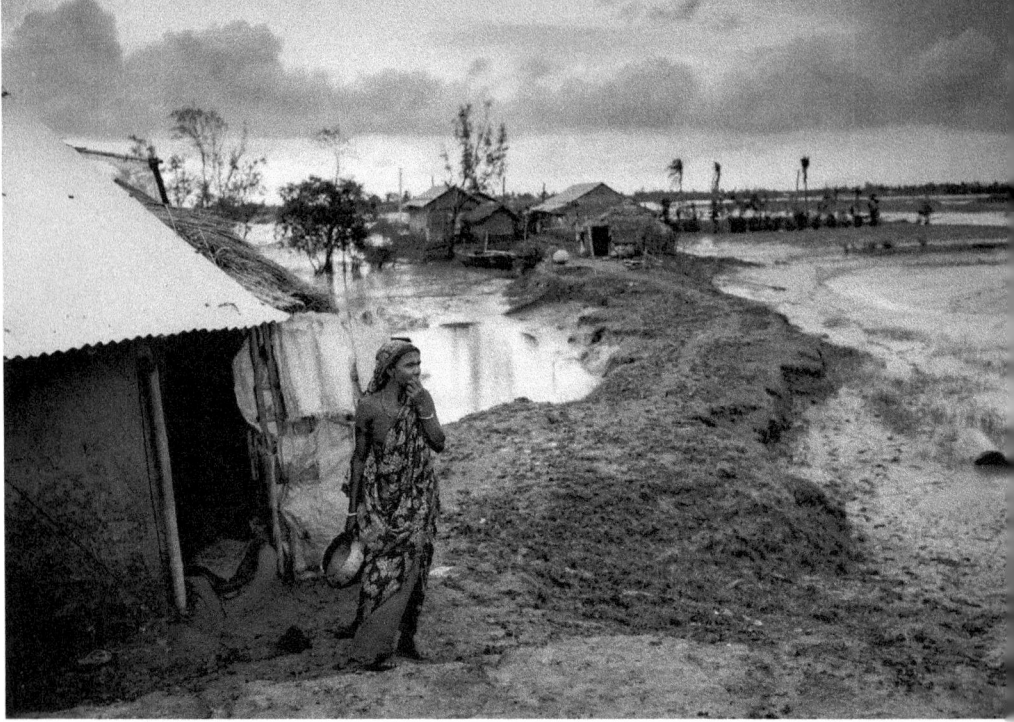

Figure 11.1 In Jaliakhali village a woman stands outside her home which was rebuilt along an embankment after being destroyed by cyclone Aila in 2009.

Figure 11.2 Françoise has been a mother with the SOS Childrens Village for 20 years. Françoise and her children sit outside in the evening and eat their meal due to the lack of electric power in Central African Republic. Power is very inconsistent and lasts only a few hours a day.

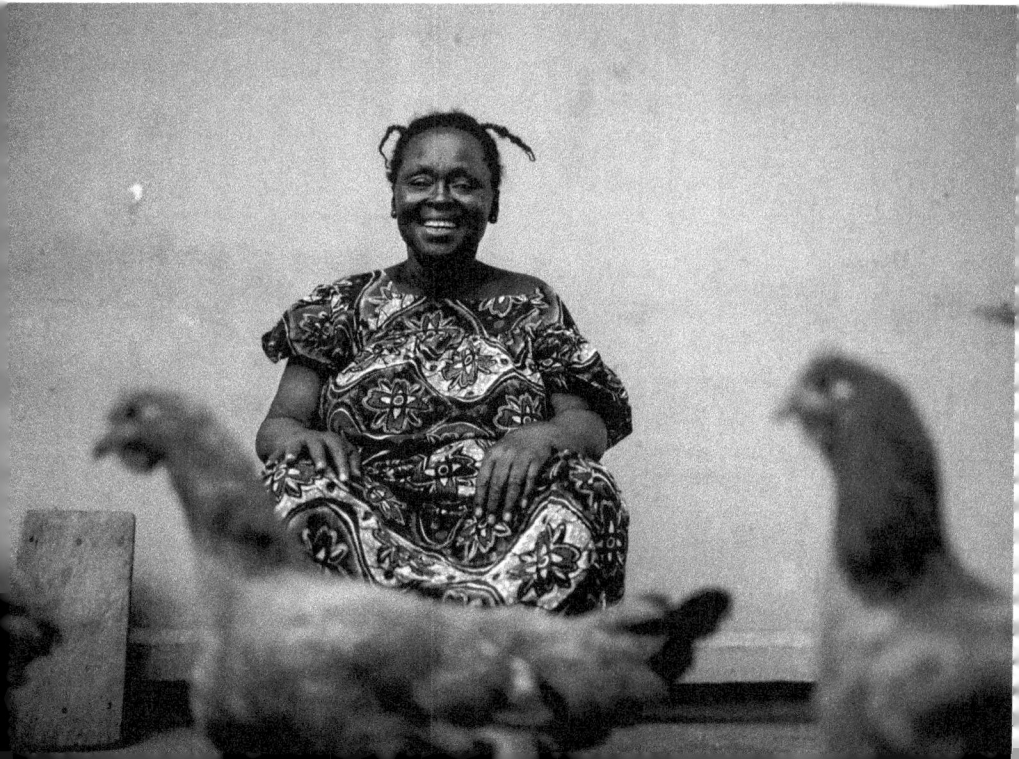

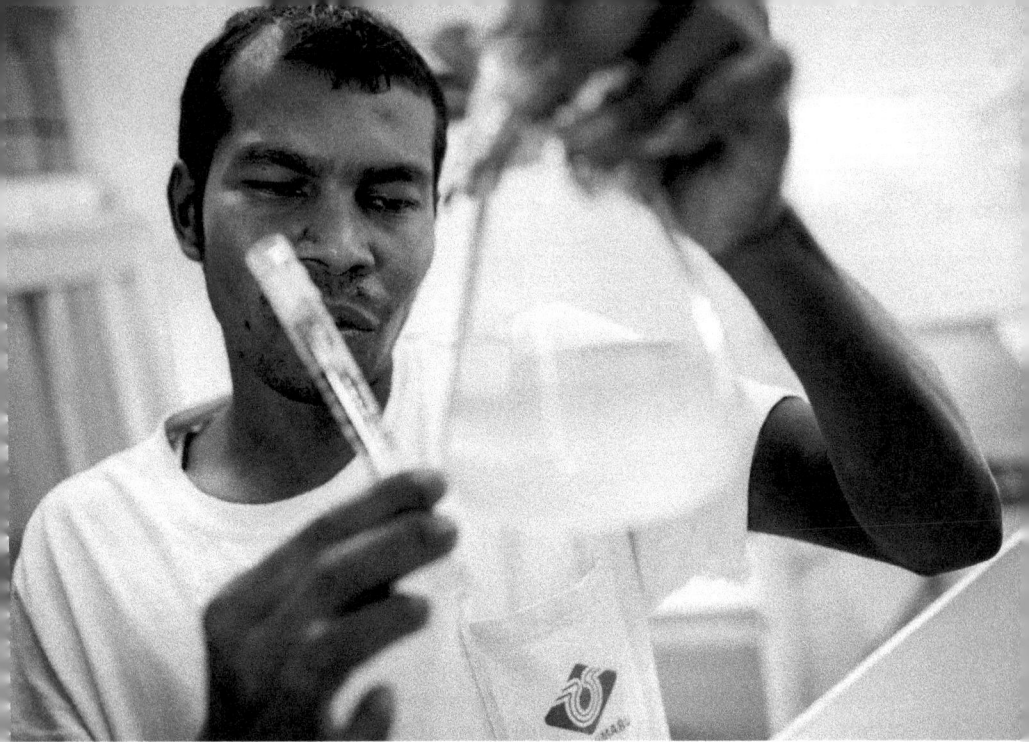

Figure 11.3 Sachin Deo works at the J. Hunter Pearls hatchery outside SavuSavu, Fiji. Sachin holds a test tube of muelleri algae before pouring it into a 500 ml flask containing seawater and nutrients; the final product will be liquid algae used to feed oyster larvae. The Australian Centre for International Agricultural Research (ACIAR) supports a pearl project in Fiji.

Figure 11.4 Children ride bikes along a road shadowed by large limestone rock formations in Maros District, Makassar, Indonesia.

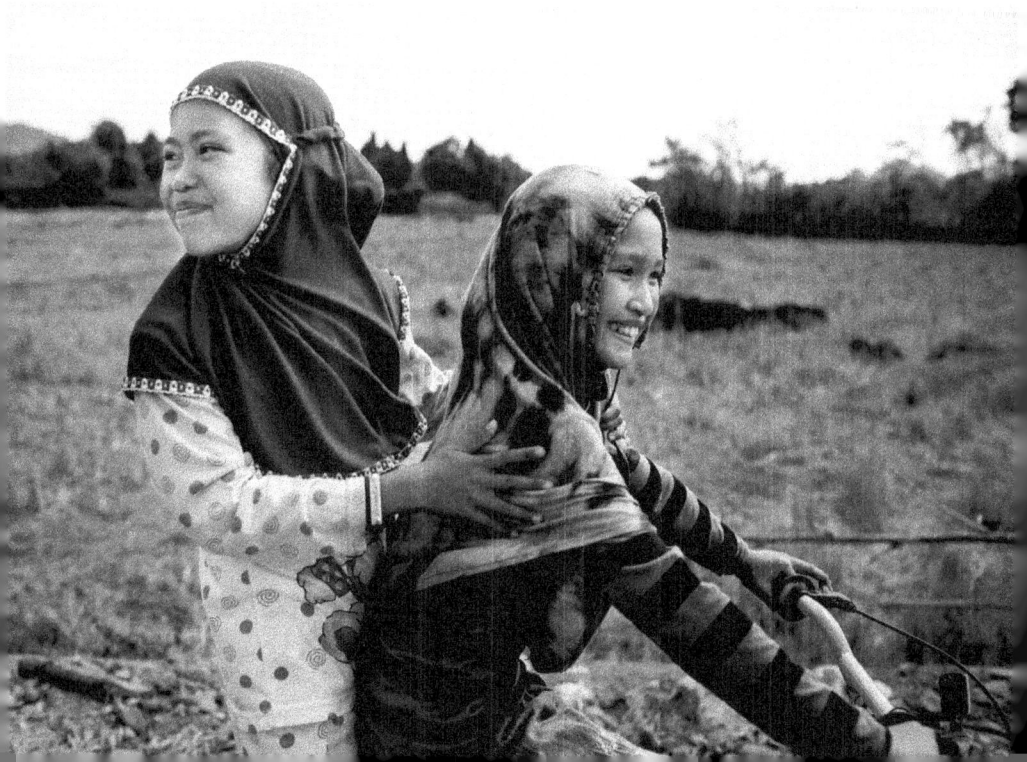

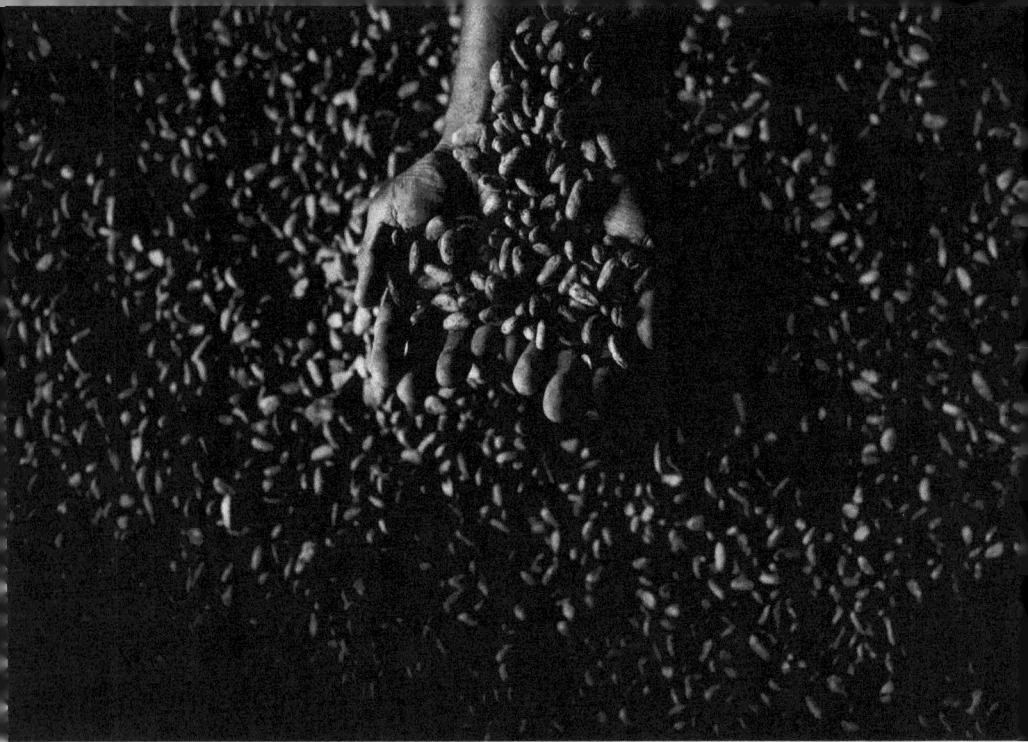

Figure 11.5 The cocoa growers co-operative help to evenly spread cocoa beans during drying. ACIAR is funding a cocoa livelihood program working with cocoa farmers to improve pre- and post-harvest techniques to ensure a higher quality of cocoa beans can be sold to niche chocolate markets. As part of the project a chocolate competition in Port Vila was held during October. Ten chocolates from ten different cocoa co-operatives around Vanuatu were tasted by a panel of judges including Australian chocolate makers. Rory Village was awarded the best chocolate and Dennis Nambith the co-operative's president was present on behalf of his community.

Figure 11.6 Litamat Benua, mother of four, is a proud female farmer from Bremway village on Malakula Island, Vanuatu. Litamat talked passionately about the role of female farmers with cocoa farmers. 'Not the heavy lifting of cocoa sacks, but all other things we women can do everything men do.' ACIAR is running two key programs in Vanuatu: the first one works to improve the livelihoods of cocoa farmers; a key part of this is to increase pre- and post-harvest farming techniques which will lead to an increased yield. The second project is focused on access to markets and aims to align Vanuatu cocoa farmers with niche chocolate makers in order to secure a higher return for their cocoa.

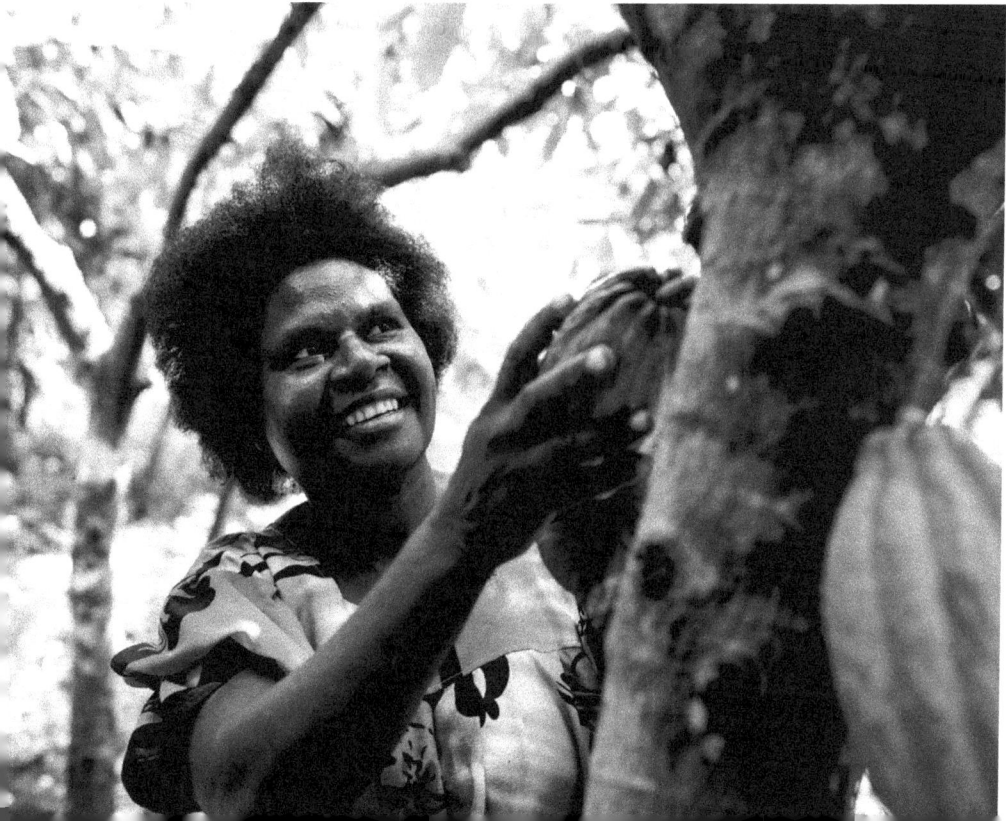

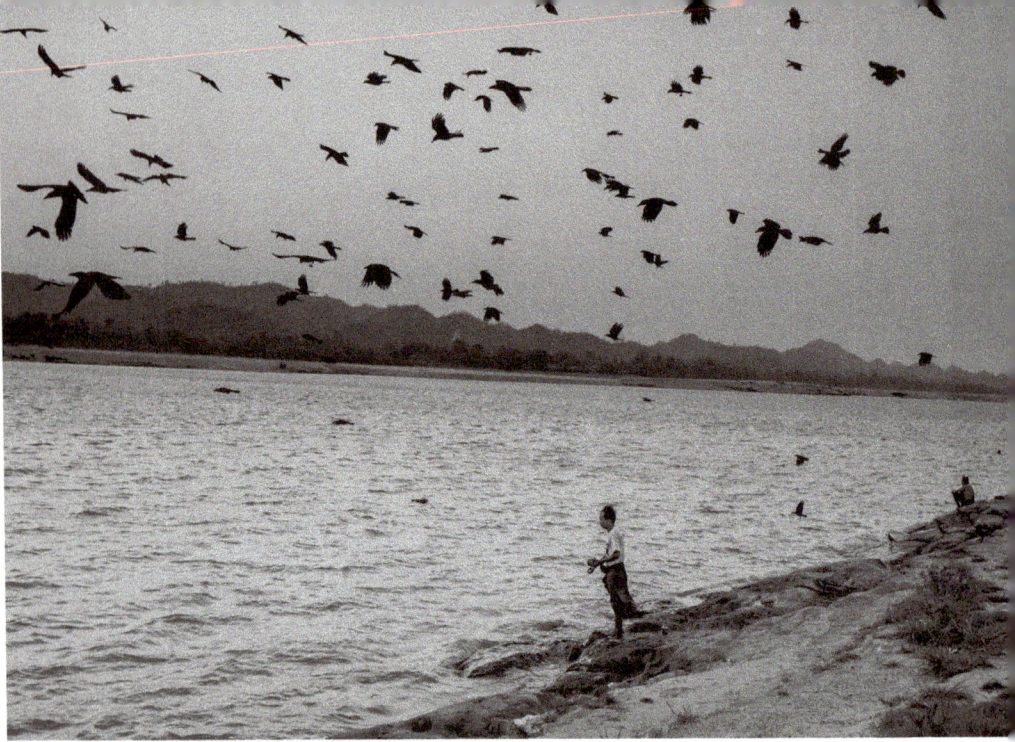

Figure 11.7 In the small city of Pyey the sun sets over the Irrawady River as a man casts another fishing line and a pack of crows fly overhead.

Figure 11.8 U Pho Pyae (white shirt), 74 years old, collects water from a communal water point close to his home. The Australian Red Cross in partnership with Myanmar Red Cross has been carrying out a Community Based Health & Resilience project in Yin Ywa and a number of other villages in central Myanmar, an area known as the Dry Zone, known as one of the driest and food insecure areas in the country. The CBHR project is working to educate and ensure sustainable changes to water and sanitation practices in these communities. A major part of the project is community education. After ensuring quality community education, the project then installs physical hardware, taps, tanks, toilets etc. When considering where to place communal water points the project consults the community to identify vulnerable members such as the elderly and disabled who may struggle to travel distances with heavy loads of water.

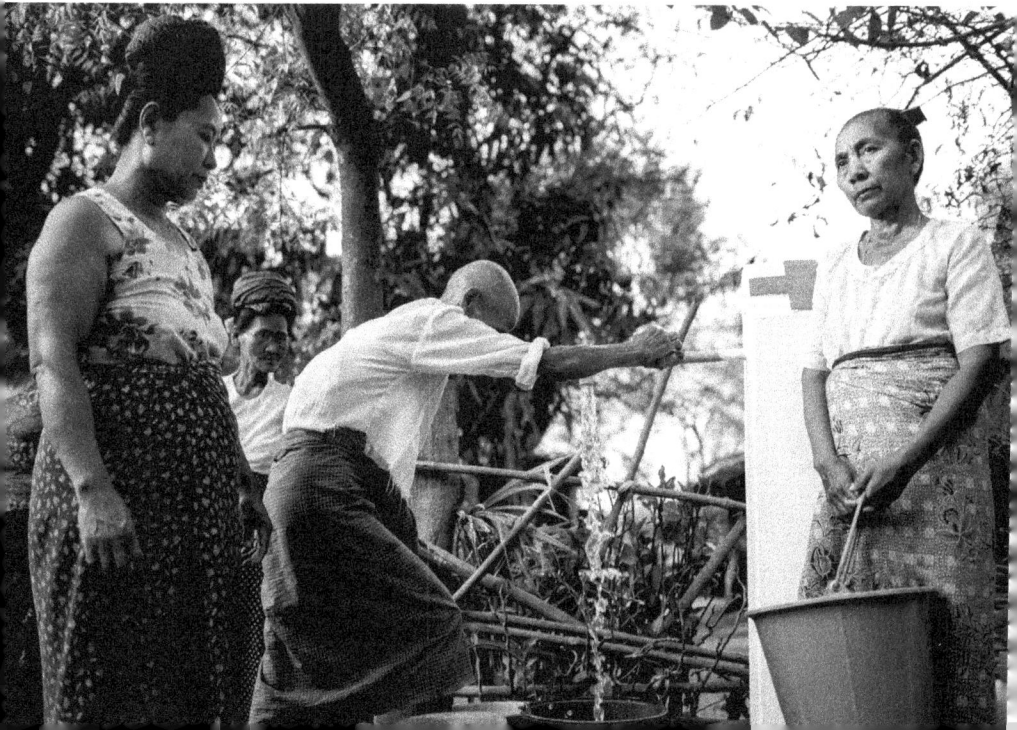

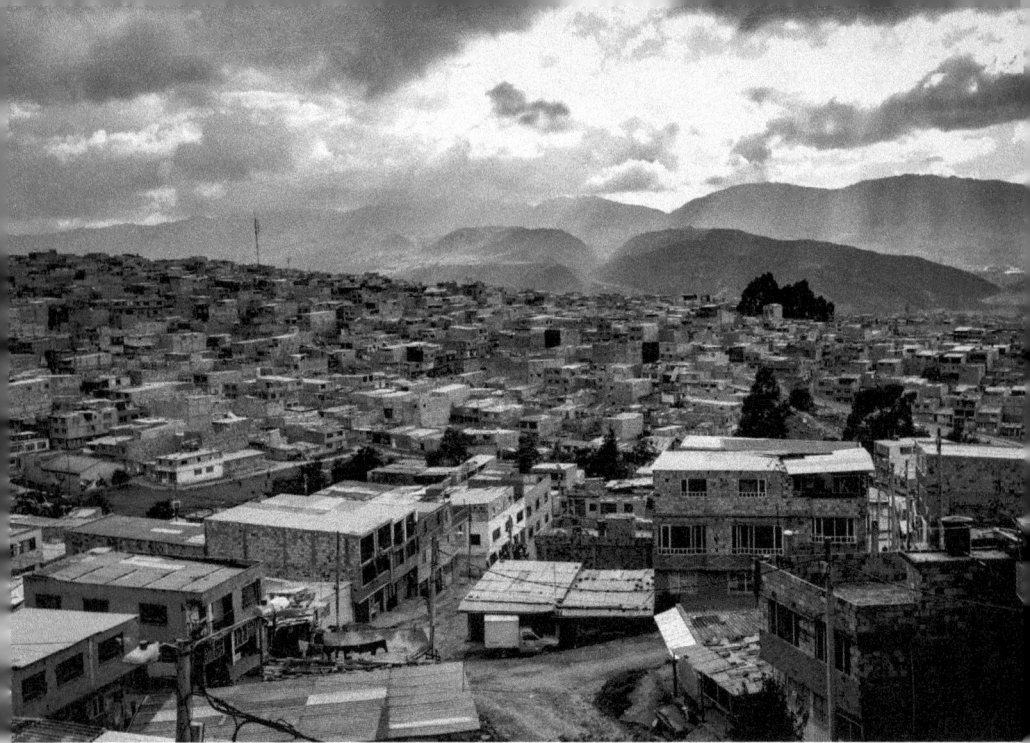

Figure 11.9 A view over the Casa Loma barrio outside Bogota, Colombia.

Figure 11.10 A man pulls a net catching small fish along the bank of the Hooghly River in Canning, West Bengal, India, with a half-constructed bridge crossing the river behind.

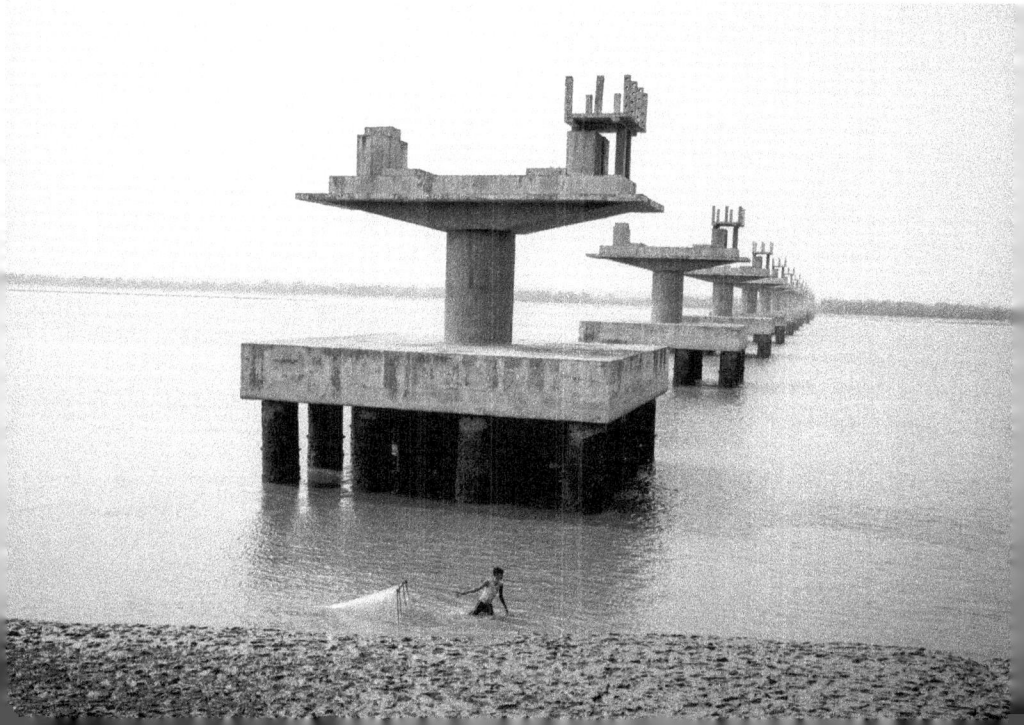

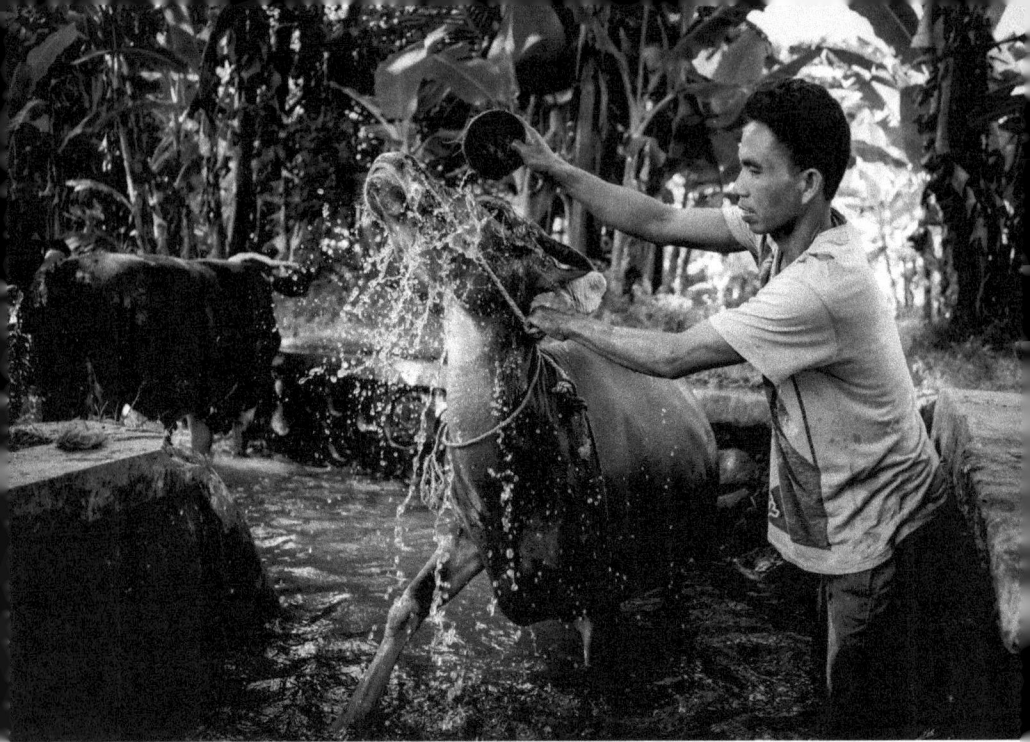

Figure 11.11 Hardiyanto, the treasurer of the cattle group in Karang Kendal hamlet, washing one of his cows in a small creek. Hardiyanto was involved with the group for six years. Hardiyanto was asked about the state of the village before the project began encouraging farmers to keep all the cattle in a communal area; he answered, 'Oh, it was a mess before, the manure was scattered everywhere and when it rained, manure was carried by the rains everywhere, it even went to other houses. It was really messy during rainy days.' Now that the cattle are kept in one place, breeding is also much easier, 'We didn't have a bull before as the cattle were scattered, not inside the cowshed; we faced difficulty in finding a mature bull for breeding. If some people had a bull, whether it was in the farm or field, we would take our cow there, so they could breed. However, now, if breeding time comes, thank God I just need to take it to the breeding shed. It was challenging before.'

About the contributors

Dr **Obijiofor Aginam** is Deputy Director and Head of Governance for Global Health at the United Nations University-International Institute for Global Health (UNU-IIGH) in Kuala Lumpur. He has served as a consultant for WHO and FAO on aspects of trade, food safety, and globalisation of public health. He represents United Nations University in the UN Inter-Agency Taskforce on the Prevention and Control of Non-Communicable Diseases, and currently serves on the editorial board of *Global Health Governance: The Scholarly Journal for the New Health Security Paradigm*. He is the author of *Global health governance: international law and public health in a divided world* (2005).

Associate Professor Robyn Alders AM is a Senior Scientific Advisor with the Centre for Global Health Security within Chatham House, Director of the Kyeema Foundation and a Visiting Fellow with the Development Policy Centre within the Australian National University. For over 25 years, she has worked closely with family farmers in sub-Saharan Africa, South-East Asia and Australia and as a veterinarian, researcher and colleague, with an emphasis on the development of sustainable infectious disease control in animals in rural areas in support of food and nutrition security. Her current research and development interests include domestic and global food and nutrition security/ systems, One Health/Planetary Health, gender equity and science communication. In 2002, Robyn was the recipient of the Kesteven Medal, awarded by the Australian Veterinary Association and the Australian College of Veterinary Scientists in recognition of distinguished contributions to international veterinary science in the field of technical and scientific assistance to developing countries. In 2011, she was invested as an Officer of the Order of Australia for distinguished service to veterinary science as a researcher and educator. In 2017, she was the recipient of the Inaugural Mitchell Global Humanitarian Award which recognises Australians and others supported by Australian aid who have made an outstanding contribution to the cause of international development.

Andi Imam Arundhana currently works at the Department of Nutritional Science, Universitas Hasanuddin. He does research in public health, nutrition and dietetics, and nutritional biochemistry.

Professor Kerry Arabena is President of the International Association in Ecology and Health, the Chair for Indigenous Health and Director of the Indigenous Health Equity Unit at the University of Melbourne, and Executive Director of First 1000 Days Australia, an intervention-based pre-birth cohort study designed with and for Aboriginal and Torres Strait Islander families. With an extensive background in public health, administration, community development and research, her work has made significant contributions in areas such as sexual and reproductive health, family empowerment, service provision, ecological health and harm minimisation. Her professional experience has seen her recognised as an Australian of the Year Finalist in 2010 and recipient of the prestigious JG Crawford Prize for Academic Excellence at Australian National University in 2011.

Conor Ashleigh is a visual storyteller and development communications practitioner. He has maintained a strong interest in documentary photography and filmmaking, and his stories have been published in media outlets including *The New York Times*, *Le Monde* and *The Guardian*. His projects have been exhibited internationally. As a visual communications specialist, he primarily works in the areas of international development, humanitarian response and research for agricultural development.

Dr Brigitte Bagnol is an independent consultant working in Africa and Asia for different national and international agencies to give training, design or evaluate projects and conduct research in the areas of development, anthropology of ecology, communication, sexuality, anthropology of health, One Health, and nutrition with a gender lens. She currently works mainly on gender, nutrition and infectious diseases from a One Health perspective. She was co-scriptwriter and co-director on several documentaries and fiction films. She is currently involved in collaborations with the University of the Witwatersrand, (South Africa), the University of Sydney (Australia), Tufts University (USA) and the University of São Paulo (Brazil).

Associate Professor Kirsten Black is an academic gynaecologist at the Royal Prince Alfred Hospital and Joint Head of the Discipline of Obstetrics, Gynaecology, and Neonatology at the University of Sydney. She is a fellow of the Royal Australian and New Zealand College of Obstetricians and Gynaecologists and a Member of the Faculty of Sexual and Reproductive Healthcare (UK) who works clinically in the fields of early pregnancy care, ultrasound, general gynaecology, menopause and contraception. She is an associate editor on the college's journal. Her research focuses on sexual and reproductive health in low resource settings and she is committed to clinical and research capacity building in the Asia Pacific region.

Thomas Betitis lives and works on Bougainville. He is the Secretary of the Department of Primary Industries and Marine Resources in the Autonomous Government of Bougainville. He is a soil scientist who has worked with the oil palm and cocoa industries in Papua New Guinea. In his current role he aims to nurture the development of sustainable and profitable agriculture in Bougainville.

Yngve Bråten is an advisor in gender and sustainable economic development. He is a social scientist with a specialisation in gender, sexual and reproductive health and rights, energy, and agriculture. Since 2017, he has been working at the KIT Royal Tropical Institute on projects focused on gender mainstreaming and inclusive value chain development, often in agricultural settings. His experience includes qualitative research, policy making, project implementation and workshop facilitation.

James Butubu lives on Bougainville where he works on an ACIAR project (HORT 2014/094) as the project co-ordinator. He has an agriculture science background specialising mostly in cocoa breeding, cocoa husbandry and pathology. He is also experienced in horticultural production and floriculture.

Professor Anthony Capon is professor of planetary health in the School of Public Health at the University of Sydney. A former director of the global health institute at United Nations University (UNU-IIGH), he is a public health physician and authority on environmental health and health promotion. His research focuses on urbanisation, sustainable development and population health. He is a member of the Rockefeller Foundation–Lancet Commission on Planetary Health and has served in numerous honorary leadership roles with professional and not-for-profit organisations in Australia and internationally.

Dr Sean C.P. Coogan is an interdisciplinary researcher with major interests in understanding the relationships between nutrition, ecology, and behaviour. His research on the nutritional ecology of urban Australian white ibis in Sydney received widespread media attention, and was voted in the top 10 Sydney science discoveries for 2017. His postdoctoral research on the population performance of grizzly bears focuses on integrating data from a wide range of modalities (e.g. remote sensing, nutritional, and physiological data) to produce novel approaches to understanding the ecology of wild carnivores in multi-use landscapes.

Professor Angus Dawson is Director of Sydney Health Ethics at the University of Sydney. His research has mainly focused on ethical issues in public and global health, particularly relating to infectious disease and so-called lifestyle choices (e.g. eating, drinking and smoking). More recently he has been exploring more socially embedded concepts such as trust, community and solidarity and topics involving collective action problems such as climate change and antimicrobial resistance.

He has been involved in ethics and policy work for many organisations including the World Health Organization and Médecins Sans Frontières. Most recently he was one of the editors of *Public health ethics: cases spanning the globe* (2016), a collection containing cases from 23 different countries.

Dr Chris Degeling is a health social scientist, philosopher, and practising veterinarian who works in the social studies and ethics of public health. He is currently a Senior Fellow at the Australian Centre for Health Engagement, Evidence and Values at the University of Wollongong where he leads the NHMRC funded project: Can One Health strategies be more effectively implemented through prior identification of public values?

Dr Keith Eastwood is a microbiologist and epidemiologist with Hunter New England Population Health, New South Wales, Australia. He has a particular interest in disease surveillance, emerging diseases, zoonoses and One Health. He co-ordinates the Regional One Health Partnership, a large and diverse network of professionals working in animal, human and environmental health operating in northern NSW and southern Queensland. This informal group has collaborated in many successful research projects and activities showing the practical value of working within a One Health approach.

Professor Stan Fenwick is a veterinarian involved in veterinary public health and capacity building in South-East Asia. He joined the Department of Infectious Disease and Global Health, Cumming's School of Veterinary Medicine, Tufts University in 2010 and since then has been based in Bangkok as regional technical advisor for USAID's EPT 1 and EPT2 programs. A major part of his work in South-East Asia is providing support for SEAOHUN, the South-East Asia One Health University Network, whose aim is to build capacity among university graduates, government employees and other stakeholders to respond to outbreaks of emerging and re-emerging diseases using the One Health approach.

Professor Lyn Gilbert AO is an infectious disease physician and clinical microbiologist. She is a senior researcher at the Marie Bashir Institute for Emerging Infections and Biosecurity and at Sydney Health Ethics at the University of Sydney. Her main research interests are prevention, surveillance, control and ethics of communicable diseases of public health importance. Currently, her research focuses on the ethics and politics of hospital infection prevention and control and antimicrobial resistance, including responsibilities of healthcare professionals and healthcare organisations; and One Health approaches to prediction and management of emerging infectious diseases.

Professor David Guest is plant pathologist in the Faculty of Science, Theme Leader for Development Agriculture in the Sydney Institute of Agriculture, executive member of the Sydney South-East Asia Centre, and a member of the self-assessment team for the SAGE Gender Equity project at the University of Sydney. While he has over 30 years' experience investigating mechanisms of plant disease resistance and developing integrated disease management strategies for horticulture and natural environments, his current research goal is to cultivate interdisciplinary approaches to improve the livelihoods of smallholder farmers in tropical horticulture by developing market incentives combined with improved soil, plant, livestock, human and environmental health. His fieldwork activities involve partnerships with research institutes and farming communities around the Asia-Pacific and in Latin America.

Dr Grant Hill-Cawthorne is a medical microbiologist and the head of the Parliamentary Office of Science and Technology for the UK Parliament, while remaining as an adjunct at the University of Sydney. His research focuses on the use of molecular epidemiology for public health policy, particularly on emerging infections, drug resistance and the impact of mass gatherings.

Dr Lenny Hogerwerf is an epidemiologist and disease ecologist with the Centre for Infectious Disease Control at the National Institute for Public Health and the Environment of the Netherlands. She has consulted for the Food and Agriculture Organization, was president of the international network Vétérinaires Sans Frontières Europe, and researcher at the Université Libre de Bruxelles, Brussels, Belgium. She has also developed a variety of models for explaining the dynamics of HPAI H5N1 and infectious disease landscapes more generally.

Professor Martin Jeggo is a veterinary surgeon and has worked in research and research management of infectious diseases. During his 18 years at the UN, he managed programs of support for animal health in the developing world with research-related projects in 150 countries. In 2002–2013 he was Director of the Australian Animal Health Laboratory. He now works on a part-time basis with the Geelong Centre for Emerging Infectious Diseases – a One Health consortium. He is also chair of the governing body of AUSGEM, a One Health partnership between the University of Technology Sydney and the Elizabeth Macarthur Agricultural Institute in New South Wales. He has edited a number of books on the concepts underpinning One Health and is an executive editor of both *Ecohealth* and *One Health* journals.

Tammi Jonas is a former vegetarian academic and resident at Jonai Farms and Meatsmiths, where she and her family raise pigs and cattle in the central highlands of Victoria, Australia. Tammi and husband Stuart brought the value chain into their control by crowdfunding and building a butcher's shop, commercial kitchen and curing room, where Tammi crafts a range of fresh cuts, smallgoods, charcuterie and air-cured products for the local community. Tammi is also the current President of the Australian Food Sovereignty Alliance where she advocates for everybody's right to access nutritious and culturally appropriate food grown in ethical and ecologically sound ways, and their right to democratically determine their own food and agriculture systems. Tammi has been writing about food culture, politics, and ethics since 2006 on *Tammi Jonas: food ethics*, and has been widely published in both academic and popular texts.

Professor Richard Kock is a wildlife veterinary ecologist, infectious disease researcher and conservationist, and professor of wildlife health and emerging diseases at the Royal Veterinary College, University of London. He received an FAO international medal in recognition of his work on morbilliviruses in 2010. Much of his work has been on ecological perspectives of disease at the livestock–wildlife interface with considerable reflection on agricultural impacts and biodiversity loss on disease emergence. He has over 150 peer-reviewed publications in books and journals, and principal investigator on a number of research projects on wildlife disease in Africa and Asia and co-investigator on a number of other programs. He is an expert member of the International Health Regulation and a Senior Fellow at Chatham House UK, and adjunct professor at the University of Tufts, USA.

Jessica Hall is a PhD student at the School of Public Health at the University of Sydney. Her research applies a One Health approach to examine the links between health, nutrition and productivity of cocoa farmers in Bougainville. Jessica has extensive experience in designing and implementing quantitative household surveys across South-East Asia and the Pacific, most recently a large-scale livelihood survey in Bougainville. Jessica has also worked with several research projects to transition from paper-based to mobile data collection systems in low resource settings.

Dr Anna Laven is a senior advisor in sustainable economic development at the KIT Royal Tropical Institute. She is a political scientist with a specialisation in sustainable development. She holds a PhD in development studies from the University of Amsterdam, where she specialised in governance and upgrading in value chains. Since 2008 she has been working on inclusive value chain development, looking specifically at gender in value chains and at sustainability in the cocoa sector. Her experience includes qualitative research, facilitation of multi-stakeholder processes, policy making and social entrepreneurship.

Professor John Mackenzie AO, FTSE, retired in 2008 after holding professorial appointments at Curtin University, the University of Queensland and the University of Western Australia. He is currently an Emeritus Professor of Curtin University, a part-time Senior Scientist-in-Charge at PathWest, Perth, and holds honorary positions at the University of Queensland and the Burnet Institute, Melbourne. He was elected

Secretary-General of the International Union of Microbiological Societies from 1999 to 2005. He has served on various committees for the World Health Organization, including the Steering Committee of the Global Outbreak Alert and Response Network, as Chair of the WHO IHR Emergency Committee for Influenza H1N1, and is currently a member of the Emergency Committee for Polio. He is a co-founder and Vice-Chair of the One Health Platform, a foundation based in Belgium, and editor-in-chief of the journal, *One Health*. In 2002, he was appointed as Officer in the Order of Australia for services to public health research and to education. In 2005 he was the inaugural recipient of the Academy of Science Malaysia's Mahathir Science Award for Excellence in Tropical Research. His recent research interests have included mosquito-borne viral diseases, emerging zoonoses, and aspects of global health security.

Professor Ben Marais works in paediatric infectious diseases at the Children's Hospital at Westmead. He is Co-Director of the Marie Bashir Institute for Infectious Diseases and Biosecurity and helps to lead the Centre for Research Excellence in Tuberculosis at the University of Sydney. His research has focused primarily on how children are affected by the global tuberculosis epidemic and the spread of drug resistant *M. tuberculosis* strains. He also has a strong interest in the environmental dimensions of health and the Marie Bashir Institute is committed to the One Planet – One Health concept. As a paediatrician he feels strongly about the 'neglected third dimension' of medical ethics, since the right of future generations to inherit a liveable planet and live a healthy life is rarely considered in medical decision making.

Dr Peter McMahon is a Research Fellow at the University of Sydney. He has worked in field agricultural research at the Entomology Branch, Queensland DPI and on Australian-funded projects in Indonesia concerned with sustainable production of tree crops and community livelihood. His main research focus has been integrated pest and disease management of smallholder cocoa and improvement of farmer livelihoods.

Dr Peter Massey is a clinical nurse consultant and program manager for Health Protection with Hunter New England Population Health. He has worked in public health in rural Australia for about 30 years and has expertise in immunisation, communicable disease control, zoonoses, public health emergencies and Aboriginal health. He brings a strong rural and equity focus to all aspects of public health and experience in research capacity building and community-based research. He has published than 75 publications, including 16 on One Health. He has worked for many years in a number of countries in the Pacific on TB programs, public health research capacity strengthening and disease control.

Professor Paul Memmott is an anthropologist and architect, and the director of the Aboriginal Environments Research Centre at the University of Queensland. He has dedicated his more than 45-year career to establishing a research and teaching field centred on the topic of Aboriginal people–environments relations. His scholarly research output includes over 275 publications, 240 applied research reports and 70 competitive grants. He won a number of prestigious teaching awards in Indigenous education (including an Australian Award for University Teaching – AAUT). One of his books, titled *Gunyah, Goondie + Wurley: Aboriginal architecture of Australia*, received three national book awards in 2008, including the prestigious Stanner Award from the Australian Institute of Aboriginal and Torres Strait Islander Studies. Most recently he has been awarded with a Vice Chancellor's Strategic Grant for the establishment of an Indigenous Design Place initiative to engage transdisciplinary research teams with Indigenous community collaborators.

Dr Siobhan Mor is an epidemiologist, with expertise in both medical and veterinary methods and applications. She is currently senior lecturer in epidemiology (One Health) at the University of Sydney. Her research focuses on the epidemiology of zoonotic, emerging and tropical infectious diseases of global health importance, with particular regional focus on sub-Saharan Africa. She is a member of the Australian College of Veterinary Scientists by examination in veterinary epidemiology and an adjunct assistant professor at Tufts University, USA.

Dr Sudirman Nasir is senior lecturer and researcher at the Faculty of Public Health, Universitas Hasanuddin in Makassar. He has conducted research on various issues related to drug use and HIV-AIDS in Indonesia, including the social context of HIV risk-taking behaviours among young people who inject drugs in low-income neighbourhoods in Makassar. Besides publishing articles in academic journals, he frequently writes essays for Indonesian and international media. He also serves as a vice-president of the Indonesian Young Academy of Sciences (ALMI), whose mission is to empower mid-career scientists for building a strong science community in Indonesia.

Dr Nunung Nuryartono is associate professor and Dean of Faculty of Economics and Management at Bogor Agricultural University. He has more than 20 years' experience in research, especially in development economics, public sector reform, financial inclusion, microfinance, poverty and economic growth, and has published many scientific papers and other publications. He is an active member of Indonesia Economists Association, Indonesia Regional Science Association and the Australasians Agricultural and Resource Economics Society. He also became a visiting associate at the School of Economics at the University of Adelaide.

Professor David Raubenheimer is a nutritional ecologist, with 25 years of experience in applying ecological and evolutionary theory in the study of animal and human nutrition. His work includes laboratory and field studies on species from insects to reptiles, fish, sharks, birds, giant pandas, grizzly bears, monkeys, gorillas, orangutans and chimpanzees, as well as pets and production animals. He also applies the perspectives of nutritional ecology to the health problems of humans in modern environments. In 2013 he took up his current position as Chair in Nutritional Ecology and Nutrition Theme Leader in the Charles Perkins Centre, the University of Sydney. He is co-author of *The nature of nutrition: a unifying framework from animal adaptation to human obesity* (2012), and has published over 250 peer-reviewed papers.

Dian Sidik Arsyad is an epidemiologist at the Faculty of Public Health, Universitas Hasanuddin in Makassar. He is a lecturer in the Department of Epidemiology. His research focuses on both communicable and noncommunicable diseases surveillance, and on the development of public health information systems.

Dr Darryl Stellmach is a postdoctoral associate in medical anthropology, food and nutrition security at the University of Sydney. His research focuses on the social and political aspects of epidemics, food security and nutritional crises as well as expertise in field research planning and methods. Prior to academia Darryl spent ten years as field manager for medical humanitarian aid operations.

Dr Kim-Yen Phan-Thien is a senior lecturer in food science at the University of Sydney, where she helped to develop the Food and Agribusiness curriculum. She undertakes research on diverse topics related to food quality and food safety in the Sydney Institute of Agriculture.

Associate Professor Jenny-Ann Toribio is an epidemiologist in the School of Veterinary Science at the University of Sydney. She has a career-long interest in small-scale livestock production systems in South-East Asia and the Pacific, with research on integrated mixed farming and on animal and zoonotic infectious diseases in these settings.

Clement Totavun lives and works on Bougainville where he is the Secretary of the Department of Health in the Autonomous Government of Bougainville. He has nursing qualifications. He previously worked for the Australian High Commission in Port Moresby, Papua New Guinea and the World Health Organization in the PNG Country Office, Port Moresby.

Grant Vinning works in cocoa in the Pacific and Indonesia. He finds new markets then works with local people to develop their skills to exploit new market opportunities. He is the author of *Cocoa in the Pacific: The First Fifty Years* (2017) and a bi-monthly cocoa market newsletter that goes to cocoa growers, chocolate makers, researchers, and policy makers in 10 countries. He is the Judges' Coordinator at the Bougainville Chocolate Festival and the adjudicator of the Festival's Big Bean Competition.

Robert G. Wallace is a public health phylogeographer presently visiting the University of Minnesota's Institute for Global Studies. His research has addressed the evolution and spread of influenza, the agro-economics of Ebola, the social geography of HIV/AIDS in New York City, the emergence of Kaposi's sarcoma herpesvirus out of Ugandan prehistory, and the evolution of infection life history in response to antivirals. He is co-author of *Farming human pathogens: ecological resilience and evolutionary process* (2009) and *Neoliberal ebola: modelling disease emergence from finance to forest and farm* (2016), and author of *Big farms make big flu: dispatches on infectious disease, agribusiness, and the nature of science* (2016). He has consulted for the Food and Agriculture Organization on bird flu and the Centers for Disease Control and Prevention on ecohealth.

Rodrick Wallace is a research scientist in the Division of Epidemiology of the New York State Psychiatric Institute at Columbia University. He received an undergraduate degree in mathematics and a PhD in physics from Columbia University, worked a decade as a public interest lobbyist, and is a past recipient of an Investigator Award in Health Policy Research from the Robert Wood Johnson Foundation. He is the author of numerous books and papers relating to public health and public order.

Professor Merrilyn Walton AM is a professor of medical education at the University of Sydney. She is a researcher and leader in global health, health service development and patient safety; most of her current work is in low- and middle-income countries. Her international work has involved patient safety and workforce development in Vietnam, Indonesia, Myanmar, Timor Leste and China. She has published over 65 peer-reviewed journal articles, 18 chapters in books and three books, 17 major government reports and 22 newspaper articles. Over the last five years she has been involved in cross-disciplinary work with agriculture to develop One Health approaches to improve livelihoods of rural farming communities in Papua New Guinea and Indonesia. She was made a Member of the Order of Australia in 2015 for 'significant service to the health care sector, particularly through policy development and reform, and to professional medical practice and standards'. In 2016 she accepted an honorary professorship at the Hanoi Medical University Viet Nam.

Dr Anke Wiethoelter is a veterinarian with interest in epidemiology, risk assessments and infectious diseases at the wildlife–livestock–human interface. As a Postdoctoral Research Associate at the University of Sydney and Western Sydney University, Anke investigated risk perception and mitigation strategies for the Hendra virus by Australian horse owners. Her current role as lecturer in veterinary epidemiology (One Health) at the University of Melbourne involves research into zoonotic diseases as well as teaching in the areas of epidemiology, veterinary public health, and One Health.

Dr Josephine Yaupain Saul-Maora gained her PhD from the University of Sydney in 2009 studying the genetic diversity of Phytophthora palmivora, the cocoa black pod pathogen. She was the Research Leader for Crop Protection at the former PNG Cocoa and Coconut Institute, Kerevat, East New Britain, Papua New Guinea. She is currently active in Women and Youth in Agriculture, East New Britain, and as a trainer for the Family Farm Teams projects across PNG. She has been involved in a number of research projects with the Australian Centre for International Agricultural Research (ACIAR). She is married with two children and currently lives in East New Britain.

Index